PHONETIC ANALYSIS OF NORMAL AND ABNORMAL SPEECH

Ralph N. Ohde
Vanderbilt University

Donald J. Sharf
Professor Emeritus
University of Michigan

MERRILL, an imprint of
MACMILLAN PUBLISHING COMPANY
New York

Maxwell Macmillan Canada
Toronto

Maxwell Macmillan International
New York Oxford Singapore Sydney

RNO wishes to acknowledge the faithful and continued support of his wife, Kathleen.

DJS wishes to acknowledge the encouragement and support of his wife, Rhoda, son Dan, and daughter Ellen.

Editor: Ann Castel
Production Editor: Linda Hillis Bayma
Art Coordinator: Vincent A. Smith
Text Designer: Anne Flanagan
Cover Designer: Robert Vega
Production Buyer: Pamela D. Bennett

This book was set in Century Old Style by Carlisle Communications, Ltd. and was printed and bound by Book Press, Inc., a Quebecor America Book Group Company. The cover was printed by Lehigh Press, Inc.

Printed in the United States of America

Macmillan Publishing Company
866 Third Avenue, New York, NY 10022

Macmillan Publishing Company is part of the Maxwell Communication Group of Companies.

Maxwell Macmillan Canada, Inc.
1200 Eglinton Avenue East, Suite 200
Don Mills, Ontario M3C 3N1

Library of Congress Cataloging-in-Publication Data
Ohde, Ralph N.
Phonetic analysis of normal and abnormal speech / Ralph N. Ohde, Donald J. Sharf.
p. cm.
Includes bibliographical references and indexes.
ISBN 0-675-20681-2
1. Speech disorders. 2. Phonetics. I. Sharf, Donald J. II. Title.
RC423.044 1992 91-8092
616-85'5—dc20 CIP

Printing: 1 2 3 4 5 6 7 8 9 Year 2 3 4 5

PREFACE

This book is designed for use in phonetics courses or other courses that include the study of the descriptive analysis of speech sounds, particularly those that constitute part of the education of speech and language pathologists. As such, the text covers the subject matter of the usual introductory phonetics course plus the phonetic and phonologic aspects of speech and language disorders and a phonetic system for transcribing them.

In many universities students take courses dealing with the anatomy and physiology of the speech mechanism, with speech science, and with linguistics before their phonetics course. Although such a background is ideal for this phonetics book, it is not absolutely necessary. Sufficient background information is presented so that students can easily follow the development of the subject matter, especially if they delve into the reference sources.

As pointed out in Chapter 1, there are good reasons for having a phonetics text oriented to the training needs of speech and language pathologists. These professionals will require: (1) a skill in analyzing children's speech patterns equal to if not better than that required for adults, (2) proficiency in analyzing abnormal as well as normal speech patterns, (3) competence in using phonetic knowledge in the rehabilitation of articulatory and phonologic disorders, and (4) the ability to make accurate, valid, and reliable judgments of the correctness of clients' speech sounds for diagnosis and for therapy.

Chapter 1 develops the premise that descriptive phonetics is firmly founded on studies from perceptual, acoustic, and physiologic phonetics, with particular emphasis on acoustic phonetics and the objective analyses of speech sounds provided by spectrograms. This emphasis is appropriate since the perceptual analysis of speech is based on speech acoustics and acoustic correlates of sound features. Starting with an introduction to the physical basis for acoustic analysis of adult and child speech, the book lays the groundwork for the presentation of spectrograms of normal and abnormal speech patterns of children and adults.

The discussion of speech begins in Chapter 2 with a description of the common types of syllable structures in English. Included in that chapter is a description of the concept of phonological processes with particular regard to those that influence the development of syllable patterns in children's speech.

Because vowels function as the basic carrier of the speech signal, the coverage of speech sounds begins with vowels in chapters 3 and 4. Chapter 3 covers normal allophonic variations of vowels, glides, and liquids, and Chapter 4 covers abnormal variants of the same sounds. Beginning with chapters 3 and 4, transcription practice, to be used in conjunction with the tapes that accompany this book, is included at the end of each chapter. The practice is designed to teach students to identify and/or discriminate normal and abnormal variations of the sounds covered in each chapter.

The articulatory potential for consonants is presented in Chapter 5. This chapter includes descriptions of the different types of sounds that the speech structures can produce, including those that occur in English, in other languages, and in abnormal speech.

Stop, fricative, affricate, and nasal consonants are covered in chapters 6, 7, 8, and 9. For each class of sound, normal productions are compared with those of individuals with articulatory disorders and with those of children who use phonological processes (see Chapter 1 glossary). The differences are illustrated by spectrograms and by the transcription practice on the tapes.

The contextual patterns of speech are covered in Chapter 10 with a discussion of the relationship between coarticulation and assimilation. Not only are numerous examples given of assimilations occurring in adult speech, but these patterns are compared with the assimilations occurring in the speech of children who use phonological processes. The transcription practice at the end of Chapter 10 includes examples of assimilation processes found in children's speech.

Suprasegmental features, or the prosody of speech, are covered in Chapter 11, which includes discussion of variations in intonation, stress, juncture, and timing. Normal patterns of these features are treated as well as abnormal ones that occur in the speech of children and dysarthrics, adults with motor speech disorders. Contrasts between basic intonation and stress patterns appear in the transcription practice at the end of this chapter.

Chapter 12 ties all the information together in terms of the application of phonetics to the diagnosis and rehabilitation of speech disorders. Included are considerations of: (1) types of articulatory and phonological assessment tests, (2) accuracy, validity, and reliability of phonetic transcription on such tests, (3) prognostic factors of consistency and stimulability, and (4) the use of phonetic modification techniques in articulation therapy.

Because review and summarizing are important for learning, each chapter includes a glossary and a review exercise. The glossary includes definitions of the new terminology introduced in each chapter so that students can review the important concepts presented. The review exercises feature short-answer questions with self-scoring keys so that students can assess how well they are absorbing the essential information given in each chapter. All terms in each glossary are listed in the defined terminology index at the end of the text.

Since glossaries are included at the end of each chapter, the terminology of articulatory disorders and phonological processes is scattered throughout the book wherever terms relate to particular sounds. Appendix A offers a synthesis of the definitions of these terms.

Throughout the book, symbols and diacritics are presented for transcribing normal and abnormal speech. This system is based on IPA (IPA, 1979), PRDS (Grunwell, 1988), and the American tradition of transcription (Pullum & Ladusaw, 1986). The complete system is summarized in Appendix B, with its descriptions of terminology, table of symbols, and figure describing a model for the systematic location of diacritics. It should be noted that in the interest of reducing repetition and saving space, nonphonetic symbols such as commas, hyphens, and capital letters are used in virgules and brackets. This practice should not be construed as condoning such usage in actual phonetic transcription.

The tapes that accompany the book help fulfill its purpose by providing adult and child models of normal and abnormal speech patterns. As indicated in Appendix D, the speech samples were obtained with a high quality recording system, including an IAC booth, Revox tape recorder (Model B77 MKII), Neumann microphone (Model TLM 170i), and Ampex 456 tape. All speech samples were transferred to a PDP 11/73 computer for final preparation of tapes. These samples were digitized at a 22 kHz sampling rate with a 10 kHz low-pass filter setting and a 12 bit quantization. The generation of stimulus orderings and temporal separations between speech samples was performed with an output program on the PDP 11/73 computer.

End-of-chapter exercises correspond to the tapes and provide response forms for transcribing stimuli. Their locations on the four cassettes are indicated by the tape log in Appendix C. The exercises are designed to present speech sounds systematically in increasingly complex contexts ranging from nonsense syllables to words in sentences. Systematic practice is provided so that students can learn to discriminate such differences as /ɪ - ɛ/, /ɑ - ɔ/, voice onset time (VOT) for voiceless unaspirated and voiced stops, vowel duration preceding voiceless and devoiced final consonants, normal and distorted (derhoticized) /r/, normal and distorted /l/, normal and lisped /s, z/, and oral and nasalized vowels.

Appendix D provides suggestions for achieving greater accuracy and reliability in phonetic transcription. Appendix E, which contains a series of tests for assessing the reliability of one's transcription, is divided into sections about vowels and consonants, /r/ misarticulations, /l/ misarticulations, /s, z/ misarticulations, and phonological processes. Each of these reliability tests is recorded on the accompanying tapes.

The tapes (ISBN: 0-675-22313-X) that accompany the exercises in the text may be obtained by contacting your local sales representative or by calling Macmillan's customer service department in Riverside, New Jersey at (609) 461-6500.

ACKNOWLEDGMENTS

We are grateful to the following people for the contributions they made toward the completion of this book:

To Vicki Knight, for selling the idea of a clinical phonetics book to the publisher;

To the following reviewers, for providing critical and insightful reviews of the manuscript: Milton Blue, The University of Georgia; Michael J. Clark, Western Michigan University; Robert Allen Fox, The Ohio State University; Thomas W. Robinson, The University of Texas at Austin; Carol Stoel-Gammon, University of Washington; and Bradford L. Swartz, Central Michigan University;

To the students, particularly Susan Corr, in the fall 1988 and 1989 articulation disorders classes at Vanderbilt University, for their evaluation of the prepublication version of the text and tapes;

To Don Riggs at Vanderbilt University, for his work on the figures;

To Julie Michie at Vanderbilt University, for her work on many facets of the project;

To Steve Camarata, who, along with the authors, transcribed the stimuli on the tapes;

To Michael McCarver, Mark Hedrick, and Katarina Haley, for assistance in figure and tape preparation;

To the clinical staff of the Bill Wilkerson Center, particularly Paulette Willie, Rod Wood, Marcy Sipes, Sara Hoffman, and Kerry Hessenthaler, for assistance in tape preparation;

To the Nashville Metropolitan School System, particularly Charles Hausman, Sandy Werth, and Larae Heil, for assistance in tape preparation;

To Mark Lehman, Holly Craig, and the staff of the West Bloomfield, Michigan library for providing computer facilities and work space during the summers of 1989 and 1990;

To the children on the tapes, particularly Gillian Klee and Laura Camarata, for their speech samples;

To Tom Klee, Wendy Love, and Steve and Mary Camarata, for their support, friendship, and permission to record their children;

To Mayhew Koellein and Mary Williams, for their superb photographic illustrations;

To Marleen Ochs, for her assiduous ear and friendship;

To Wes Grantham, for his omnifarious technical assistance and friendship; and

To the supporting staff at Macmillan, particularly Ann Castel, Brenda Rock, Vincent Smith, Linda Bayma, JoEllen Gohr, and Jeff Johnston, for guiding us through this project.

Some of the materials and data presented in this book were obtained while Ralph N. Ohde was working on a research grant from the National Institutes of Health (DC 00464-01A2HUD-3) and a Biomedical Research Support Grant (RR05424-27).

CONTENTS

CHAPTER 1

Nature of Phonetic Analysis

CLINICAL FUNCTION OF PHONETICS

Phonetics is the study of the production and acoustic properties of speech sounds as elements of language. It involves the analysis, description, and classification of sounds as they relate to each other. A major purpose of phonetics is to describe the differences among speech sounds that are important in the production and perception of meaningful utterances and the nature of variations in the production and perception of these sounds. In considering variations among sounds, one can distinguish those that occur within a language and those that occur between languages. For example, 'heat' and 'hit' differ in English because their vowel sounds are different; this vowel distinction conveys a difference in meaning between this pair and many other word pairs, for example: 'beat/bit,' 'read/rid,' 'seek/sick.'

Phonology is used to refer to the system of differences in speech sounds that convey meaning in languages. In the phonology of French, there is a vowel like the one in 'beat' but not like the one in 'bit.' As a result, French speakers of English tend to produce words with the vowel in 'bit' so that it sounds like the vowel in 'beat.' Since the focus of this book is on normal and abnormal English speech, such differences between English and other languages are not dealt with systematically. Instead, the focus is on the phonetics and phonology of English alone.

Within a language, sound differences that are meaningful, contextual, dialectal, optional, or abnormal can be identified. A meaningful difference produces distinctions between words, such as the difference between vowels in 'hat' and 'hit' and between consonants in 'pat' and 'bat.' A contextual difference involves variation of a sound in different contexts, such as the same vowel being longer in 'feed' than in 'feet,' a difference that is attributed to the influence of the final consonant. A dialectal difference occurs between the pronunciation of the same word by speakers in different parts of the United States, such as the pronunciation of 'card' with the /r/ sound deleted in New England and Southern dialects and maintained in General American dialect. An optional difference is exemplified by the way in which the final sound in 'pat' is produced, sometimes released with a burst of air at the end and sometimes unreleased, and by the pronunciation of 'palm' with or without the /l/ sound. Such differences are commonly known as **free variations.** Unlike dialectal variations, optional differences are not restricted to particular regions of the country.

Although dialectal and optional variations are of interest, the major focus in this book is on differences that are abnormal. *Abnormal* is used here to describe a sound that differs from a correct, or target, sound so as to produce a change in meaning of a word, confusion about the word intended, or an unacceptable distortion of the target sound. For example, in one type of lisp, speakers substitute a *th* sound for the /s/ sound in 'sigh' so that it cannot be distinguished from 'thigh.' A similar change in meaning occurs when /w/ is substituted for /r/ in words like 'ring.' The substitution of /w/ in a word like 'rat' still causes confusion about the intended word even though 'wat' is not a word.

In another type of lisp, speakers produce a distorted, lateral sound which sounds somewhat like a whispered /l/ sound in words like 'sigh.' This distortion is generally recognized as deviant, although it does not result in a change in meaning. The same can be said for the occurrence of the distorted /r/ sound in words like 'ring.' In children, misarticulations of this type may occur as a part of the normal development process. According to one criterion such errors are not considered abnormal unless they persist beyond the age by which 90% of children produce the sounds correctly (Sander, 1972).

Speech and language pathologists are concerned with the accurate analysis of the speech of individuals who misarticulate sounds. The information and skill required to achieve this goal forms the basis for their study of phonetics. But speech and language pathologists have special needs that require more specialized training in phonetics. Consider the application of phonetics to the diagnosis and treatment of misarticulations. In order to diagnose and design treatment, one must be able to (1) determine if a sound is produced correctly; (2) specify the differences between the intended sound and the incorrect production; (3) select the best procedure for correcting the error; (4) give the client in therapy feedback about the correctness of his/her productions of the target sound; and (5) explain the adjustments required for closer approximation to the target sound.

An important factor in specialized phonetics training for clinical purposes is that much of the articulation disorder caseload is made up of children. Phoneticians with experience in transcribing the speech of children can attest to the particular difficulties involved in the task. The preponderance of information and training in phonetics, however, is related to adult speech. Although speech and language pathologists make the transition from their predominantly adult-oriented phonetics training to predominantly child-oriented articulation therapy, there is no justification for disjunction between learning and application. In describing sounds and in transcription practice, this book emphasizes children's speech. Particular emphasis is placed on clinical phonetics by developing the student's awareness of similarities and differences between normal and misarticulated sound features in children's speech.

A second important factor in phonetics training for clinical purposes is the need for objective evidence to resolve questions about differences between sounds. Analysis of speech by listening has many shortcomings, but there are subtle acoustic cues which might help refine judgments about the speech of children (Weismer, 1984). Moreover, auditory information about differences between sounds is much more meaningful when it is integrated with physiologic and acoustic knowledge (Locke, 1979). Since most speech and language pathology students come to phonetics courses with a background in anatomy, physiology, and acoustics as these relate to speech, descriptions of normal and deviant sounds include information from these fields.

A third factor is the necessity for evaluating students as transcribers of speech sounds. Reliability tests are a means for accomplishing this goal. To diagnose misarticulations, one must have standards for normal speech. The models presented through transcription practice provide a basis for determining the correctness of variants and for the variations produced by speech and language pathologists in transcribing them. Transcribers' reliability is also important for therapy. Reliable feedback from the clinician about the correctness of sound production is vital to the client's successful rehabilitation.

PHONETICS, ORTHOGRAPHY, AND PHONOLOGY

Before learning how to analyze speech effectively, the student needs to master the system of phonetic symbols used for specifying the distinctive auditory characteristics of speech sounds. One might ask what is wrong with the alphabet, the **orthography** of English, for this. Although the alphabet is helpful in giving us some idea about how to pronounce sounds, it is not a very precise system for their description. It is deficient in three ways: (1) Each sound may be represented by a number of different letters; (2) One letter can represent a number of different sounds or even silence; and (3) The system does not provide for variations in speech sound production.

Examples of the deficiencies should be kept in mind so as to avoid the pitfall of depending on spelling to determine how words are pronounced. For the first deficiency mentioned above, consider the pronunciation of the vowel in 'feet.' This same vowel is represented in many other ways, as indicated in the following words: 'bead,' 'eve,' 'shriek,' 'pity' (second syllable). This flexibility of representation results in many **homophones,** words that are spelled differently but pronounced alike, such as 'to,' 'too,' and 'two'; 'weight' and 'wait'; 'scene' and 'seen.' For the second deficiency, representations of multiple sounds or silence by a letter, one can observe that *e* represents different vowels in 'bet' and 'we,' and silence when it is the last vowel, as in 'eve,' or that 'bow' is pronounced differently when it refers to a violin and when it refers to how one acknowledges applause. For the third deficiency, inability to show variations in sound production, many examples will emerge in the study of normal and deviant speech. Two examples: (1) The spelling does not reflect the fact that some speakers do not pronounce the /l/ in 'palm,' and (2) the alphabet does not provide a way of indicating what happens to /s/ as produced by those lispers who distort rather than substitute another sound of English for it. The potential for confusion between orthography and phonetics can be demonstrated by nonsensical orthographic strings which can produce meaningful words phonetically. For example, 'ghoti' produces the word *fish* by putting together the sounds represented by the letters in the following words: *gh* in 'laugh' = /f/; *o* in 'women' = /ɪ/; and *ti* in 'motion' = /ʃ/.

Phonetics describes and classifies sounds that are the basic units of language and the variations in the production of these sounds. Since normal language production involves a flow of continuous sound, it is not easy to identify individual units of speech. A simple procedure is used for deriving the segments of spoken language that involves **minimal pairs** of words. For example, comparison of 'bee' and 'pea' reveals that they differ only in their initial segments. Because that difference makes them two words, their initial consonants are identified as distinct units of spoken English, or **phonemes.** The set of sound segments that distinguish words in each language comprises the phonemes of that language. As part of the study of clinical phonetics, you need to learn the phonemes of English.

By analyzing English words, one can find a finite set of phonemes and a finite number of ways to combine them. For example, the initial sounds in 'seek,' 'teak,' and 'reek' can be identified as three different phonemes since, in spite of the spelling difference in the vowels, these words are the same except for the initial sounds. The initial sounds from each word can be combined to form the word 'streak.' In English *str* is a permissible combination of phonemes at the beginning of a word, but *sr* is not. Note that *sr* can be pronounced easily enough in the nonsense word 'sreek' and can be described phonetically. Initial *sr,* however, is a phonological sequence which does not fit the rules of English.

The distinction between phonetics and phonology involves the difference between describing the way language sounds are produced and the way rules are used to structure those sounds in words. In light of the current trend in the analysis of children's deviant speech sounds, the distinction is an important one. In recent years an attempt has been made to analyze children's articulatory disorders in terms of phonology (Ingram, 1976). This new focus has given rise to phonological analysis techniques for describing misarticulations (Shriberg & Kwiatkowski, 1980) and cognitive therapy techniques (Weiner, 1981) for treating them. In keeping with the new orientation and the focus on clinical phonetics, this book relates misarticulations to phonological processes whenever possible. A **phonological process** is a systematic sound change or simplification that affects a class of sounds or a sequence of sounds. For example, a phonological process, final consonant deletion, is presumed when the underlying form of 'pig' /pɪg/ takes the surface form /pɪ/. That such rules work is presumed to be corroborated by morphophonemic alternations in the speech of children. A **morphophonemic alternation** is a change in the phonemic structure of a morpheme in different contexts. For example, some children who delete final /g/ by saying /pɪ/ for 'pig' will also say /pɪgi/ for 'piggy.' The morphophonemic alternation is the use of /g/ to terminate the **morpheme** 'pig' in 'piggy' but not in the word 'pig.'

The distinction between phonological and phonetic errors may be useful in the diagnosis and treatment of children's sound errors. In traditional analysis of children who used /w/ for /r/ in 'ring,' the error was called a substitution and ascribed to articulatory difficulty in producing /r/. Phonological process analysis of the same error results in describing it as gliding (Ingram, 1976). In this analysis, saying, /w/ for /r/ follows a **phonological rule** which neutralizes the distinction between the sounds.

Errors which appear to be more clearly due to difficulty in producing a sound, such as the production of a distorted /r/, are considered phonetic. If the problem is cognitive, as may be the case for a child who substitutes /w/ for /r/ by rule, treatment would be different from that for a child who is unable to articulate /r/ correctly. It is not easy to distinguish between phonological and phonetic errors. Assuming that a child is using a phonological rule requires some evidence that the child knows the difference between the two sounds involved. In addition to morphophonemic alternations, the child might use acoustic cues to help distinguish the sounds. Children may make vowels longer in words ending in voiced consonants, for example, 'pig,' than in those ending in voiceless consonants, for example, 'pick'—even though they omit the consonants. Some researchers contend that acoustic analysis of speech is required to discover such cues (Maxwell, 1981a; Weismer, Dinnsen, & Elbert, 1981; Weismer, 1984).

PHONETICS AND PHONEMICS

In the analysis of speech sounds, there are two levels of interest. At the phonetic level, one identifies sounds that differ and the acoustic and physiologic characteristics that differentiate them. The vowels in 'bit' and 'bet' are different because 'bit' is produced with a higher tongue position than 'bet.' The vowel sounds in 'key' and 'coo' differ partly because the tongue position for the vowel of 'key' is more anterior than it is for the vowel of 'coo.' The same observation can be made about the tongue position for the initial consonants in these words, a distinction that you can feel as your tongue makes contact in pronouncing them.

The interest at the phonemic level is to identify which sounds make meaningful distinctions in our language, that is, which cues are important in distinguishing words. The same comparisons used for showing the phonetic level can be reexamined with a different question in mind. The vowels are different in 'bit' and 'bet,' but is it this difference that is responsible for distinguishing words in English, or could it be due to consonantal differences? Comparing the initial and final consonants of the two words indicates that they differ very little, if at all, between these two words. On this basis, one may conclude that the vowels in 'bit' and 'bet' are two different phonemes in English. They differentiate words. Pairs of words that differ in only one structurally analogous phoneme, like 'bit' and 'bet,' are minimal pairs, and minimal pair comparisons are basic to phonemic analysis.

Does the spelling of words serve to identify phonemes, since the spelling of the vowels in 'bit' and 'bet' is different? In many cases, spelling is a false friend when it comes to phonemic analysis. For example, *ee* and *ea* differentiate words like 'breed' and 'bread' but not words like 'reed' and 'read' (present tense), which are pronounced exactly alike.

The initial sounds of 'key' and 'coo' demonstrate another important phonemic concept. These words differ both in their vowels and in their initial consonants. Obviously there is a phonemic difference here, but is it due to the vowels or the consonants? Additional evidence shows that the difference is due to the vowels. The same vowels as in 'key' and 'coo' distinguish another pair of words, 'bee' and 'boo,' where there is no discernible difference between the consonants. Also, no words differ only because they have the same initial consonants as 'key' and 'coo,' respectively. The initial sound in 'key' always occurs before vowels made with the tongue in an anterior position, as in 'kit' and 'cat,' and the initial sound in 'coo' always occurs before vowels made with the tongue in a posterior position, as in 'caught' and 'cot.' The comparison of 'key' and 'coo,' then, results in the classification of their vowels, not their consonants, as two phonemes of English.

If the vowels in 'key' and 'coo' are meaningfully different, then what does the difference between the initial consonants represent? These sounds can be identified in other minimal pairs where they contrast with other consonants, as in 'key' and 'tea' and in 'coo' and 'too.' Such comparisons demonstrate that the initial consonants of the minimal pair words are phonemes of English. There are, however, no minimal pairs that differ solely because of the consonants of 'key' and 'coo.' These consonants are members of the same phoneme, or allophones of the same phoneme. An **allophone** is a variant of a phoneme which results from variations in context like the front vowel of 'key' and the back vowel of 'coo.'

In contrasting the status of phonemes and allophones, the emphasis is on their contextual distribution in English. For example, the (phonemic) initial sound of 'key' also appears in 'coo' and 'school.' But, in each context, the release of air for the consonant is different. The burst of air in 'key' is higher in frequency than it is in 'coo,' and it is negligible in 'school.' These differing characteristics can be attributed to context, that is, before vowels made from different tongue positions in 'key' and 'coo,' and after /s/ in 'school.' This pattern of contextual variations is called **complementary distribution;** one allophone does not occur in the same context as another allophone. But phonemes by definition must contrast. For example, the initial phonemes of 'sat,' 'bat,' 'cat,' and 'fat' contrast before the identical *at* context to produce different words.

The concepts of the phoneme and the allophone are not only important in descriptive phonetics but also in clinical phonetics. Use of minimal pairs has become an integral part of therapy for children with phonological disorders (Weiner, 1981). Allophonic analysis helps explain why some children say 'wook' for 'look' but 'yady' for 'lady' (Stoel-Gammon & Dunn, 1985).

On the basis of phonemic distinctions, transcription of speech can be described as broad or narrow. Broad, or phonemic, transcription includes only those distinctions between sounds that differentiate minimal pairs. Such transcriptions are generally set off between slant lines (virgules). Narrow, or phonetic, transcription includes allophonic variations and misarticulations. Such transcriptions are set off between brackets.

DESCRIPTIVE AND EXPERIMENTAL PHONETICS

Descriptive Phonetics

Descriptive phonetics is the study of how speech sounds are produced, how they differ, and how symbols are used to describe the differences. This study depends on individuals' skill at perceiving the important distinctions between sounds and transcribing them accurately. Three experimental areas of phonetics provide information and objective methods for resolving questions about the nature of variations in speech sounds: physiologic phonetics, acoustic phonetics, and perceptual phonetics.

Physiologic phonetics is the study of the formation of speech in terms of the contacts, configurations, and movements of the articulatory structures that distinguish speech sounds by means of X-ray, palatography, electromyography, airflow and air pressure measuring devices, and other procedures. **Acoustic phonetics** is the study of the physical nature of speech in terms of the frequency, duration, and intensity of speech sounds. Acoustic analysis is carried out with the help of spectrographs, oscilloscopes, sound level meters, and digital signal processing techniques, and other instrumentation and procedures. **Perceptual phonetics** is the study of the auditory cues of speech. It uses tests of identification and discrimination of real speech, synthesized speech, and speech distorted by such procedures as filtering and masking.

Physiologic Phonetics

In physiologic phonetics, X-ray and palatography techniques have been used to visualize the position of the tongue during sound production. Figure 1–1 is a midsagittal section of the **vocal tract** which shows important parts of the articulatory system, or speech mechanism. In the upper part of the tract, the upper lip is relatively inactive except in

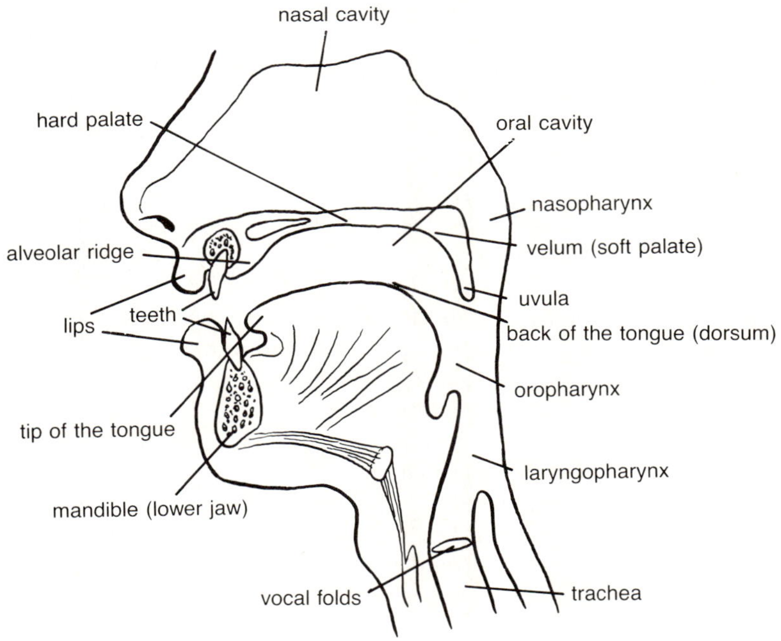

Figure 1–1
Midsagittal section of the vocal tract illustrating various articulators and cavities.

the production of rounded vowels in words like 'two.' Directly posterior to the upper lip are the upper teeth, which the tongue tip and the lower lip touch in speech production. Directly posterior to the upper teeth is the **alveolar ridge,** which is the bony prominence that you can feel by drawing the tip of your tongue backward along the roof of your mouth. This is an important location for tongue contact or approximation in the production of the initial sounds in 'sue,' 'zoo,' 'to,' and 'do.'

If you continue pulling your tongue tip backward along the roof of your mouth, you will feel soft tissue that does not give way to the pressure of your tongue because it is backed by the maxilla and palatine bones of the skull. This portion of the roof of your mouth is the **hard palate.** If you continue drawing your tongue tip backward, it will reach a point where the bony structure ends and the soft tissue can be pushed upward. This is the **soft palate,** or **velum.** The most posterior part of the velum is the **uvula,** which you can see moving to a raised position if you look in a mirror and say "ah." As you look into your mouth, you can see the **pharyngeal wall** just posterior to the uvula. Just posterior to the uvula is the part of the pharynx called the oropharynx. Superior to the oropharynx is the nasopharynx. The opening between the nasal cavity and the oral cavity is formed by these two parts of the pharynx. This opening is closed off by elevation of the velum (through the action of the **velopharyngeal muscles**) during speech production.

Everything identified so far is a location on the upper surface of the vocal tract. All are contacted or approximated by articulators of the **mandible** or lower jaw—the lip, teeth, and tongue. The velum plays an active role in the production of nasal consonants by moving up and down to assist in closing off or opening up the channel between the oral and nasal cavities.

Figure 1–1 shows the articulators of the lower jaw or mandible on the inferior surface of the vocal tract. First is the lower lip, which, along with the upper lip, purses in the production of rounded vowels. With the assistance of the upward movement of the lower jaw, the lower lip contacts the upper teeth in producing the sounds that begin 'fine' and 'vine.' Directly posterior to the lower lip are the lower teeth, which, with the assistance of upward jaw movement, are articulators in the production of the sounds that begin 'sue' and 'zoo.'

The tongue is the most active articulator. For purposes of specifying the articulation of speech sounds, it is divided into the somewhat arbitrary parts indicated in Figure 1–1. First is the **tongue tip,** or **tongue apex,** which is the part that makes contact when you touch the back of your upper teeth. Immediately posterior to the tip is the **tongue blade,** or **tongue lamina,** which is the part that makes contact with the alveolar ridge when you raise the whole tongue to the roof of your mouth. In this raised position, the front part of the tongue contacts the hard palate, and the back part, or **tongue dorsum,** contacts the soft palate, or velum.

Basic to the entire speech mechanism are the **vocal folds,** located at the upper end of the **trachea.** Air from the lungs passes through the trachea and between the vocal folds into the vocal tract. Superior to the vocal folds and inferior to the oropharynx is the laryngopharynx. For voiced sounds, the folds are approximated so that the air pressure built up beneath them makes them vibrate.

The terminology used for consonant articulation distinguishes between lower jaw and upper jaw articulators. For example, *apico-alveolar* describes the position for the /t/

sound produced by placing the tongue tip (apical part or apex) against the alveolar ridge. In combinations like apico-alveolar, the first element is always the lower jaw articulator and the second is always the upper jaw articulator.

Contact with the palate during consonant production has been inferred from tongue contact impressions obtained by means of **palatography.** Over the years a number of different procedures have been used, but most involve a dental appliance that fits in the roof of the mouth much like a retainer for orthodontic work. Recent techniques employ prostheses with embedded electrodes which generate electrical signals in response to tongue contacts during the production of consonants. The electrical signals the contacts make provide a picture of tongue contact during consonant production. Figures 1–2 and 1–3 show the tongue contacts for the initial sounds in words like 'see,' 'she,' 'tea,' and 'key.' What you see is an outline of the margins of the upper teeth and the hard palate. The contacts for 'tea' and 'see' are more anterior than those for 'she' and 'key.' In addition, the channel, or groove, for 'see' is narrower than it is for 'she' (Fletcher, 1989). **Palatograms** (figures 1–2 and 1–3) do not indicate which part of the tongue is making contact.

Although palatography is helpful in visualizing tongue contact for consonants, one must keep in mind its limitations. Tongue position must be inferred, the contour of the palate is usually lost in most procedures, and much of the dynamics of speech is missing. Since most vowels involve little contact with the palate, palatography is not useful for vowel analysis.

Acoustic Phonetics/Acoustics of Speech

In this text, differences among normal sounds and between normal and abnormal productions of the same sounds are illustrated by means of acoustic analyses. For the most part these analyses were made by a **spectrograph** on printouts called **spectrograms.** In order to read them one must be aware of the relationship between the acoustics of speech and spectral analyses.

The connection between sound and its visual representation may be considered by using a tuning fork. A vibrating tuning fork produces a pure tone; that is, it vibrates at a constant frequency like 125 Hz, 250 Hz, 500 Hz, 750 Hz, or 1000 Hz. The vibration of a tuning fork as a source of sound can be represented by the diagram in Figure 1–4, which shows time along the ***x* axis** (abscissa) and amplitude along the ***y* axis** (ordinate). **Amplitude** refers to how far a vibrating body moves from its resting position. Figure 1–4 plots the movements of a tuning fork vibrating at 125 Hz through two complete cycles of vibration. This type of display is a **waveform analysis.** The same kind of analysis can represent not only the displacement of the tines of a tuning fork but also the positive and negative changes in air pressure produced by the vibration of the tuning fork. The air pressure variations are perceived as sounds.

Figure 1–4A provides a basis for understanding the relationship between the period and the frequency of vibration. The waveform in the figure represents two complete cycles of vibration, or air pressure variation, produced by a tuning fork. As the diagram shows, each cycle occurs in .008 second or 8 milliseconds (msec). The duration of one cycle of vibration is called the **period of vibration.** In one second a 125 Hz

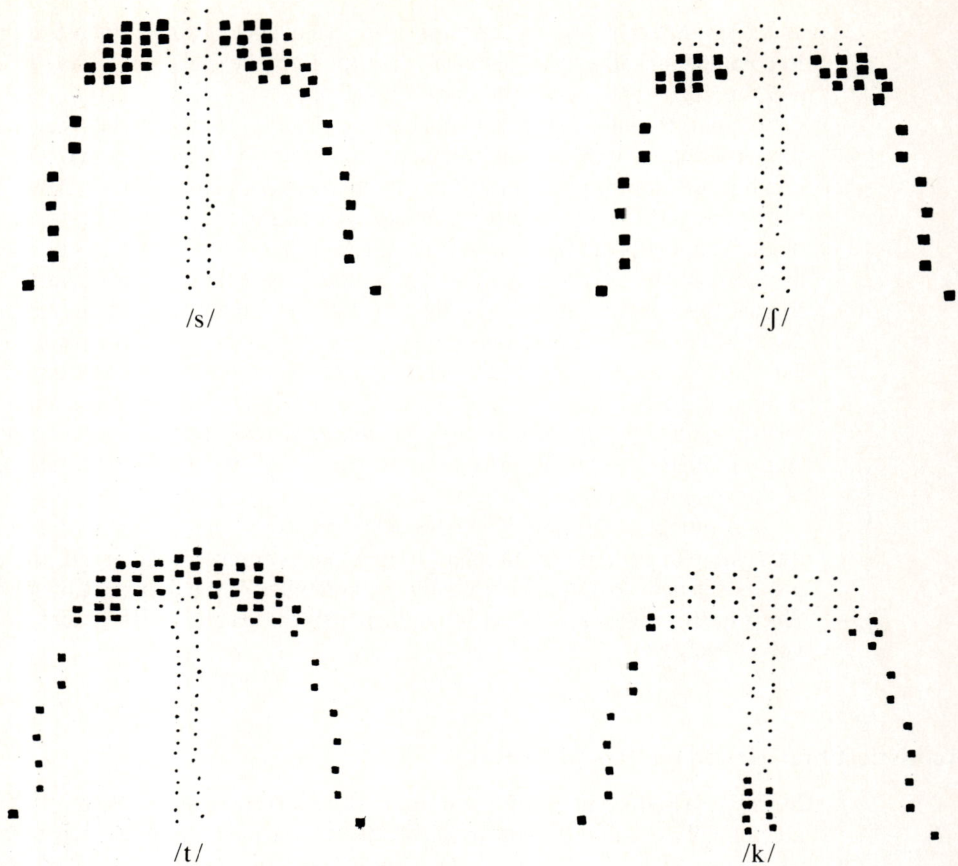

Figure 1–2
Palatograms for a child's productions of /s/, /ʃ/, /t/, and /k/ in prevocalic position. These palatograms were produced using a pseudopalate containing the palatometric sensors connected to a light array system. The dots show the placement of the sensors. Darker dots indicate palatal contact by the tongue. In each palatogram, the front of the hard palate is at the top and the back is at the bottom.
Source: "Palatometric Specification of Stop, Affricate, and Sibilant Sounds" by S. G. Fletcher, 1989, *Journal of Speech and Hearing Research, 32,* p. 741. Copyright 1989 by the American Speech-Language-Hearing Association. Adapted by permission.

tuning fork completes 125 cycles, which is the **frequency** of vibration. (Formerly this was specified as cycles per second, but is now simply called Hertz and abbreviated Hz.)

The vibration of the tuning fork can be illustrated by means of another type of display, shown in Figure 1–4B. In this diagram frequency is shown along the *x* axis and amplitude along the *y* axis. The display reflects the sound produced by a 125 Hz tuning fork by a vertical line positioned to correspond to its frequency and made long enough to correspond to the sound's amplitude. This type of display is the result of a **spectral analysis,** which is referred to as a *line spectrum,* and it is not limited to portraying the

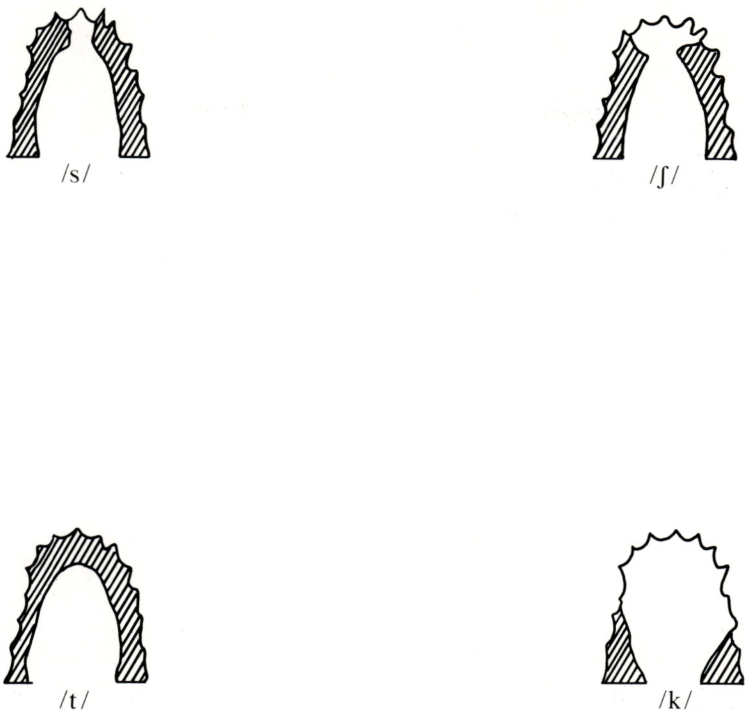

Figure 1–3
Palatograms for an adult's productions of /s/, /ʃ/, /t/, and /k/ in prevocalic position. These palatograms were produced in the classic manner by examining areas where a color-contrasting powder was removed from a pseudopalate after a particular production. Areas where tongue contact was made are highlighted by bold lines. In each palatogram, the front of the hard palate is at the top, the back of the hard palate is at the bottom, and the scalloped line shows the inner margins of the upper teeth.

action of just one tuning fork. If tuning forks with frequencies of 125 Hz, 250 Hz, and 375 Hz are simultaneously set into motion, they produce a more complex waveform than that for any single pure tone (see Figure 1–5). Even **complex sounds** can be subjected to spectral analysis. The complex waveform (Figure 1–5d) repeats itself at periodic intervals which correspond to the period of its lowest frequency component (125 Hz). The lowest frequency component is the **fundamental frequency** (f_0). The higher frequency components in this example are whole-number, or integral multiples of f_0, which means they are harmonically related to it. Harmonically related frequency components of a complex sound are also referred to as **harmonics.** In the example, 125 Hz, 250 Hz, and 375 Hz are the first, second, and third harmonics. Spectral analysis (Figure 1–5e) shows that 125 Hz, 250 Hz, and 375 Hz are the frequency components of the complex sound.

In speech production there are no simple vibrating systems like a tuning fork. The basic sound for vowel and vowel-like sounds is produced by the vocal folds, which are

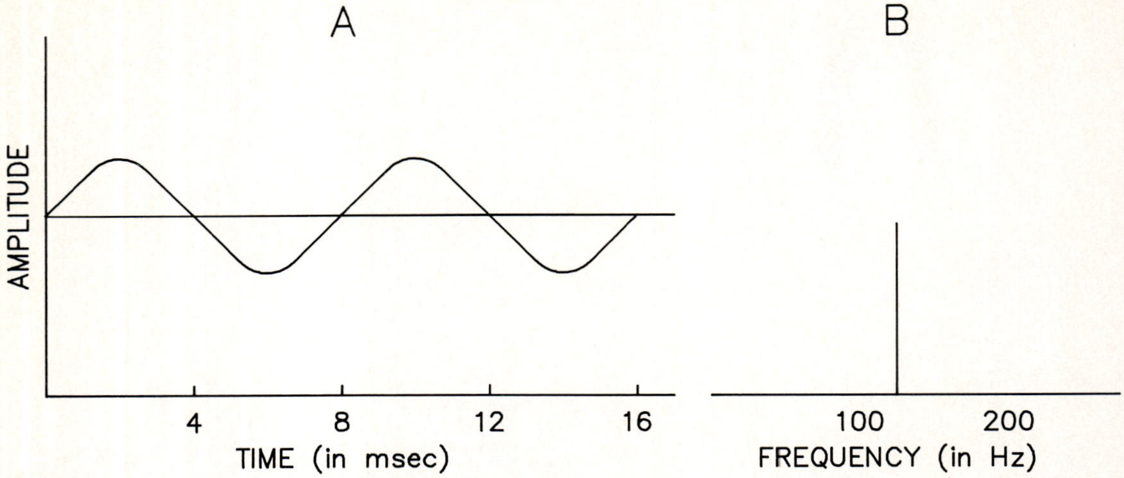

Figure 1–4
A waveform analysis (amplitude × time) of the vibration of a 125 Hz tuning fork (panel A) and a spectral analysis (amplitude × frequency) of the pure tone produced by it (panel B).

set into vibration by the air flowing out of the lungs. The vocal folds do not produce a pure tone but a complex sound made up of a fundamental frequency and a series of harmonics. The fundamental frequency is the basic vibratory period of the vocal folds, the rate at which they open and close, and the harmonics are the vibratory periods of their complex wavelike motions as they open and close.

Since the sound output, or **glottal tone,** from the vocal folds is not heard until it has traveled through the vocal tract, its original acoustic characteristics can only be inferred. Spectral analysis for an adult with a 125 Hz f_0 and a child with a 250 Hz f_0 might look like those in the two left panels of Figure 1–6. The vertical lines represent f_0 and the harmonics. The diagram shows (1) vertical lines for an adult, the first five of which correspond to a f_0 of 125 Hz and harmonics of 250 Hz, 375 Hz, 500 Hz, and 625 Hz, which are two, three, four, and five times the f_0, and (2) vertical lines for a child, the first five of which correspond to a f_0 of 250 Hz and harmonics of 500 Hz, 750 Hz, 1000 Hz, and 1250 Hz, which are two, three, four, and five times the f_0. Figure 1–6 shows many higher harmonics than these, but the actual number of harmonics in the glottal tone is greater than shown in the diagrams, since it contains harmonics up through the whole range of human speech. Note that the tone for the child has a higher f_0 and fewer harmonics than that for the adult. The amplitude of harmonics successively decreases, which is an acoustic characteristic of the glottal tone.

As it is transmitted through the vocal tract, the glottal tone is affected by that resonance system. Certain frequencies are reinforced. Like other resonators, the vocal tract has resonance frequencies to which it responds with a greater amount of vibration and other frequencies which elicit a minimal response. In general, the larger vocal tract

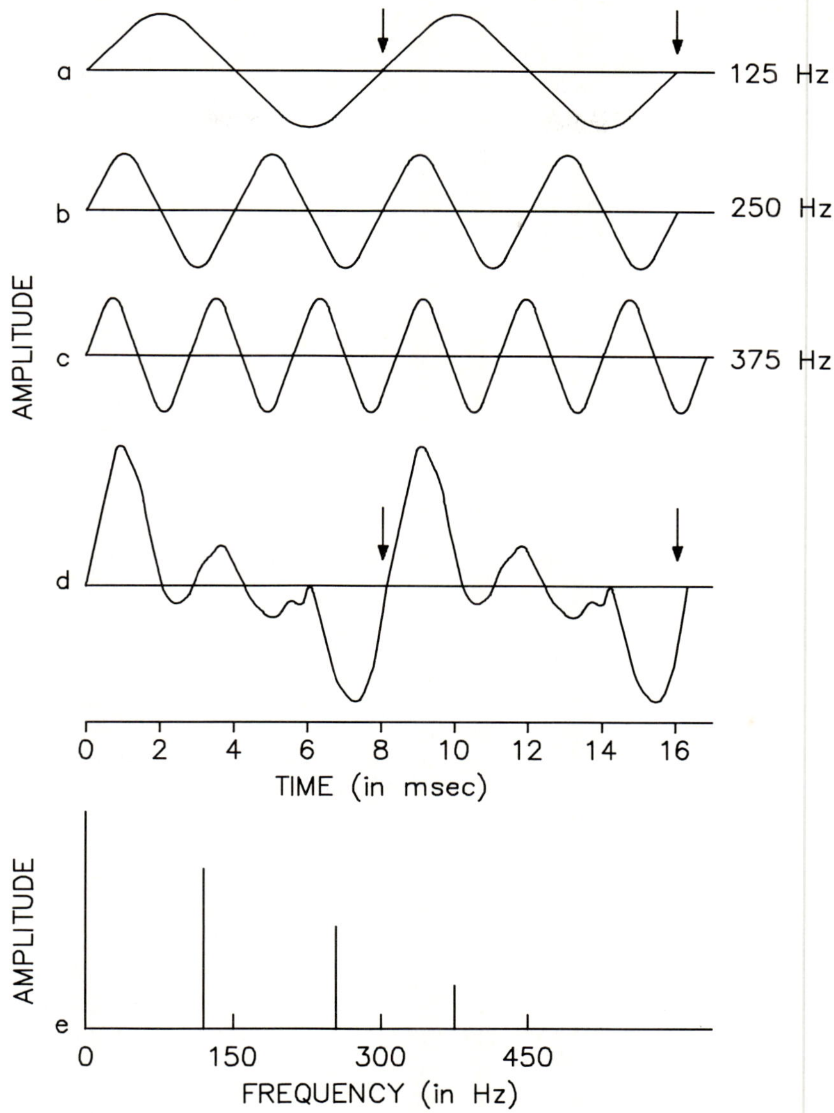

Figure 1–5
Waveform analyses (amplitude × time) of pure tones with frequencies of (a) 125 Hz, (b) 250 Hz, (c) 375 Hz, (d) the complex sound they produce when vibrating at the same time, and (e) spectral analysis (amplitude × frequency) of the complex sound. Arrows indicate the correspondence between the periods of vibration of the lowest component of the complex sound and the waveform analysis of the complex sound.

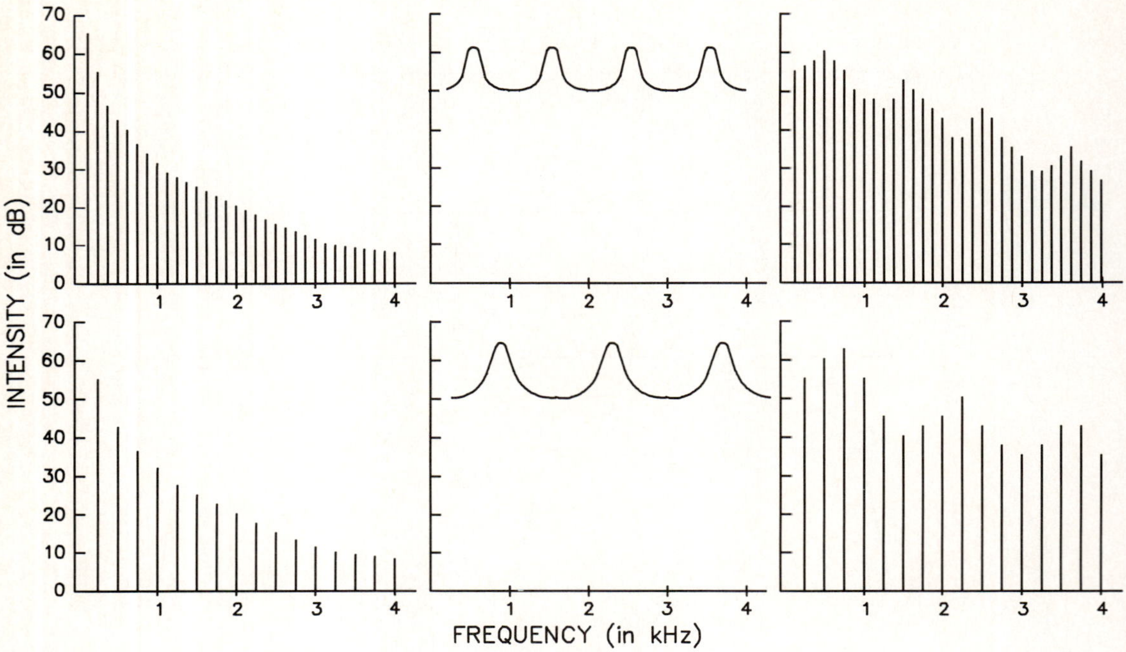

Figure 1–6
Spectral analyses of the glottal tone (left panels) for an adult (upper panel) and a child (lower panel); hypothetical resonance characteristics of the adult and child vocal tracts (middle panels) producing a vowel like that in the second syllable of 'above'; spectral analyses of the vowel (right panels) in the second syllable of 'above' as produced by an adult and a child. Note that an additional formant, F_4, occurs in the adult analysis within the 4000 Hz range shown.

of an adult has lower resonance frequencies than a child's smaller vocal tract. The vocal tract is a complex system, and it is difficult to show its resonance characteristics simply. The simplest pattern is obtained from the production of a neutral vowel, as in the second syllable of 'above.' In this position the vocal tract is most like a long tube, open at the mouth end and with no significant constrictions or side cavities along its length.

The resonance characteristics of the vocal tract in the position for a neutral vowel are illustrated in the middle panels in Figure 1–6. Frequency is shown along the *x* axis and amplitude along the *y* axis. The adult's vocal production shows four peaks corresponding to frequencies of 500 Hz, 1500 Hz, 2500 Hz, and 3500 Hz; the child's has three peaks at 750 Hz, 2250 Hz, and 3750 Hz. These peaks are the resonance frequencies of the vocal tract, commonly called **formants.** For a neutral vowel the vocal tract reinforces the frequency components of sound that correspond to its resonance frequencies much more than other components. Of course, the vocal tract by itself cannot produce a vowel sound, and so it must be activated by the input from the vocal folds, which are set into motion by the airflow between them.

If a glottal tone with the frequency components shown in Figure 1–6 activates the vocal tract in the position for a neutral vowel with the resonance characteristics also shown there, only the harmonics of the glottal tone that correspond to the peaks will be reinforced. The spectrum analysis looks like those in the two right panels of Figure 1–6. The frequency components at 500 Hz, 1500 Hz, 2500 Hz, and 3500 Hz are much greater in intensity than the others for the adult, and those at 750 Hz, 2250 Hz, and 3750 Hz are much greater in intensity than the others for the child.

Using a spectrograph, analyses like those illustrated in Figure 1–6 can be made. The spectrograph makes an analysis of speech sounds by filtering. A **filter** is a resonator that transmits selected frequencies. The bandwidth of the filter is the range of frequencies that are at least 70% of the amplitude of the frequency passed with maximum amplitude. These center frequencies passed through the filter with maximum sound energy are referred to as formant frequencies.

Figure 1–7 (lower left panel) shows a narrow band spectrogram of the /ʌ/ vowel; the spectrogram is called **narrow band** because the filter used transmits frequencies within a relatively narrow range of 45 Hz, for example, 550 Hz to 595 Hz. Actually, the spectrograph filter is continuously varied in the narrow range of frequency as a speech signal is played back repeatedly from a recording. As a result, the entire frequency range of speech can be scanned to determine where the greatest intensity is. In spectrograms, time is shown from left to right along the *x* axis, frequency from bottom to top along the *y* axis, and intensity is shown by the darkness of the pattern. The equally spaced horizontal lines in Figure 1–7 correspond to the f_0 (125 Hz) and the harmonics, 250 Hz, 500 Hz, 750 Hz, 1000 Hz, and higher. Notice that the lines representing the 500 Hz, 1500 Hz, and 2500 Hz harmonics are much darker than the others.

The relative darkness of the horizontal lines in the spectrograms in Figure 1–7 represents the relative intensity of the harmonics—the darker the line the greater the intensity. **Intensity** is a measure of sound energy that is more analogous to our judgment of the loudness of sounds than is amplitude since it is influenced by both amplitude and frequency. Intensity is proportional to the square of the amplitude and the frequency of sounds. In simple terms, greater amplitude, which reflects greater displacement, produces more sound energy than lower amplitude, and higher frequency of vibration, which reflects more frequent displacement, also produces more sound energy than lower frequency of vibration.

The concentration of sound energy in the 500 Hz, 1500 Hz, and 2500 Hz harmonics shown in the narrow band analysis of Figure 1–7 indirectly reflects the formants of the /ʌ/ vowel illustrated in Figure 1–6 (upper middle and right panels). In order to display the filter characteristics of the vocal tract more clearly, spectrograms of speech are usually made using a **wide band** analysis, where the filter has a range of 300 Hz. Such a filter transmits frequencies within a wider range than a narrow filter, for example, 300 Hz to 600 Hz. A wide band analysis of the /ʌ/ vowel is shown in Figure 1–7 (lower right panel). The discrete horizontal lines seen in a narrow band spectrogram do not appear in a wide band spectrogram, which does not show individual harmonics. The wide, dark horizontal bars centered around 500 Hz, 1500 Hz, and 2500 Hz, however, provide a prominent display of the energy present in those regions for the /ʌ/ vowel. These bars are referred to as formants although, more accurately, they are the spectrographic manifestation of the formants of the vocal tract during vowel production. The

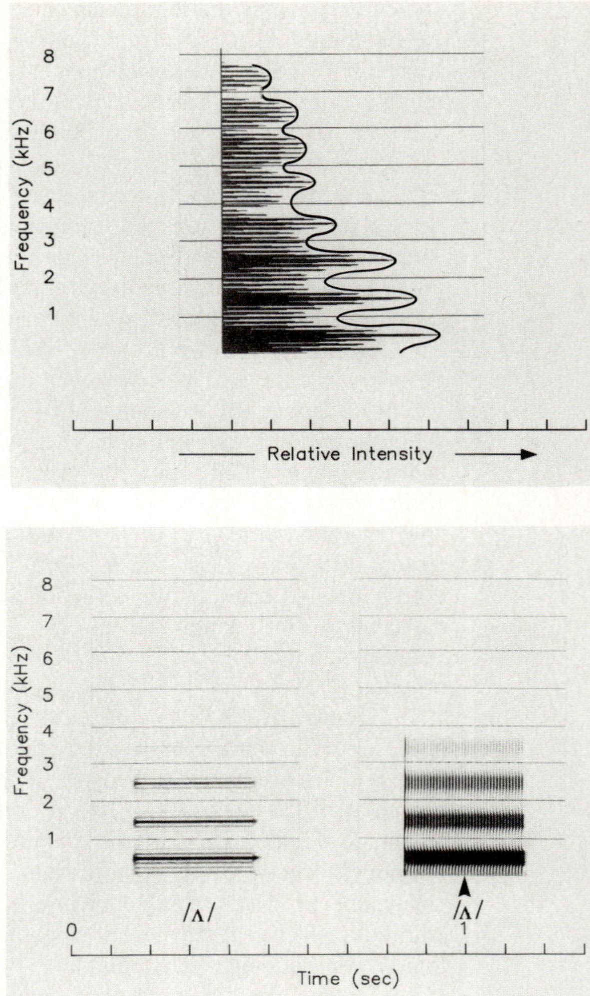

Figure 1–7
A narrow band spectrogram (bottom left panel) and a wide band spectrogram (bottom right panel) of a vowel like that in the second syllable of 'above' as produced by an adult male. A power spectrum or amplitude section taken at the point indicated by the arrow below the wide band spectrogram is shown in the upper panel. An envelope curve marks the upper limits of the harmonics.

bars are usually identified as F_1, F_2, F_3, and F_4, from lowest to highest frequency formant. Formants higher than F_4 may also be observed in spectrograms.

Although wide band analysis does not include the harmonic information obtained in narrow band analysis, it does reflect the activation or pulsing of the vocal tract each time the vocal folds open and close. If you look at the wide band pattern in Figure 1–7 (lower right panel), you will notice that there are vertical lines, or **striations,** closely spaced throughout the pattern. Each vertical line represents a glottal **pulse,** and the interval between any two lines indicates the period of vibration of the vocal folds.

The spectrograph can be used to take a closer look at the spectrum of a sound at a specific point. In Figure 1–7, a point has been selected in the middle of the /ʌ/ vowel for such an analysis, which is called a **power spectrum** or **amplitude section.** The section produced for the /ʌ/ vowel is shown in the upper panel of Figure 1–7. Here frequency is shown along the vertical axis and intensity along the horizontal axis. The lines represent f_0 and higher harmonics, and the peaks indicate reinforced harmonics. As you would expect, the peaks are at 500 Hz, 1500 Hz, 2500 Hz, and 3500 Hz, as is characteristic of an adult male /ʌ/ vowel. A line called an **envelope curve** has been drawn marking the upper limits of the harmonics. The peaks of this curve correspond very closely in frequency to those in Figure 1–6 for the resonance characteristics of the vocal tract in the position for /ʌ/.

Since the production of vowels and consonants is different, they look different in sound spectrograms. Unlike vowels, consonants are characterized by noises, in particular, pulse, **frication noise,** and **aspiration.** Frication noise is produced when the vocal cavity is constricted at some point so that the airstream from the lungs undergoes turbulence. This turbulence results in noise at the point of constriction and is a characteristic of fricative sounds like those in 'foe,' 'so,' and 'show.'

If a complete closure rather than a constriction is produced in the vocal cavity, air pressure builds up behind the articulators responsible for the stoppage. When the articulators separate and the air is released from the oral cavity, a **burst** is produced, which consists of pulse and frication noises. This type of noise is characteristic of the release of stop sounds, like those in 'pea,' 'tea,' and 'key.' In addition, voiceless stops generally have a period of aspiration noise produced by air passing between the open vocal folds.

Unlike vowels, pulse, frication, and aspiration noises have no glottal tone, so no fundamental frequency or harmonics are produced for them. As a result, the energy of these sounds is not organized by frequency components but spreads across the frequency range. This type of acoustic pattern is shown in Figure 1–8, which is a spectrogram of the /s/ and /ʃ/ sounds produced in isolation. There are no harmonics or formants in the patterns for these sounds. Instead, the patterns are made up of random vertical lines, called **fill,** across a wide range of frequencies.

Although frication noises do not activate the vocal tract resonator as vowels do, the oral cavity anterior and posterior to the constriction acts as a resonator, and certain frequency ranges of the noise are reinforced. As a result, the range of frequencies characteristic of fricatives that differ in articulatory position like /s/ and /ʃ/ also differ, as can be seen from Figure 1–8.

The burst noise associated with stops is very brief, varying from about 10 to 30 msec. Like frication noise, burst noise is not made up of an f_0 and harmonics but of sound energy spread across a range of frequencies. Figure 1–9 includes spectrograms of bursts produced as the /p/, /t/, and /k/ sounds are released in the pronunciation of 'pea,' 'tea,' and 'key.' The brevity of the pulse may be observed from the initial vertical line that represents it in each of these utterances. In some cases the pulse may be so weak that it does not appear on a spectrogram, as appears to be the case for /p/ in Figure 1–9. Following the pulse is a short period of frication noise caused by the narrow

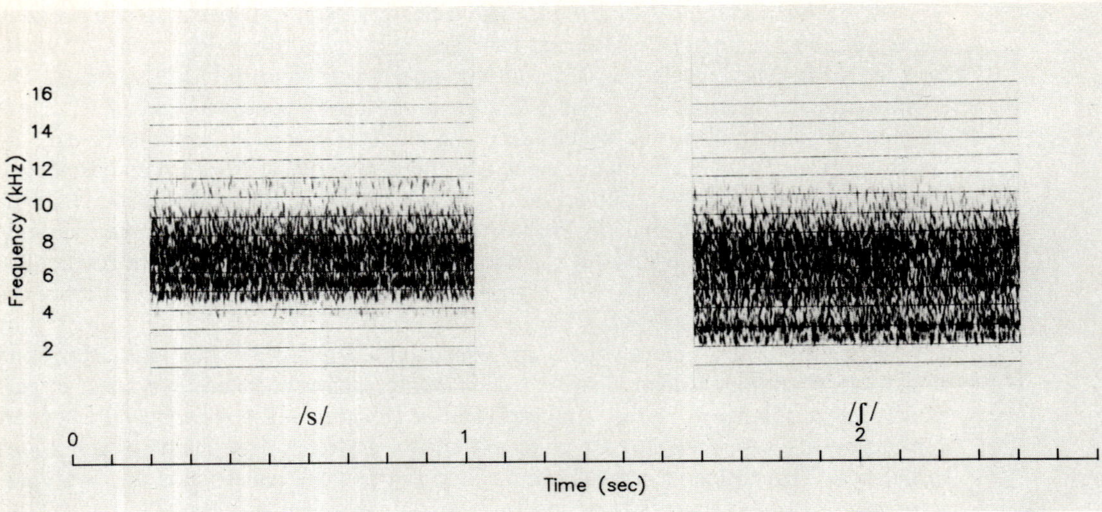

Figure 1–8
Wide band spectrograms of the /s/ of 'see' and the /ʃ/ of 'she' produced in isolation by an adult male.

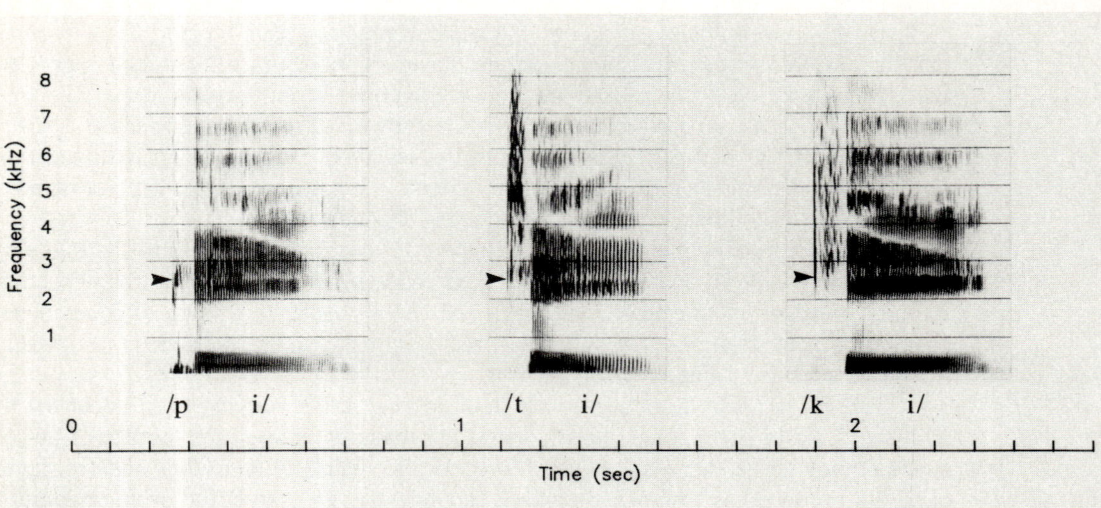

Figure 1–9
A wide band spectrogram of the /p/ of 'pea,' the /t/ of 'tea,' and the /k/ of 'key' produced by an adult male. The pulses of the stop bursts are marked by initial vertical lines (spikes), most evident between 2 and 3 kHz, as indicated by the arrows.

opening between two articulators. Since the closures responsible for these bursts are at different points of articulation, the different shapes of the vocal cavity reinforce different frequencies. As a result the vertical lines representing the pulses vary in the range of frequencies they cover. A period of aspiration following the frication is also shown in these patterns.

In speech, consonants are produced by various combinations of systems. For example, stops and fricatives may be produced with a glottal tone, and these sounds can be expected to include various combinations of sound types. Figure 1–10 shows spectrograms of the word 'syntax' produced by a child and an adult male. Sounds that are produced with vocal fold vibration, such as the vowels of the first and second syllables of 'syntax,' show formants which reflect the resonances of the vocal tract as it changes length and shape during speech production. For the vowel in the first syllable of 'syntax,' for example, the first formant (F_1) and second formant (F_2) levels are different from those for the vowel of the second syllable. The formant frequencies of the child's vowels are higher than the adult's because of the child's shorter vocal tract. Changes in the formant pattern as vocal tract size and shape change are further demonstrated in Chapter 3.

Many consonants, like the initial and final /s/ sound in 'syntax,' are characterized by frication noise. In Figure 1–10 the frication noise for /s/ is reflected by the fill at the beginning and end of 'syntax.'

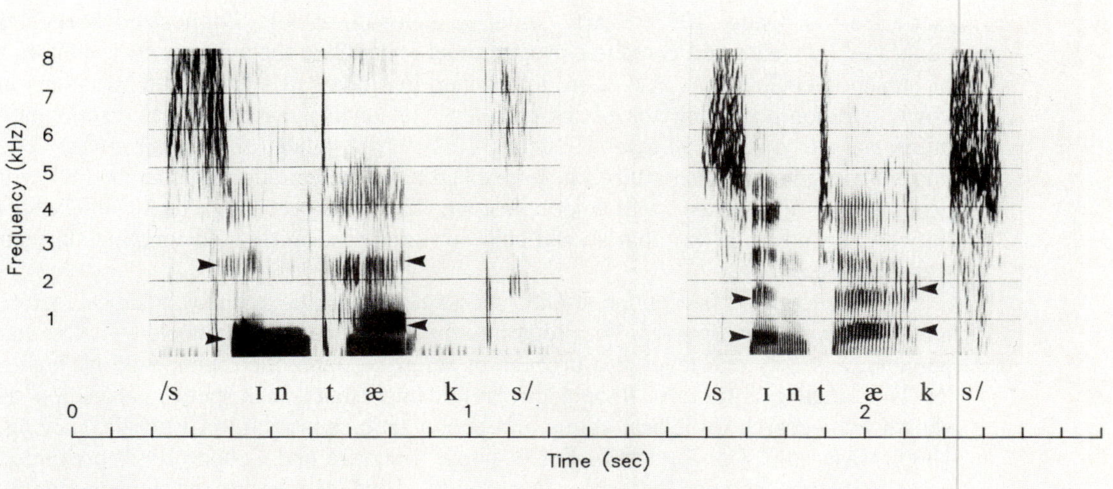

Figure 1–10
Spectrograms of the word 'syntax' produced by a child (left panel) and an adult male (right panel). Arrows along the *y* axis indicate the approximate positions of the first (F_1) and second (F_2) formants of vowels. The filter bandwidth was 300 Hz for the adult male and 500 Hz for the child. Unless noted otherwise, these bandwidths are used for spectrographic analyses throughout the book.

Some consonants, like the /n/ of 'syntax,' also display formants reflecting the resonance of the oral and nasal cavities in nasal consonant production. Other consonants, like /t/, are produced by momentarily stopping the flow of air and then releasing it. During the stoppage, no sound occurs, but with the sudden opening of the vocal tract comes a pulse of air pressure followed by frication noise as the air escapes between the articulators. In Figure 1–10 these acoustic cues are shown for the /t/ of 'syntax.' The **gap** or blank space following /n/ reflects the pressure buildup for /t/, during which no sound is produced. The vertical line or **spike** immediately following the gap reflects the pulse or puff of air produced at the release of the /t/, and the fill following the spike reflects the frication noise produced as the air escapes from the vocal tract.

Perceptual Phonetics

Although the evidence regarding perceptual phonetics is not as definitive as it is for physiologic or acoustic phonetics, it still is of considerable interest. In considering this evidence, one must examine the relationships both between the acoustic characteristics of speech and speech perception and between levels of language processing and speech perception.

Listeners are able to differentiate sounds on the basis of their frequency and duration (acoustic characteristics). It has been determined in studies of synthesized child speech that speech and language pathology students can differentiate distorted /r/ from normal /r/ and /w/ sounds on the basis of small changes in the F_2 and F_3 frequencies (Sharf & Ohde, 1983; Sharf, Ohde, & Lehman, 1986). Synthesized speech is generated by means of a computer programmed to simulate the acoustic characteristics of human speech. It has also been determined in studies of synthesized variations in vowel duration preceding voiced and voiceless consonants that adults can discriminate differences as small as 50 msec (Lehman, 1988; Sharf, Ohde, & Lehman, 1988). The information given in such studies helps explain how one can identify sounds and what acoustic cues are needed for their identification. This book presents acoustic differences between sounds in a way that should help you capitalize on these distinctions in your transcription efforts.

Evidence from perceptual studies shows that linguistic and psychological factors influence sound identification. With regard to the linguistic factor, it should be noted that phonology is only one level in a process of language perception influenced by higher levels of language structure. Phonology plays an important role in speech perception, as shown by research on lexical status and phonotactic constraints in English (Ganong, 1980; Massaro & Cohen, 1983). For example, Massaro and Cohen (1983) presented listeners with utterances that varied between /s l i/ and /s r i/ and asked them to identify the sounds as /l/ or /r/. The listeners heard significantly more of the sounds as /l/ than as /r/. This finding was presumably due to the fact that initial /s/ is permissible before /l/ but not before /r/ in English.

In some cases, interaction between language levels is useful, as, for example, when context enables you to understand what is said in a noisy listening environment even though portions of the speech signal are masked by the noise. But the linguistic factor can also interfere with accurate perception, and you should be aware of this when you make phonetic transcriptions. Such conditions include context, language or phonological structure, and linguistic function.

Context

Just as context may assist in making a correct judgment about what is said, it may also interfere with a correct judgment. The context 'she put a ________ on her finger' leads one to expect that 'ring' is the missing word even when someone, say a child with an /r/ problem, actually says something more like 'wing.'

Language or Phonological Structure

Individuals tend to hear differences in their own language but not those that occur in other languages. For example, Japanese speakers have difficulty differentiating 'late' and 'rate' because the initial consonants do not produce meaningful distinctions (are not phonemic) in Japanese. Of greater significance for speech and language pathologists is the evidence that adults may not perceive differences in sounds produced by children because they are not analogous to those of adult phonology. For example, adults frequently hear young children produce the initial sound in 'cold' so that it sounds like 'gold.' Actually, children's distinction between such words differs from that expected by adults (Macken & Barton, 1980).

Linguistic Function

According to the categorical model of speech perception, an individual's ability to discriminate sounds is constrained by the identification of sounds in his/her language (Liberman, Cooper, Shankweiler, & Studdert-Kennedy, 1967; Liberman & Mattingly, 1985). For example, it is possible to synthesize sounds that vary between /w/ and /r/ by varying the formant frequencies in a series of equal steps (Sharf & Benson, 1982). As indicated in Figure 1–11, individuals listening to the stimuli will identify those at one end of the series (stimulus 1) as /w/, those at the other end (stimulus 9) as /r/, and those in the middle (stimulus 5) about 50% as each (Sharf & Benson, 1982). In other words, listeners tend to put the stimuli into two phonetic categories. The categorical perception model predicts that listeners presented with pairs of such stimuli that differ by the same magnitude of formant frequency will be able to discriminate sounds that belong to different categories (stimuli 4 and 6), but not those that belong to the same category (stimuli 1 and 3, or 7 and 9). The model appears to predict that distorted /r/, which speech pathologists identify as a type of abnormal sound, cannot be discriminated from normal /r/, since both of these sounds fall within the /r/ end of the continuum (Locke, 1979). But evidence from studies of synthesized child distorted /r/ sounds shows that speech and language pathologists can make such distinctions (Sharf & Ohde, 1983; Sharf, Ohde, & Lehman, 1986).

This chapter covered the similarities and differences between clinical phonetics and general phonetics. Clinical phonetics is the study of phonetics as applied to the diagnosis and treatment of articulatory and phonological disorders. It differs from general phonetics as follows: (1) the focus of the study is on speech sound contrasts

Figure 1–11
Percent /r/ identification of a nine-step /we/ to /re/ synthetic speech continuum for child and adult listeners. 1 is canonical /w/; 9 is canonical /r/.

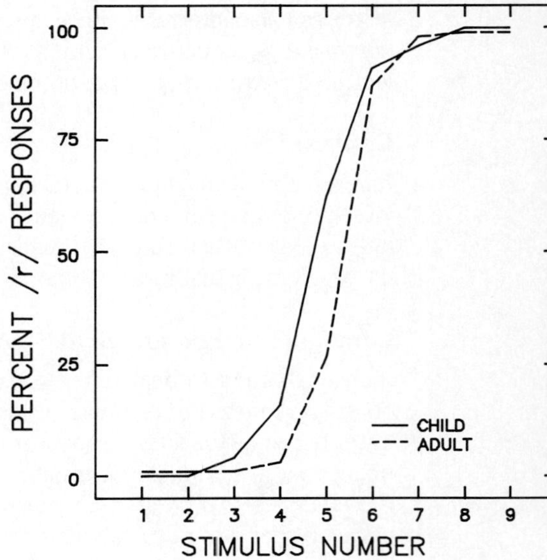

between normal and abnormal productions; (2) the primary model for sound analysis is the speech of children; and (3) standards for reliability are an integral part of transcription training.

GLOSSARY

Acoustic phonetics. The study of the physical nature of speech in terms of the characteristics of frequency, duration, and intensity that distinguish speech sounds. The study is carried out by using spectrographs, oscilloscopes, sound level meters, digital signal processing techniques, and other instrumentation and procedures.

Allophone. One of two or more variants of the same phoneme.

Alveolar ridge. The bony prominence just posterior to the upper teeth.

Amplitude. The extent of movement or displacement of a vibrating body from its rest position.

Amplitude section. *See* Power spectrum.

Aspiration. The final noise portion of a stop burst that results from air passing between the open vocal folds. Represented by fill on spectrograms.

Burst. The noise produced when a stop sound is released. Includes a pulse, frication and aspiration noise.

Complementary distribution. The mutually exclusive occurrence of allophones of one phoneme in different contexts.

Complex sound. A sound, such as that produced by the human voice, characterized by a fundamental tone and a number of harmonically related tones.

Envelope curve. A line drawn to mark the upper limits of harmonics in a power spectrum.

Fill. Random vertical lines on a spectrogram that represent the frication or noise energy of fricatives and stops.

Filter. A resonator that transmits selected frequencies.

Formants. The resonances of the vocal tract that change as it changes length and shape during speech production. Most often identified as wide horizontal bars on spectrograms.

Free variation. Optional variation in the production of sounds, e.g., 'palm' said with and without the /l/.

Frequency. The number of complete cycles of vibration of a sound-producing mechanism like a tuning fork in one second (125 cycles per second = 125 Hz).

Frication noise. The noise following the pulse in a stop burst and characteristic of fricatives. Represented by fill on a spectrogram.

Fundamental frequency. The lowest frequency component or repetitive frequency of a complex sound, such as that produced by the human voice. Abbreviated f_0.

Gap. The absence of markings on a spectrogram. Indicates the pressure buildup phase of a stop consonant.

Glottal tone. The complex sound produced by vibration of the vocal folds. Includes a fundamental frequency and harmonics.

Hard palate. The anterior part of the palate or roof of the mouth.

Harmonic. One of a number of frequency components of a complex sound. Harmonics are whole-number or integral multiples of the fundamental frequency.

Homophone. One of two or more words pronounced alike but different in meaning, e.g., 'to,' 'too,' and 'two.'

Intensity. A measure of sound energy, analogous to loudness, which is proportional to the square of the amplitude and frequency of sounds. Increases with greater amplitude and higher frequency.

Mandible. The bone that forms the lower jaw.

Minimal pair. Two words which are alike in all but one phoneme, e.g., 'pat' and 'bat.'

Morpheme. A meaningful linguistic unit, e.g., 'cat' and 's' in 'cats.'

Morphophonemic alternation. A change in the phonemic structure of a morpheme, as in the use of /g/ in 'piggy' but not in 'pig.'

Narrow band. Spectrogram made with a narrow band filter (45 Hz). The fundamental frequency and harmonics of complex sounds are displayed as horizontal lines.

Orthography. The representation of the sounds of a language by written or printed letters; spelling.

Palatogram. A record of tongue contact obtained by means of palatography.

Palatography. Procedures for visualizing tongue contact with the roof of the mouth during sound production.

Perceptual phonetics. The study of the auditory cues of speech. Includes identification and discrimination of speech sounds.

Period of vibration. The duration (in milliseconds) of one complete cycle of vibration of a sound-producing mechanism like a tuning fork.

Pharyngeal wall. The surface of the back of the throat, behind the nasal, oral, and laryngeal cavities.

Phoneme. A group of sounds, similar acoustically and in articulation, which contrast with other groups to produce meaningful distinctions in a language.

Phonetics. The study of the production and the acoustic properties of speech sounds as elements of language.

Phonological process. A systematic sound change or simplification that affects a class or a sequence of sounds.

Phonological rule. The specification of a change regularly observed in speech, with the exact conditions for its occurrence.

Phonology. The sound structure of language. Characterized by a finite set of phonemes and specific arrangements in which they are combined into syllables.

Physiologic phonetics. The study of the formation of speech in terms of the contacts, configurations, and movements of the articulatory structures that distinguish speech sounds, using X-ray, palatography, electromyography, airflow and air pressure measuring devices, and other instrumentation and procedures.

Power spectrum. A spectrographic analysis that displays complex sounds as a series of lines representing the fundamental and higher harmonics along the *y* axis and their intensity along the *x* axis.

Pulse. The very brief initial portion of a stop burst. Represented by a spike on a spectrogram.

Soft palate. The posterior part of the roof of the mouth.

Spectral analysis. A procedure for obtaining a graphic representation of a sound with frequency on the *x* axis and amplitude or intensity on the *y* axis.

Spectrogram. A record of the analysis of sounds obtained by means of a spectrograph.

Spectrograph. An instrument for obtaining analyses of the frequency, intensity, and duration of sounds.

Spike. A long vertical line in a spectrogram. Marks the release of a stop sound.

Striations. On a wide band spectrogram, a series of vertical lines that represent glottal pulses; the interval between any two lines indicates the period of vibration of the vocal folds.

Tongue apex. *See* Tongue tip.

Tongue blade. The portion of the tongue posterior to the tip.

Tongue dorsum. The portion of the tongue posterior to the blade.

Tongue lamina. *See* Tongue blade.

Tongue tip. The most anterior part of the tongue.

Trachea. The tube through which the lungs exhale air between the vocal folds.

Uvula. The most posterior portion of the soft palate.

Velopharyngeal muscles. Muscles of the velum and pharyngeal wall that function to open and close the velopharyngeal port between the oral and nasal cavities.

Velum. The posterior portion of the palate; the soft palate.

Vocal folds. The two bands of muscle tissue that vibrate to produce voicing for speech.

Vocal tract. The structures that make up the speech mechanism, from the vocal folds to the lips.

Waveform analysis. A graphic representation of the vibration of a sound-producing mechanism or the sound produced by it, with time shown along the *x* axis and amplitude or intensity along the *y* axis.

Wide band. Describes a spectrogram made with a wide band filter (300 Hz) so that the formants are displayed as horizontal bars.

***x* axis.** The horizontal dimension or abscissa of a graph.

***y* axis.** The vertical dimension or ordinate of a graph.

REVIEW QUESTIONS

A. Give one homophone for each word.

1. rows ________________	6. plane ________________
2. blue ________________	7. way ________________
3. freeze ________________	8. scene ________________
4. clothes ________________	9. size ________________
5. reed ________________	10. main ________________

****

Key: 1. rose; 2. blew; 3. frees; 4. close; 5. read; 6. plain; 7. weigh; 8. seen; 9. sighs; 10. mane

B. Check Yes or No if the following letters are pronounced alike in both words of each pair.

	Yes	*No*
1. oo in 'pool' and 'foot'	________	________
2. o in 'prove' and 'move'	________	________
3. ou in 'out' and 'coupe'	________	________
4. ew in 'sew' and 'new'	________	________
5. oi in 'coin' and 'boil'	________	________
6. ei in 'deceive' and 'rein'	________	________
7. ai in 'said' and 'rain'	________	________
8. o in 'dog' and 'bone'	________	________
9. ea in 'bead' and 'bread'	________	________
10. ou in 'cough' and 'rough'	________	________

****

Key: 1. No; 2. Yes; 3. No; 4. No; 5. Yes; 6. No; 7. No; 8. No; 9. No; 10. No

C. Select a minimal pair for each word by inserting the correct letter.

1. suite ________	a. brought
2. bread ________	b. blood
3. cried ________	c. road
4. rode ________	d. sweat
5. flood ________	e. trees
6. wade ________	f. pride
7. mail ________	g. raid
8. freeze ________	h. floor
9. rope ________	i. meal
10. brute ________	j. broad

****

Key: 1. d; 2. j; 3. f; 4. g; 5. b; 6. g; 7. i; 8. e; 9. c; 10. a

D. Indicate whether the following are true (T) or false (F).

1. ________ A waveform analysis shows time along the abscissa.
2. ________ A spectral analysis shows amplitude along the ordinate.
3. ________ The second harmonic of a complex sound with a 150 Hz fundamental is 300 Hz.
4. ________ A wide band spectrogram reflects pulsing of the vocal folds.
5. ________ A narrow band spectrogram shows harmonics as vertical lines.
6. ________ A power spectrum or amplitude section shows time along the abscissa.
7. ________ A spike represents the frication portion of a stop burst.
8. ________ Frication is due to air passing between the open vocal folds.
9. ________ Aspiration is the final portion of the stop burst.
10. ________ Intensity increases with greater amplitude and lower frequency.

****

Key: 1. T; 2. T; 3. T; 4. T; 5. F; 6. F; 7. F; 8. F; 9. T; 10. F

CHAPTER 2

Syllabic Structure of Speech

SYLLABLE PATTERNS OF ENGLISH

Before analyzing speech phonetically, it is necessary to select a unit for analysis. Ideally we would like to transcribe large units of speech like phrases or sentences. Practically, however, much of the analysis done in clinical phonetics is of words. If possible, it is desirable to have the word in a phrase or sentence so as to capture pronunciation in the most natural context. Acoustic analysis reveals that speech is a continuous signal with no clear-cut basis for segmenting sentences or phrases into smaller units. Words tend to be run together with no clear boundaries between them, and sounds that we perceive do not have clearly marked beginnings or endings. The poor segmentation characteristics of speech have long been recognized as a basic problem in speech perception (Pisoni, 1981). Figure 2–1 presents a spectrogram of the sentence 'Did you hit it to Tom?' as spoken by a child and by an adult. As the spectrograms illustrate, there are no boundaries marking each word. The acoustic pattern is somewhat analogous to seeing the sentence printed without spacing, as 'DidyouhitittoTom?'

Despite the difficulties in segmenting acoustic analysis into units that correspond to those of auditory analysis, phoneticians have successfully analyzed speech by using the **syllable** as an easily identifiable unit. Even a naive English listener can identify the number of syllables pronounced in most words. Spelling can be a confusing factor, as in the case of 'hire,' which looks as if it ought to be one syllable but is usually pronounced the same as 'higher,' which looks as if it ought to be two syllables.

Identifying the number of syllables in most words is easy compared with defining the syllable. Syllables have been described as thrusts of the chest muscles of respiration (Stetson, 1951), peaks of sonority (Heffner, 1952), pulses of sound energy (Tiffany &

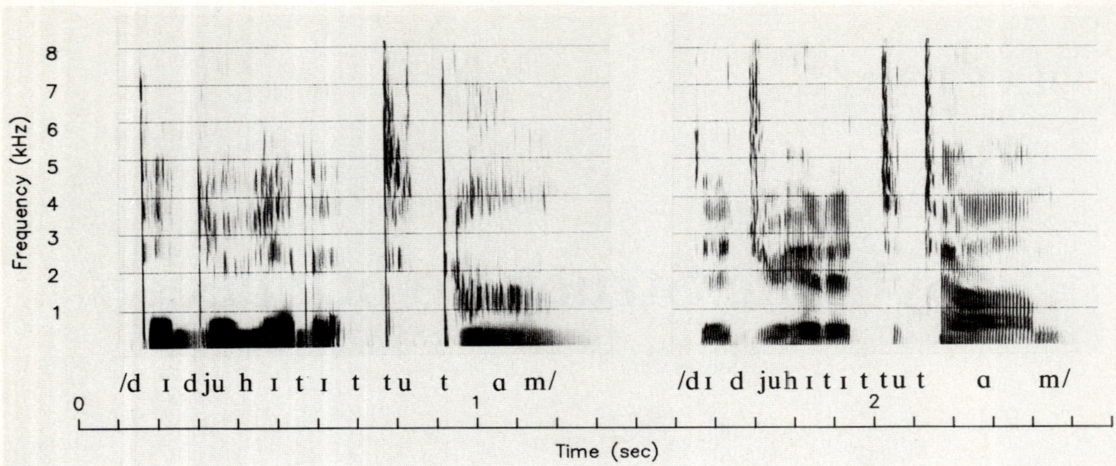

Figure 2–1
Spectrograms of the sentence 'Did you hit it to Tom?' produced by a child (left panel) and an adult male (right panel).

/Carrell, 1977), necessary units in the mental organization and production of speech (Ladefoged, 1975), a group of speech movements (Shriberg & Kent, 1982), and a basic unit of speech perception (Miller & Liberman, 1979). Although the syllable is difficult to define precisely, in listening to speech, we can identify periods when the signal is louder or relatively higher in intensity and other periods when it is softer or relatively lower in intensity. These loud and soft intervals may be described as maxima, or peaks, of sound energy and minima, or valleys, of sound energy. **Sonority** is an auditorily based term that is used by some phoneticians as analogous to sound energy. Peaks of sonority may be thought of as the result of pulses of sound energy. For example, in 'pea,' the vowel /i/ is a maximum of sonority which is preceded by the consonant /p/, a minimum of sonority. This unit is a CV syllable (C = consonant; V = vowel). With few exceptions, every syllable must include at least a vowel sound, which is its nucleus and may include one or more consonant sounds. One exception is the exclamation 'pst' /pst/, which has no vowel but still has a peak of sonority produced by the /s/. Frequent exceptions involve syllabic consonants in the second syllable of words like 'cotton' [kɑtn̩] and 'bottle' [bɑtl̩] that are produced with no vowel. Syllabic consonants like [n̩] and [l̩] form the nucleus of syllables in words like 'cotton' and 'bottle,' and the peaks of sonority in the second syllables occur on these consonants.

Acoustic evidence does not usually make syllable determination easier than it is in perception. In Figure 2–2, spectrograms of a child's and an adult's productions of 'the big rockets' are shown with illustrations of amplitude contours above them. In general, consonants are characterized by relatively low amplitude because their production results from constriction, whereas amplitude is at a maximum for vowels. Exceptions occur, such as the frication noise of the /s/ at the end of 'rockets.' Although one would

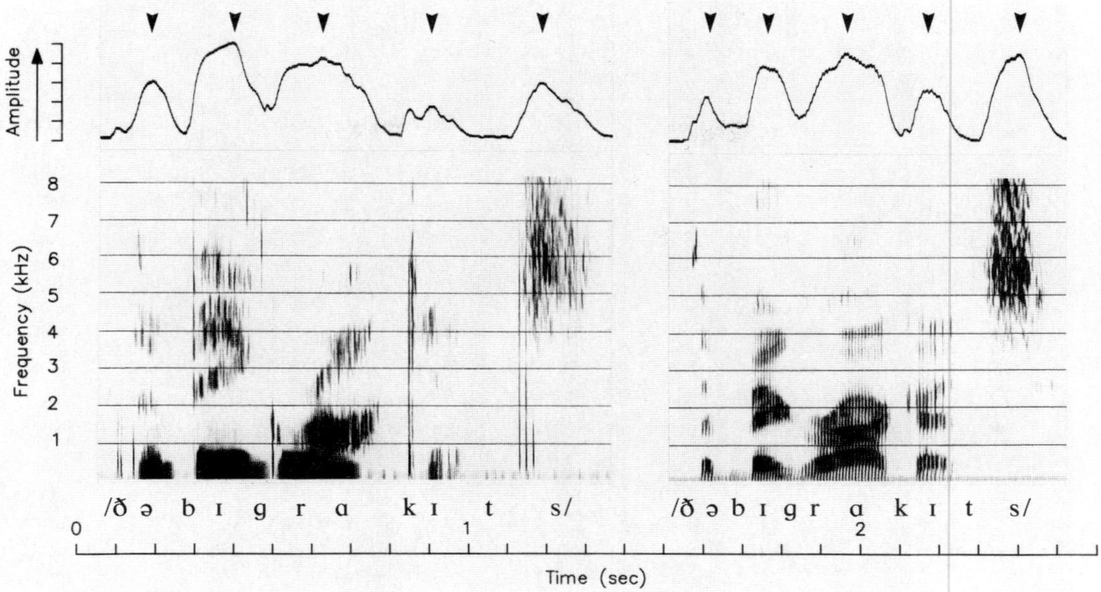

Figure 2–2
Spectrograms of a child (left panel) and an adult (right panel) saying 'the big rockets.' A waveform analysis (amplitude × time) appears above each spectrogram. Arrows indicate amplitude peaks.

have no difficulty deciding that there are four syllables in 'the big rockets,' the amplitude contour makes it look as if there are five because of the amplitude peak of the final /s/.

The basic syllable patterns of English are as follows: (1) a V type, like 'I' /ɑɪ/; (2) a CV type, in which the consonant is prevocalic, that is, it precedes the vowel, like 'my' /mɑɪ/; (3) a VC type, in which the consonant is postvocalic, that is, it follows the vowel, like 'I'm' /ɑɪm/; and (4) a CVC type, like 'mime' /mɑɪm/. It is possible to have a minimum of sonority that includes more than one consonant in CV, VC, and CVC syllables (using C to represent a cluster); that is, the minimum can be a consonant cluster. Syllables can include as many as three consonants in the prevocalic position, as in 'stray' /stre/, and as many as four consonants in the postvocalic position, as in 'glimpsed' /glɪmpst/. Thus, we can have the following types of monosyllabic words: V, as in 'I' /ɑɪ/; CV, as in 'my' /mɑɪ/; VC, as in 'on' /ɑn/; CCV, as in 'tray' /tre/; VCC, as in 'elm' /ɛlm/; CCCV, as in 'stray' /stre/; VCCC, as in 'elms' /ɛlmz/; CCVCC, as in 'steps' /stɛps/; CCVCCC, as in 'blinks' /blɪŋks/; CCCVCCC, as in 'strands' /strændz/; and CCVCCCC, as in 'glimpsed' /glɪmpst/.

Table 2–1 contains examples of words that fit the different monosyllabic patterns of English. These examples provide interesting insights into the orthographic, phonetic, and phonological structure of English. First, spelling is not a reliable indicator of the number of syllables in words: 'toe' /to/, 'oak' /ok/, and 'soup' /sup/ have two ortho-

Table 2–1
Examples of monosyllabic word patterns of English, including consonant clusters frequently reduced by children by omitting one or both consonants (C = consonant; V = vowel; CC = consonant cluster).

	V	CV	VC	CVC	CCV	CCVC	CCVCC	VCC	CVCC
/i/	—	bee	eat	beat	free three	sleep	sleeps	eats	beats field
/e/	a	day	ate	date rain	clay pray	plane train	planes trains	apes	rains makes
/æ/	—	—	at	hat	—	grass bran	plant gland	ant ask	gasp talc
/u/	ooh	do	ooze	soup	glue grew	glues smooth	blooms	oops	soups
/o/	oh	toe	oak	soap	crow flow	stone store	stones stores	oaks	bolt
/ɑ/	ah	pa	—	mom pop	spa	stop scar	stops spark	odds art	barb sharp
/ʌ/	—	—	—	cup	—	drum	drums	ump	dump bulb

graphic vowels but only one spoken one. Second, there are many fewer examples of the more complex syllable types, those with consonant clusters, than of the less complex ones. This is not because the phonology of English does not permit more complex patterns but because there are no words that fit the pattern. For example, it should be possible to have a CCCVCCC pattern for the /o/ vowel, since /s t r o/ is permissible in 'stroke' /strok/, and so is /o n t s/ in 'don'ts' /d o n t s/. However, 'stronts' is not a word in English.

Table 2–1 also includes examples of some of the consonant cluster patterns that children frequently simplify by omitting one or more consonants. These are: (1) /s/ plus /m, n, p, t, k/ in prevocalic position and /s/ plus /p, t, k/ in postvocalic position; (2) stop /p, t, k, b, d, g/ plus liquid /l, r/ in prevocalic position and liquid plus stop in postvocalic position; (3) fricative /f, θ/ plus liquid /l, r/ in prevocalic position; and (4) nasal consonant /m, n/ plus stop /p, t, d/ in postvocalic position. Since cluster simplifications are dealt with specifically later in the chapter, only the following unpermitted monosyllabic cluster patterns should be noted: (1) /s/ plus nasal consonants in postvocalic position; (2) stop /t/ or /d/ plus liquid /l/; (3) fricative /θ/ plus /l/; (4) nasal consonant /m/ plus /t/, except in a word like 'prompt' when it is pronounced with the second /p/ sound omitted; (5) nasal consonant /n/ plus /p/.

Table 2–2 presents patterns for two-syllable words, all of which derive from the basic VCV pattern, with stress on the first or second syllable. The pattern and the structure of clusters become very complex, and examples become harder to find as the number of consonants increases. The structural pattern and the complexity of words are determined primarily by the morphemes that can be strung together to form

Table 2–2
Examples of two-syllable English word patterns (V = vowel; C = consonant; n. = noun; v. = verb). Note that the spellings 'aw,' 'ay,' 'er,' 'ew,' 'ey,' 'oa,' 'ow,' and 'oy' each represent one vowel or diphthong, the spellings 'dd,' 'ng,' and 'pp' each represent one consonant, and the spelling 'x' represents two consonants.

Pattern	First Syllable Stressed	Second Syllable Stressed
VCV	owner	away
CVCV	teddy	below
VCVC	owners	along
CVCVC	teddys	believe
VCCV	only	apply
VCCVC	in-laws	applies
VCCCV	osprey	astray
VCCCVC	ospreys	astride
CVCCV	toaster	reply
CVCCVC	toasters	replies
CCVCV	story	prefer
CCVCVC	stories	prefers
CCVCCV	prosper	–
CCVCCVC	prospers	prestige
CVCCCV	sixty	destroy
CVCCCVC	thankful	describe
CCVCVCC	protest n.	prevent
CCVCVCCC	protests n.	prevents
CVCCCVCC	contract n.	contract v.
CVCCCVCCC	contracts n.	contracts v.

English words. For example, 'ts' is a frequent cluster in postvocalic position in words like 'cats' and 'bets,' in which 's' is a plural or person indicator, but 'ts' is rare in prevocalic position, occurring in 'tsetse.'

Descriptions of syllable patterns and variants of consonant sounds make frequent reference to the consonant's position in relation to the vowel. **Prevocalic** consonants precede the vowel, like /t/ in 'tea,' **intervocalic** consonants come between vowels, like /t/ in 'eating,' and **postvocalic** consonants follow the vowel, like /t/ in 'eat.' Some phoneticians also use syllable-releasing and syllable-arresting for prevocalic and postvocalic, respectively.

In a few two- or three-syllable words like 'neon,' 'piano,' and 'aorta,' two contiguous vowels are produced in different syllables with no apparent intervening consonants. These examples seem to be exceptions to the rule that consonants are needed to separate peaks of sound energy formed by vowels. In most cases, however, either a glide like the prevocalic sound in 'you' or a glottal stop is inserted between the vowels when such words are pronounced. Listeners have no difficulty determining that there are two syllables in 'neon' and three syllables in 'piano' and in 'aorta.'

SIMPLIFICATION OF SYLLABLE STRUCTURES

Consideration of the syllable as a unit of speech production and speech perception provides a basis for examining the misarticulations of children. Many errors in children's speech involve the simplification of syllable structures through the omission of consonants or vowels. These simplifications are phonological processes. Three are commonly used by children.

Cluster Reduction

Table 2–3 includes examples of **cluster reduction,** which involves simplifying consonant clusters by deleting one or more consonants or by substituting another consonant for one member of the cluster (Ingram, 1976; Edwards & Shriberg, 1983). Greenlee (1974) has proposed that children pass through four stages as they develop the ability to produce clusters. As indicated in Table 2–3, the first stage involves omission of the entire cluster, so that 'stop' /s t ɑ p/ would be 'op' /ɑ p/. In the second stage, one of the consonants is produced, so that 'stop' would be 'top' /t ɑ p/. In the third stage, the previously omitted consonant is replaced by another consonant, so that 'stop' would be 'thtop' /θ t ɑ p/. Finally, in the fourth stage, the correct cluster is produced. Figure 2–3 shows spectrograms of a child's productions of 'stop' characterizing the four stages of cluster development. Observe the differences in consonant noise from stage 1 to stage 4. It is clear that some children do not reach the final stage as soon as they should, but it is not clear that all children go through both intermediate stages.

There is some question as to the likely outcome of stage 2 in the reduction process on a cluster like /s t/ in 'stop' when the /s/ is deleted, as illustrated spectrographically in Figure 2–3. One might expect cluster-reduced 'stop' to sound no different from 'top' (Weismer, 1984). According to another view, though, the /t/ will sound like

Table 2–3
Examples of prevocalic (CV) and postvocalic (VC) consonant cluster reduction patterns of children. Target words are given in the Stage IV row. (S = stop; L = liquid; N = nasal; F = fricative; N/S = nasal or stop)

	/s/ + N/S		S + L / L + S		F + L	N + S
Stage	**CV**	**VC**	**CV**	**VC**	**CV only**	**VC only**
I	all	de	ing	mi	ow	bu
II	mall	dek	bing	mik	fow	bup
III	thmall	dethk	bwing	miuk[a]	fwow; thwow	bu*p[b]
IV	small	desk	bring	milk	throw	bump

[a]Many adults pronounce 'milk' this way.
[b]Asterisk indicates nasalized vowel.

a /d/ in the nonsense word 'dop' to the untrained ear but like a voiceless unaspirated stop to the phonetician. (This stop variant is described in Chapter 6.) According to acoustic evidence, children produce both variants (Bond & Wilson, 1980). The distinction could be important to understanding the nature of phonological processes. The basic question relates to the degree to which the presumed **neutralization rule** (a neutralization rule is a specification for the pronunciation of sounds that results in a loss

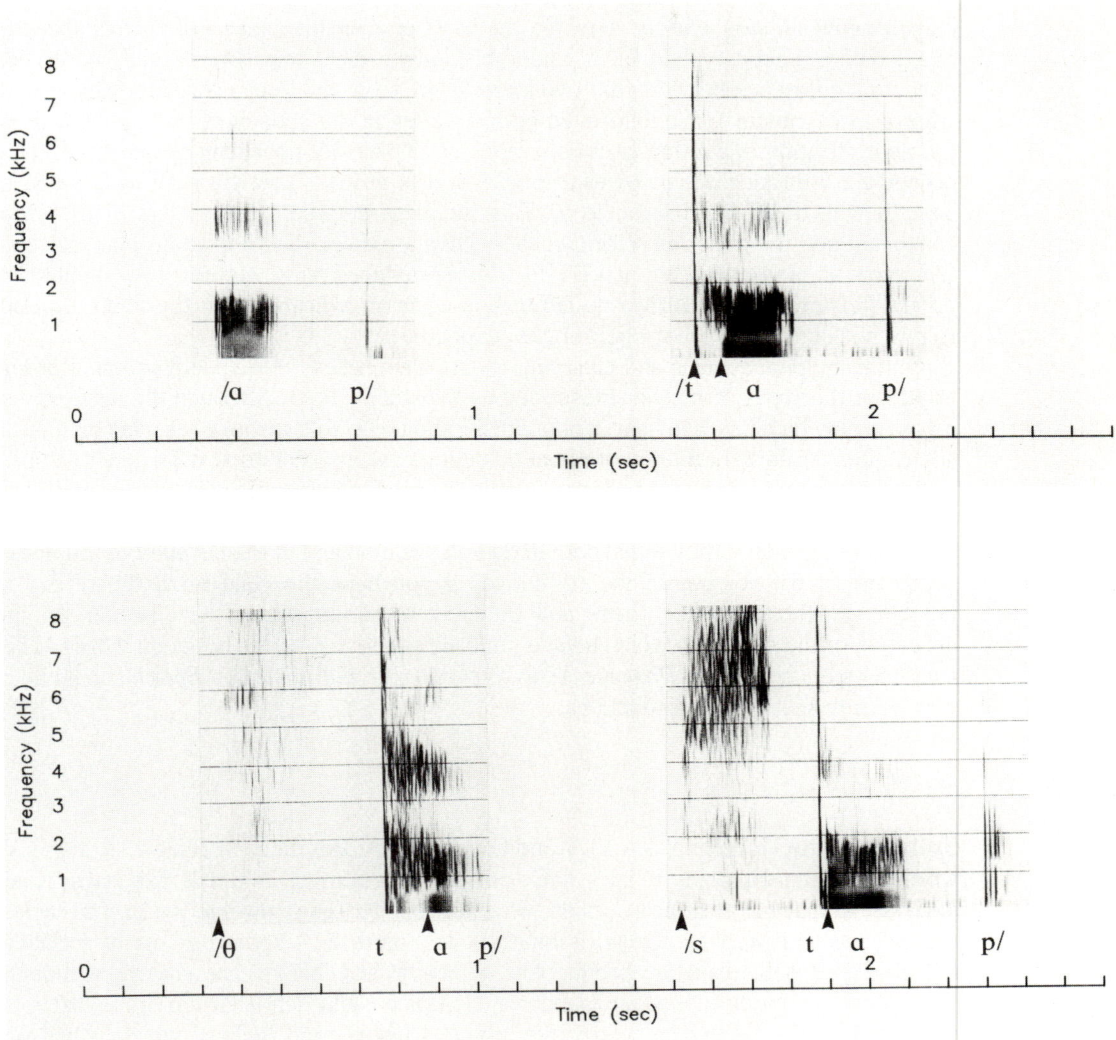

Figure 2–3
Spectrograms of the four stages of cluster development for a child speaker: /ɑp/, /tɑp/, /θtɑp/, and /stɑp/. Prevocalic consonant intervals are indicated by arrows for the stages in which they are present.

of differentiation between them) that changes the underlying form 'stop' /s t ɑ p/ to the surface form 'top' /t ɑ p/ also neutralizes the distinction between the words 'stop' and 'top.'

Weismer (1984) proposes using spectrographic analyses to deal with this problem under the assumption that clinicians may not be able to differentiate speech sounds produced by children accurately enough. Each analysis involves a measurement of duration. The first measure is the duration of the prevocalic consonant intervals for cluster-reduced 'stop' and for 'top.' On the basis of acoustic analysis of normal speech, one would expect 'stop' to be considerably longer than 'top.' One would, however, expect no difference between the two intervals in 'stop' and 'top' as produced by a child who reduces clusters. If a difference persists even in the speech of such a child, then the neutralization rule either is not operating at all or is not operating as expected. The second acoustic approach involves measurement of **voice onset time (VOT),** which is described in detail in Chapter 5. VOT is the time between the release of the stop consonant and the onset of voicing of the following vowel. The important point here is that acoustic measurements of VOT for cluster-reduced 'stop' and for 'top' should not differ (Weismer, 1984). If they do differ, it is again an indication that the neutralization rule is not operating or not operating as expected.

Ideally, phoneticians and clinicians should have access to a spectrograph in order to pursue the types of analyses described by Weismer (1984). Although the distinctions involved may be difficult to hear, a phonetician should be able to make reliable judgments about differences in durations of phonetic segments. In order to test for such distinctions, try asking a child who reduces clusters to produce utterances like 'stop' and 'top' in short phrases like 'This is a ________.' Compare cluster-reduced 'stop' with 'top' in order to determine if they differ both in overall duration and in the duration of the noise produced on the release of the /t/ sound. If you have the child randomly record a number of utterances like these and then try to identify them, you should get an indication of the extent to which he/she neutralizes the distinction between words. The audiotapes to accompany *Phonetic Analysis of Normal and Abnormal Speech* should help you learn to make such distinctions.

Syllable Reduction

Syllable reduction simplifies VCV and CVCV words, like those in Table 2–2, into CV words by eliminating the initial syllable, or the vowel in it, in words like 'away' and 'believe' so that they are pronounced 'way' and 'blieve.' The vowel in the first syllable, the syllable with weaker stress, is omitted. In Figure 2–4 spectrograms of a child's normal and syllable-reduced productions of 'away' and 'blieve' are shown. Although word stress is not discussed until Chapter 11, it is easy to hear that the first syllable is weaker than the second in words like 'above,' 'below,' and 'police,' which would be shortened to 'bove,' 'blow,' and 'plice.' Syllable reduction may also influence VCV and CVCV words with weak stress on the second syllable, as in 'ted' for 'teddy,' or in polysyllabic CVCVCV words like 'banana,' shortened to 'nana.'

Final Consonant Deletion

Final consonant deletion reduces VC and CVC syllables to V and CV syllables. For example, 'eat' and 'beat' would be simplified to 'ea' and 'bea.' Spectrograms of these examples in Figure 2–5 show little evidence of a final consonant except the abrupt

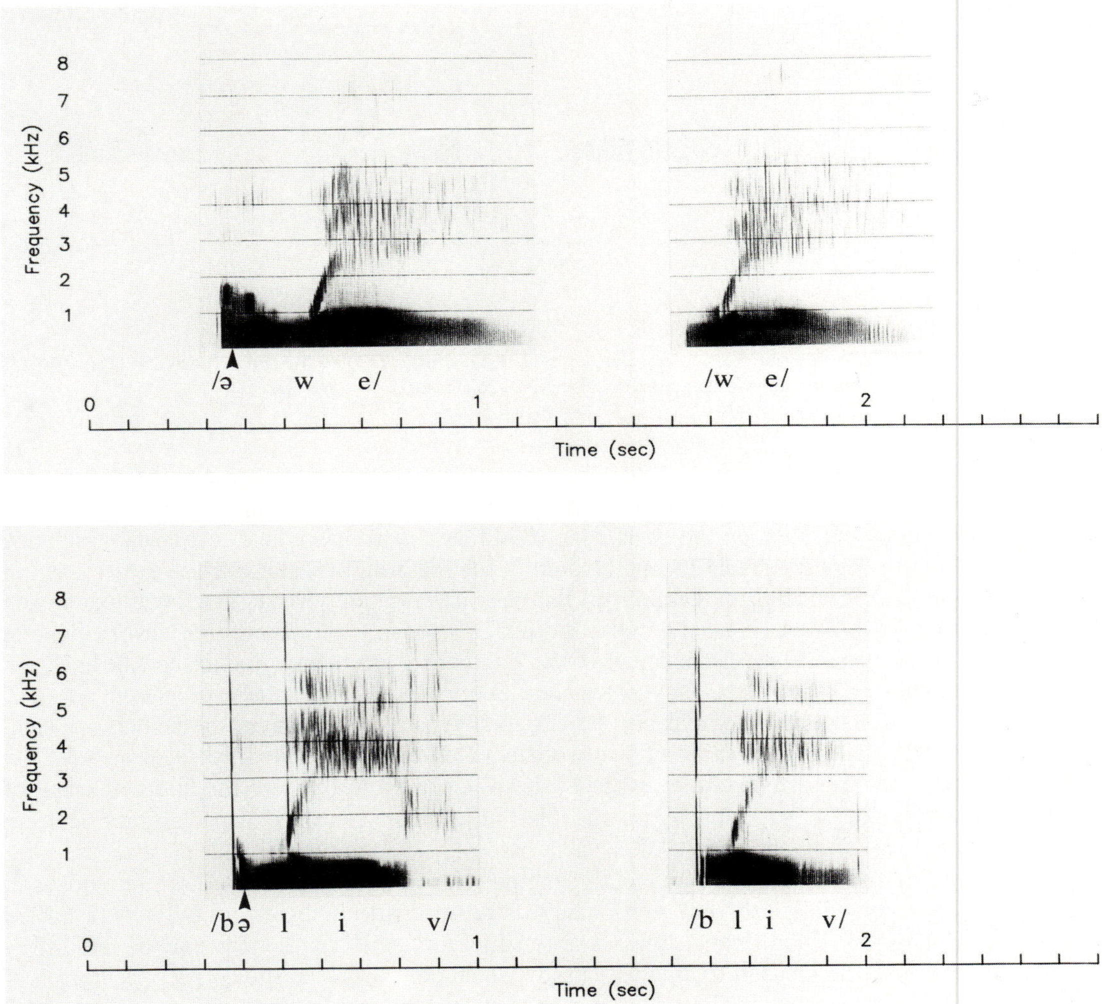

Figure 2–4
Spectrograms of a child's normal and syllable-reduced productions of 'away,' /ə w e/ and /w e/, and of 'believe,' /bə l i v/ and /b l i v/. Arrows along the *x*-axis (abscissa) indicate the approximate position of /ə/ in the normal productions.

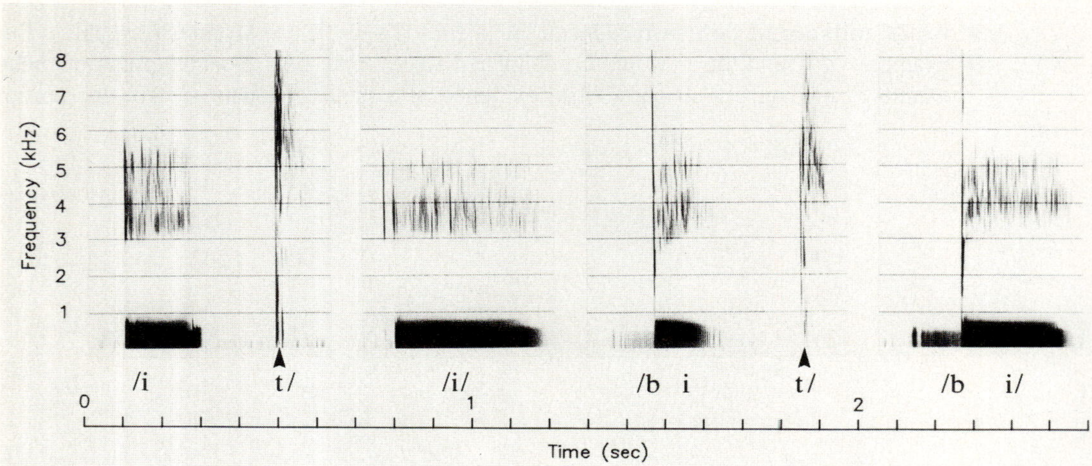

Figure 2–5
Spectrograms illustrating final consonant deletion in a child's productions of 'eat,' /i t/ and /i/, and of 'beat,' /b i t/ and /b i/. Arrows along the *x*-axis indicate the approximate position of the final consonant in /i t/ and /b i t/.

termination of the vowel. Although many children omit final consonants, it is not always clear that the omissions arise from a phonological process. Clarification requires evidence of cognition on the part of the child that a word has a final consonant. Evidence of such cognition could be one or both of the following: (1) the child deletes the /t/ in 'eat' but includes it in 'eating'; (2) the child differentiates words like 'beat' and 'bead,' from both of which he/she omits the final consonant, by making the vowel longer in 'bead' than in 'beat.' Evidence of vowel lengthening has been noted in acoustic analyses of children who delete final consonants. See Chapter 4 for details.

Consideration of syllable simplification processes should not be limited to single words. In the production of two-word phrases commonly used by children, CVCVC patterns are formed. An example is 'sit up.' Children who delete the final consonant of words like 'sit' may simplify phrases like 'sit up' /s ɪ t ʌ p/ to CVVC patterns by omitting the final /t/ of 'sit' or to CVV syllable patterns by omitting the final /t/ of 'sit' and the final /p/ of 'up.' Children frequently lengthen the vowel in the first syllable of phrases in which they delete the final consonant in order to mark the boundary between syllables (Johnson & Hood, 1988). Since a large variety of consonant sounds may be omitted in phrases, the focus in traditional therapy would be to work on the correct production of each of these sounds. The clinician who views this pattern of omissions as a phonological process of syllable structuring, however, focuses on the phonological pattern to be acquired rather than on isolated phonemes (Hodson & Paden, 1983; Johnson & Hood, 1988). In this approach the emphasis is on teaching the child to include a transition between syllables, no matter how imperfect the sound may be.

In transcribing speech, you should be aware of the target syllable structure, that is, the number of syllables in the utterance that the speaker is trying to convey. For each intended syllable, there should be a vowel or a sound that serves the same syllabic function as a vowel. If a syllable or a final consonant is deleted, or if a sound in a cluster is omitted or replaced by another consonant, the misarticulations should be noted in your transcription. Syllable simplifications are found primarily in the speech of children. Although most children do not have syllable simplifications in their speech after four years of age, they can be found in seven- and eight-year-olds with unintelligible speech (Hodson & Paden, 1981). Some simplifications occur in the rapid, informal speech of adults as, for example, in 'believe' and 'ferocious,' when they are simplified to 'blieve' and 'frocious.' Some speakers may add syllables to words, usually to simplify consonant clusters, by inserting a vowel between two consonants. This process, called **epenthesis** (the inserted vowel is an **epenthetic** vowel) results in the pronunciation of words like 'blue' and 'great' with a vowel between the first two consonants: /bəlu/ and /gəret/. Since Japanese has almost exclusively V and CV sequences, this type of addition occurs when Japanese speak English in order to make the sequence conform to the syllabic structure of their native language.

GLOSSARY

Cluster reduction. A phonological process which involves the omission of one or all of the consonants in a cluster.

Epenthesis; epenthetic. A phonological process which involves the insertion of a vowel between consonants in a cluster; the adjective used to describe such an inserted sound.

Final consonant deletion. A phonological process which involves the omission of a final consonant in a word; also called deletion of final consonants.

Intervocalic. Describes a consonant produced between vowels.

Neutralization rule. A specification for the pronunciation of sounds that results in a loss of differentiation between them.

Postvocalic. Describes a consonant following a vowel.

Prevocalic. Describes a consonant preceding a vowel.

Sonority. A term used to denote the perception of relative sound energy in the production of speech sounds.

Syllable. A perceptual unit of speech with a nucleus, usually a vowel, which is marked by a peak of sound energy or sonority and may be preceded and followed by one or more consonants, usually marked by minima of sound energy or sonority.

Syllable reduction. A phonological process that involves the omission of a weak syllable or its vowel in a word.

VOT. Abbreviation for *voice onset time,* the interval between the release of a prevocalic stop consonant and the onset of vocal fold vibration for a following vowel.

REVIEW QUESTIONS

A. Children may simplify syllables by deleting a whole weak syllable or the vowel of a weak syllable. In the following, indicate the word intended.

1. plice ____________
2. tato ____________
3. frocious ____________
4. prade ____________
5. spose ____________

****

Key: 1. police; 2. potato; 3. ferocious; 4. parade; 5. suppose

B. Children who simplify syllables by reducing prevocalic clusters often produce different words from those intended. In the following, indicate the intended word.

1. bought ____________
2. tip ____________
3. keep ____________
4. cash ____________
5. back ____________
6. mall ____________

****

Key: 1. brought; 2. trip; 3. creep; 4. crash or clash; 5. black; 6. small

C. Children who delete final consonants make it difficult to decide what word is spoken. For each deletion indicate a word that might be mistaken as intended by inserting the appropriate letter.

1. 'wa' for 'wash' ________	a. pick
2. 'ta' for 'take' ________	b. nail
3. 'wa' for 'wake' ________	c. hit
4. 'ta' for 'tag' ________	d. tape
5. 'si' for 'sit' ________	e. walk
6. 'na' for 'name' ________	f. tan
7. 'pu' for 'push' ________	g. pull
8. 'pi' for 'pit' ________	h. wait
	i. sip

****

Key: 1. e; 2. d; 3. h; 4. f; 5. i; 6. b; 7. g; 8. a

CHAPTER 3

Analysis of Vowels, Glides, and Liquids

PHYSIOLOGIC AND ACOUSTIC CHARACTERISTICS OF VOWELS

In the discussion of the syllable as the basic unit of speech in Chapter 2, the prominence of vowels in the syllable was clear. It is appropriate, therefore, to begin the discussion of sounds by noting certain characteristics of normal vowel production. First, during vowel production, the vocal folds vibrate to produce a glottal tone so that the vowels are voiced sounds. Although the vocal folds can be approximated to a lesser degree than for voiced vowels to produce whispered vowels, these do not normally occur except in whispered speech. Second, normally produced vowels involve resonance of the oral cavity, which means that the velopharyngeal muscles close off the opening into the nasal cavity from the pharynx. Although it is possible to produce nasalized vowels by leaving the valve open, these vowels do not occur normally in English, except when preceding or following nasal consonants (see Chapter 4). Third, the oral cavity is relatively open during vowel production. The lips, tongue, and jaw do not stop the flow of air out of the oral cavity or interfere with it to produce frication noise. The relative prominence of the resonance of a vowel accounts for its occurrence as the nucleus of a syllable. Briefly, a **vowel** may be defined as a speech sound produced with relatively open vocal tract resonance and functioning as the nucleus of a syllable.

Vowels can be differentiated by phonemic analysis. (Remember that phonemes are sounds that contrast in identical contexts to produce meaningful distinctions, as demonstrated by minimal pairs like 'bet' and 'bat.') Table 3–1 provides a minimal-pairs analysis for the General American dialect. More than one type of CVC syllable is included to compensate for gaps in the occurrence of minimal pairs. Each word listed for each CVC syllable represents a change in vowel phoneme, and each word is a key to the

Table 3–1
Minimal pairs analysis of the vowels of the General American dialect.

	Syllable Structures				
Vowel	**hVd**	**hVt**	**bVd**	**bVt**	**pVl**
/i/	heed	heat	bead	beat	peel
/ɪ/	hid	hit	bid	bit	pill
/e/	hayed	hate	bayed	bait	pail
/ɛ/	head	—	bed	bet	—
/æ/	had	hat	bad	bat	pal
/u/	who'd	hoot	booed	boot	pool
/ʊ/	hood	—	—	—	pull
/o/	hoed	—	bowed[a]	boat	pole
/ɔ/	hawed[b]	—	bawd	bought	pall
/ɑ/	hod	hot	—	—	—
/ə/	—	hut	bud	but	—
/ɝ/	heard	hurt	bird	—	pearl

[a]Meaning to play a violin.
[b]As in 'hemmed and hawed,' meaning to be indecisive in speech.

pronunciation of the vowel by a speaker of the General American dialect. The symbols that represent the vowels are from the International Phonetic Alphabet (IPA), as are most of those used in this book. If you use New England or Southern or foreign dialects, the key words may not help for certain vowels. Ultimate mastery of the perception of the vowels, however, depends on how well you distinguish them with the help of the audiotapes that accompany this text.

In considering the objective basis for vowel differentiation, evidence from X-rays and photographs can be used. Figure 3–1 shows tracings of midsagittal X-rays taken during the production of English vowels. These tracings show the midline position of the tongue as it relates to the walls of the vocal tract, which are formed by the hard palate, soft palate, or velum, and the upper part of the pharynx. Note that the tongue closely approximates the palate for /i, u/ but is far away from it for /æ, ɑ/. On the basis of tongue height, /i, u/ are classified as **high,** /e, o/ as **mid,** and /æ, ɑ/ as **low** vowels. The closest approximation of the tongue to the palate is more anterior for some vowels, like /i/, and more posterior for others, like /u/. On this basis, /i, e, æ/ are classified as **front** vowels and /u, o, ɑ/ are classified as **back** vowels. Actually, /ɑ/ is so far back that the tongue root, which is just posterior to the dorsum, comes close to the pharyngeal wall (Perkell, 1969; Shriberg & Kent, 1982). For some of the vowels the differences in tongue height and horizontal position may seem small. Some X-ray studies reveal that these differences are not always reliable as absolute indicators of differences between vowels. They are helpful, however, in showing relative differences. Try saying each vowel and determine for yourself if your tongue changes position as the X-rays suggest.

Some vowels are neither high or low, but are mid position in tongue height, and neither front or back, but central in horizontal position. These are the **central** vowels of the General American dialect. The /ə/ vowel, commonly referred to as **schwa,** may

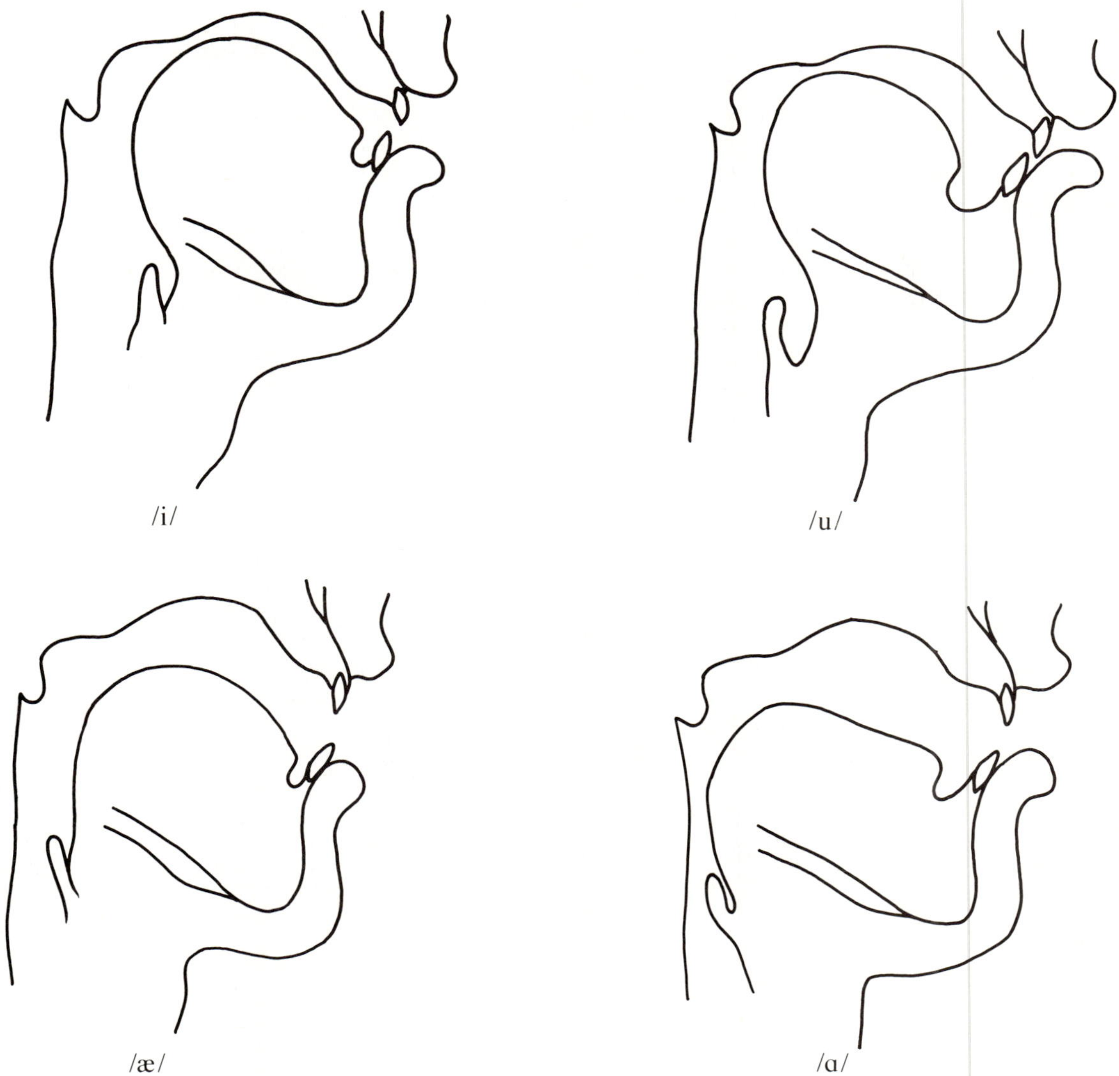

Figure 3–1
Tracings of midsagittal X-rays of /i/, /æ/, /u/, and /ɑ/.

be described as having a mid central position, but the symbol represents a wide variety of central vowels that occur in the unstressed syllables of words like 'above,' 'below,' 'today,' and 'conceive.' In words like 'cut' and 'fuss,' the first and stressed syllable of words like 'mother' and 'custard,' and the second and stressed syllable of words like 'above' and 'among,' the /ʌ / vowel occurs. This vowel is similar to /ə /, except that the tongue is retracted toward /ɑ /. Many phoneticians consider /ʌ / to be the stressed counterpart of /ə / (Bronstein, 1960; Calvert, 1980; Shriberg & Kent, 1982), but others note that it differs in quality from /ə / (Tiffany & Carrell, 1977). In IPA, /ʌ / represents the unrounded equivalent of the /ɔ / vowel.

Because the /ɝ/ vowel in words like 'hurt' and the first syllable of words like 'birthday' and the /ɚ/ vowel in the second syllable of words like 'father' are of such importance in the study of abnormal speech, their production should be examined carefully. Observations about the position for /ɝ/ and /ɚ/ also apply to the /r/ glide, which starts from the position of these vowels. Two major articulatory positions are used by speakers of the General American dialect to produce /ɝ/ and /ɚ/, the **retroflex** and the **bunched** (see Figure 3–2). Retroflex means turned back, and refers to the raising of the apex and blade of the tongue toward the palate just posterior to the upper alveolar ridge. The back portion of the tongue is not raised but remains below the level of the apex and blade (Delattre & Freeman, 1968; Figure 3–2A). In the bunched tongue position (Figure 3–2B), the tongue apex remains relatively low in the oral cavity, just posterior to the lower teeth, and the middle portion of the tongue is raised toward the hard palate. The upper surface of the tongue does not touch the palate in either the

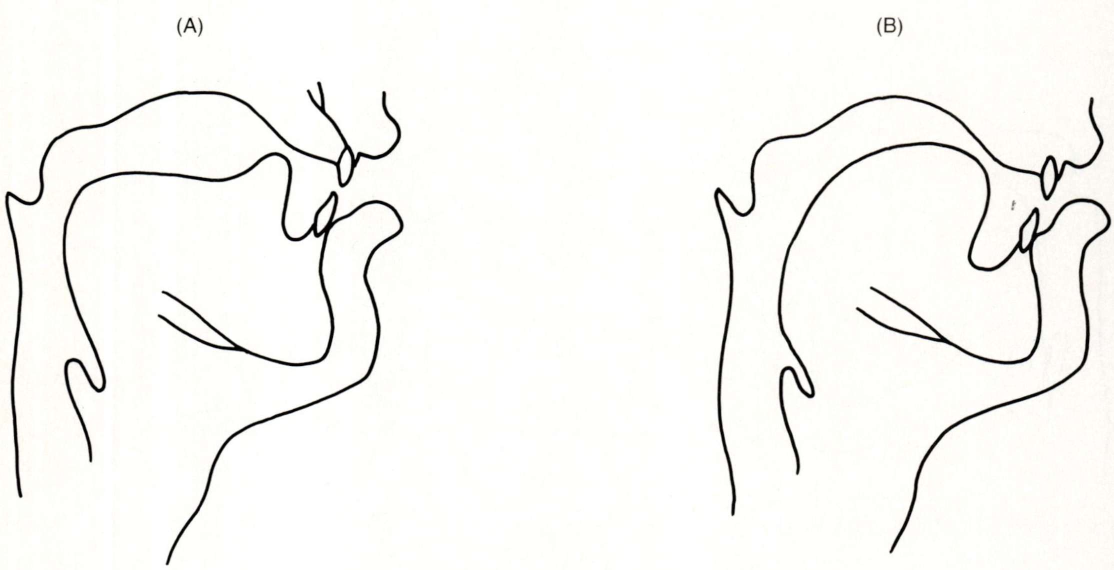

Figure 3–2
Schematized midsagittal sections of retroflex (A) and bunched (B) productions of /ɝ/.

retroflex or the bunched /ɝ/ and /ɚ/, but the sides of the tongue touch the inner surfaces of the molars. For both types the back part of the tongue closely approximates the pharyngeal wall (Delattre & Freeman, 1968; Zawadzki & Kuehn, 1980). Although some speakers round the lips in producing /ɝ/ and /ɚ/, this is not a necessary feature of their production. Unfortunately there is insufficient evidence to describe variants of /ɝ/ and /ɚ/ that apparently occur depending on the speaker and the context. According to Delattre and Freeman (1968), the bunched sound is more prevalent than the retroflex in the General American dialect.

In transcribing central vowels, some phoneticians use the /ə / symbol to represent the vowel in the unstressed first syllable and the stressed second syllable in 'abut' and the /ɚ/ symbol to represent the vowel in the stressed first syllable and the unstressed second syllable in 'murder.' They transcribe 'abut' as /ə bə t/ and 'murder' as /m ɚ d ɚ/ and use stress markers to note the stressed vowels. In the two-symbol system, /ʌ / and /ɝ/ represent the stressed equivalents of /ə / and /ɚ/. Although neither the difference between /ɝ/ and /ɚ/ nor the one between /ə / and /ʌ / produces phonemic distinctions, many phoneticians find it advantageous to use these symbols.

Lip rounding is a third dimension by which vowels are differentiated. Figures 3–3 and 3–4 include photographs of the lip opening during the production of vowels by a child and an adult. For some vowels the horizontal dimension of the lip opening is much greater than the vertical dimension; for others the dimensional difference is not as great, and the size of the lip opening is small. On this basis, the /i, ɪ, e, ɛ, æ, ɑ, ə/ vowels are classified as **unrounded,** and the /u, ʊ, o, ɔ/ vowels as **rounded.** Phoneticians disagree about the degree of lip rounding on the /ɝ/ and /ɚ/ vowels in American English. Some (Heffner, 1952; Bronstein, 1960; Singh & Singh, 1976; Calvert, 1980) indicate no rounding for these vowels, but others (Tiffany & Carrell, 1977; Shriberg & Kent, 1982) suggest that they are usually rounded or that they have some degree of rounding. It is most likely that in American English, /ɝ/ and /ɚ/ are rounded by some speakers, as evidenced by the /ɝ/ lip opening for the adult in Figure 3–4, which appears to be more rounded than the same vowel shown produced by a child in Figure 3–3.

Vowels are also divided into **tense** and **lax,** but unfortunately, the basis for the distinction is not clear. Some phoneticians suggest that the concept is related to greater tension in the tongue muscles for tense vowels than for lax vowels (Bronstein, 1960). Others propose that subglottal air pressure (Heffner, 1952), greater deviation from the neutral vowel position (Heffner, 1952), or drawing forward of the back of the tongue (Tiffany & Carrell, 1977; MacKay, 1987) makes the difference. In an electromyographic study, greater muscle activity was found for tense vowels than for lax vowels, but only in two of the twelve muscles observed (Raphael & Bell-Berti, 1975). According to some phoneticians (Jones, 1956; Bronstein, 1960), the difference in muscle tension can be felt by placing a finger on the throat between the chin and the thyroid cartilage while producing tense and lax vowels.

Two characteristics help differentiate tense and lax vowels: their phonological distribution and their diphthongization tendency. With regard to distribution, tense vowels can terminate monosyllabic words in the General American dialect, for example, /i/ in 'see,' /e/ in 'say,' /u/ in 'sue,' /o/ in 'so,' /ɔ/ in 'saw,' and /ɝ/ in 'sir,' but the lax

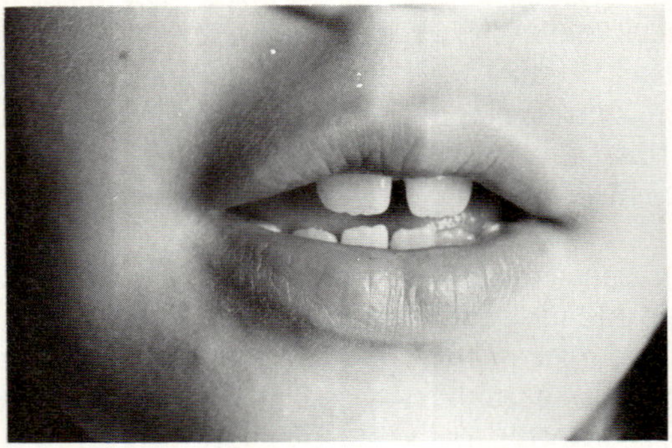

/i/

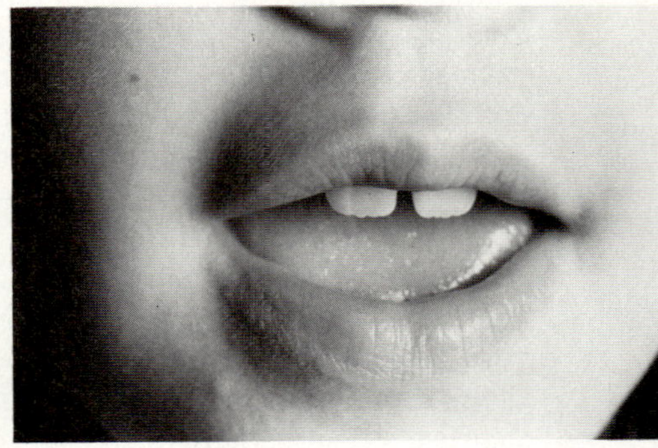

/e/

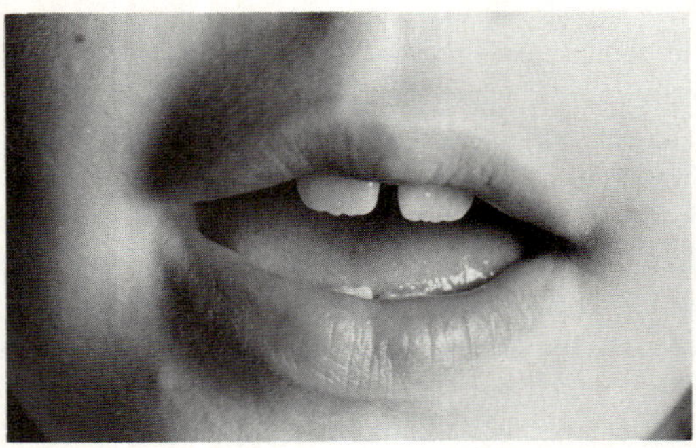

/æ/

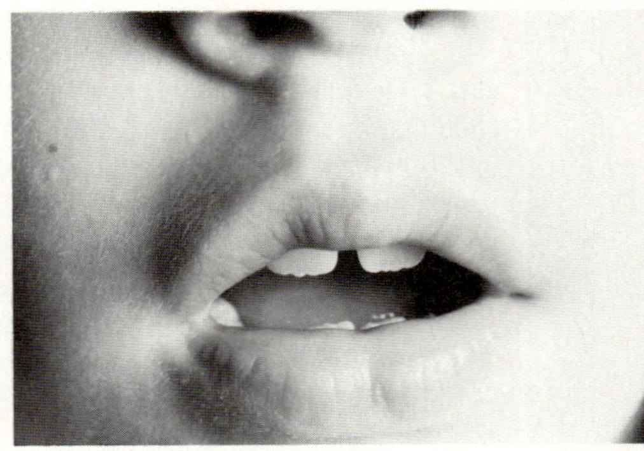

/ʌ/

Figure 3–3
Photographs of lip openings of a child saying /i/, /e /, /æ /, /ʌ /, /ɝ/, /u/, /o /, and /ɑ /. The /ʌ / and /ɝ/ views also illustrate the approximate lip rounding for /ə / and /ɚ/.

vowels, /ɪ/, /ɛ/, /æ/, /ʊ/, /ɑ/, and /ə/, cannot, except for a few words that end with /ɑ/: 'pa,' 'ma,' 'spa,' and 'blah.' There is controversy about the classification of /æ/. Some phoneticians call it tense, at least in some contexts (Bronstein, 1960; Tiffany & Carrell, 1977). With regard to diphthongizing, tense vowels tend to become diphthongs in open syllables. A **diphthong** is produced by shifting from the position for one vowel to another one in the same syllable. The /i/ of 'heat' changes to [ɪ i] in 'he'; the /e/ of 'hate' changes to [e ɪ] in 'hay'; the /u/ of 'hoot' changes to /ʊ u/ in 'who'; and the /o/ of 'hope' changes to [o ʊ] in 'hoe.' Diphthongization does not occur for the tense vowel /ɔ/ or for any of the lax vowels. Transcription of the diphthongs indicates that they either start from a laxer tongue position, as for [ɪ i] and [ʊ u], or they end with a laxer tongue position, as for [e ɪ] and [o ʊ] (Bronstein, 1960; Tiffany & Carrell, 1977).

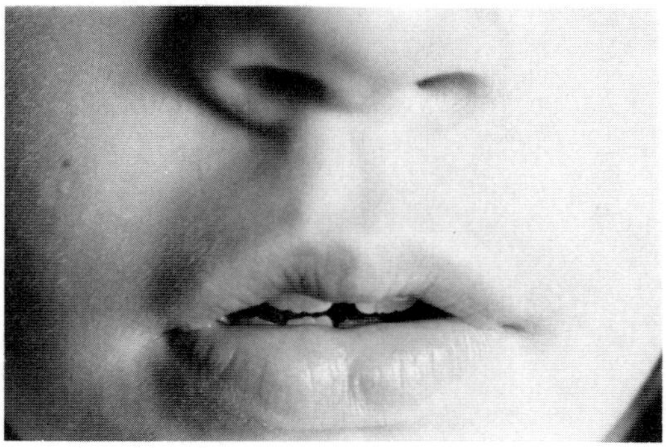

/ɝ/

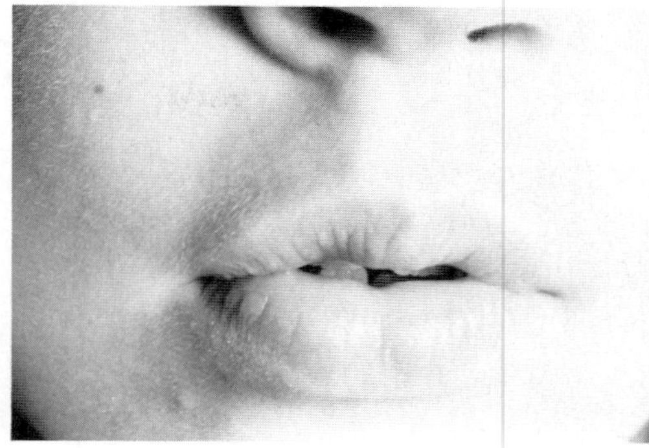

/u/

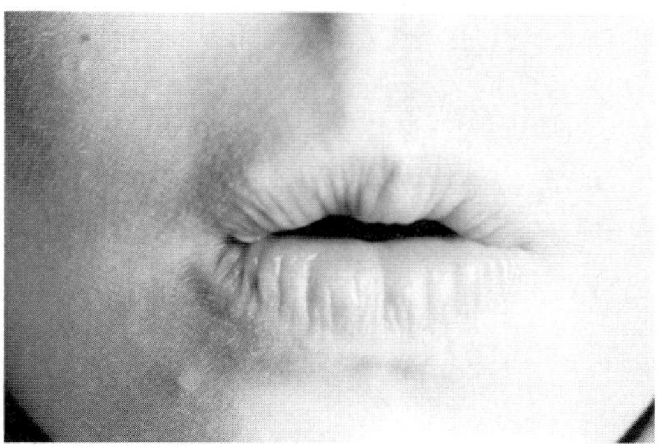

/o/

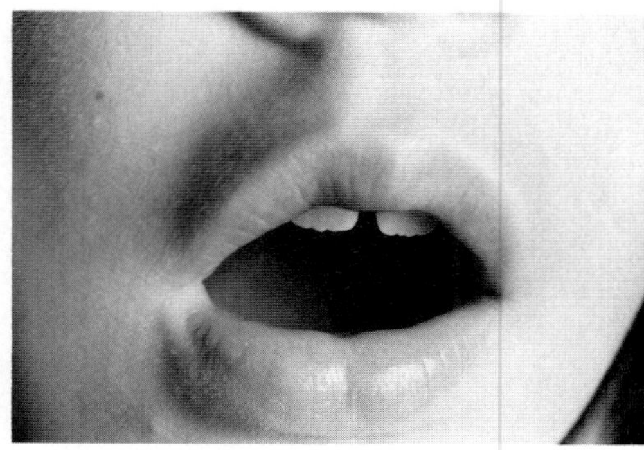

/ɑ/

A major distinction between tense and lax vowels, whether or not diphthongization occurs, is that tense vowels are longer than lax vowels. It is a robust distinction, since deaf children, for example, maintain an absolute difference in the mean duration of the /i/ and /ɪ/ vowels, with /i/ being 370 msec and /ɪ/ 238 msec (Monsen, 1974). Since vowel tension manifests itself by differences in duration and diphthongization for which there are phonetic symbols, there is no need for extra symbols to indicate variations in tenseness.

Vowels can also be differentiated on the basis of their acoustic characteristics. Figures 3–5 and 3–6 show spectrograms of the vowels of the General American dialect as produced by a child and an adult. The horizontal bars marked by arrows on the *y* axis are the formants, which reflect the varying resonances of the vocal tract arising from its unique shaping for each vowel. Note that F_1 and F_2 are relatively far apart for the front vowels and relatively close together for the back vowels. By examining the patterns for the front and back vowels separately, high and low vowels can be compared. Note that

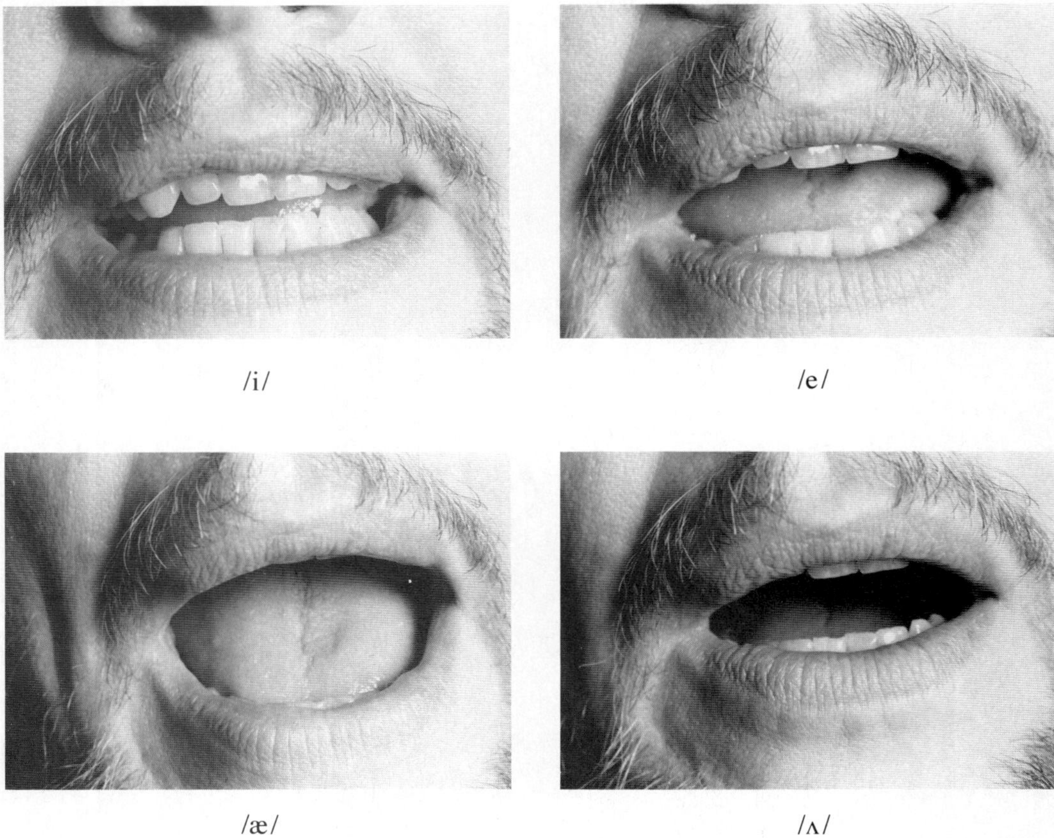

Figure 3–4
Photographs of lip openings of an adult male saying /i/, /e /, /æ /, /ʌ /, /ɝ/, /u/, /o /, and /ɑ /. The /ʌ / and /ɝ/ views also illustrate the approximate lip rounding for /ə / and /ɚ/.

F_1 is relatively low for the high vowels /i, u/ and relatively high for the low vowels /æ, ɑ/. From high to low vowels, the concentration of energy in the lowest resonance component, F_1, tends to shift from lower to higher frequencies. In examining the difference between the front vowels /i, ɪ, e, ɛ, æ/ and the back vowels /u, ʊ, o, ɔ, ɑ/, note that F_2 is relatively high for front vowels and relatively low for back ones. From front to back vowels, the concentration of energy in the next-to-lowest resonance component, F_2, tends to shift from high to low frequency. This relationship is shown more clearly in Figure 3–7, which is a plot of F_1 and F_2 for each of the vowels in figures 3–5 and 3–6.

The energy concentration for the mid central vowels is different from that for the other vowels. As shown in figures 3–5 and 3–6, F_1 and F_2 for /ʌ/ are not as close as they are for back vowels and not as far apart as they are for front vowels. The

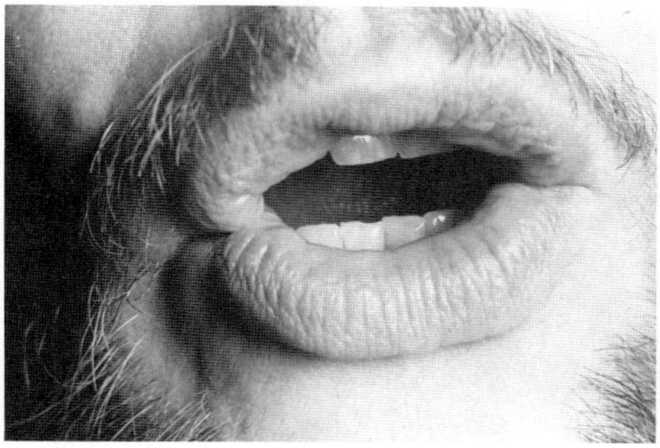

/ɝ/

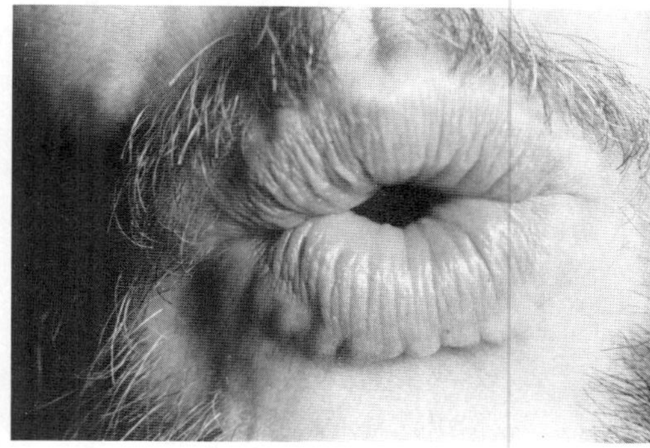

/u/

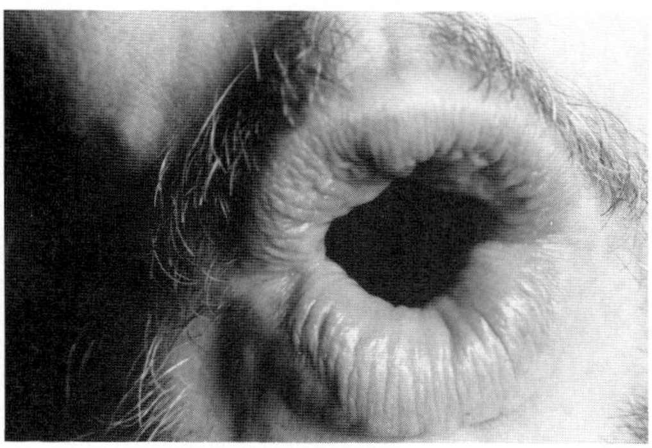

/o/

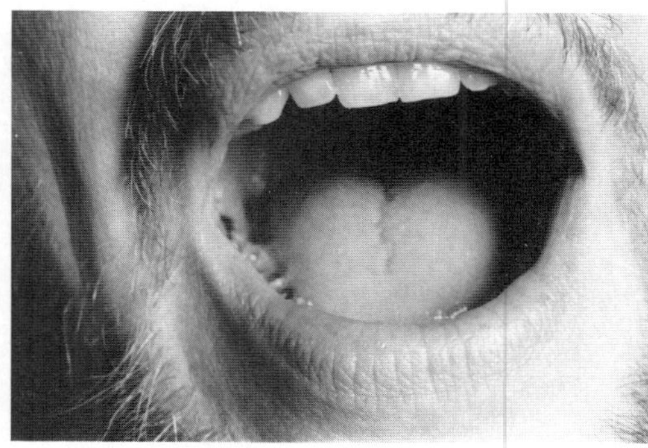

/ɑ/

unstressed equivalent of /ʌ/, commonly referred to as the schwa vowel, is /ə/. It will sound more like a back vowel when it is in the first syllable of 'abut' and more like a front vowel when it is in the first syllable of 'believe.' The mid central vowel /ɝ/ is a special case, since it is the one American English vowel that is characterized acoustically by the proximity of F_2 and F_3 (see arrows in figures 3–5 and 3–6). This vowel is sometimes referred to as **rhoticized** because of its r-coloring (Ladefoged, 1975). (*Rhoticized* was apparently first used by Ladefoged [1975] and spelled *rhotacized.* As Ladefoged [1989] acknowledged, this term should be spelled as indicated in this book by analogy with the pattern for *critic* and *criticize.*)

In phonetics the relative tongue positions of the vowels are usually presented in a diagram like the one in Figure 3–8, which includes the vowels of the General American dialect. The vertical dimension represents tongue height, and the horizontal dimension represents tongue position. Since the diagram represents tongue position only, lip rounding must be indicated by specifically marking those vowels that are rounded. Placement of the vowels in the diagram is based on X-ray studies (Russell, 1928;

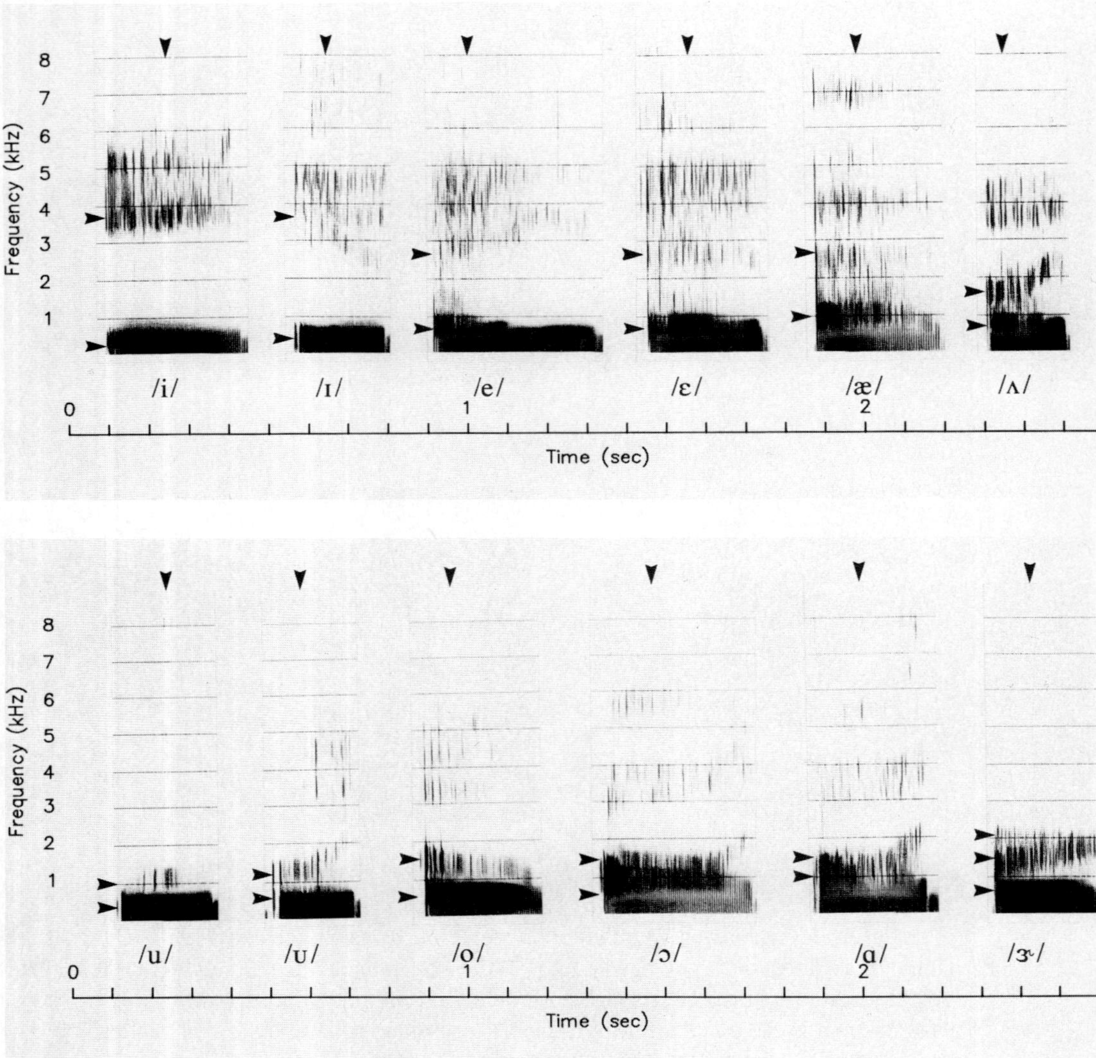

Figure 3–5
Spectrograms of front vowels and /ʌ/ (top panel), and back vowels and /ɝ/ (bottom panel) produced by a child in a /h Vd/ context. Approximate frequencies of F_1 and F_2 for each vowel, except for /ɝ/, are indicated by the lowest and highest arrows on the *y* axis (ordinate). These arrows reflect the different formant frequency patterns of the vowels plotted in Figure 3–7. For /ɝ/, F_3 is indicated by the highest arrow. Arrows along the upper *x* axis (abscissa) of each panel indicate points in time for the power spectrum analyses (amplitude sections) used to derive the formant frequencies. The analysis filter was 45 Hz for all power spectrum analyses throughout the book.

Delattre & Freeman, 1968; Perkell, 1969), but these studies show great variation in the position of vowels. This diagram can serve as a general guide to the relative tongue positions for vowels and, along with their acoustic representation in figures 3–5, 3–6, and 3–7, can help refine your perception of them.

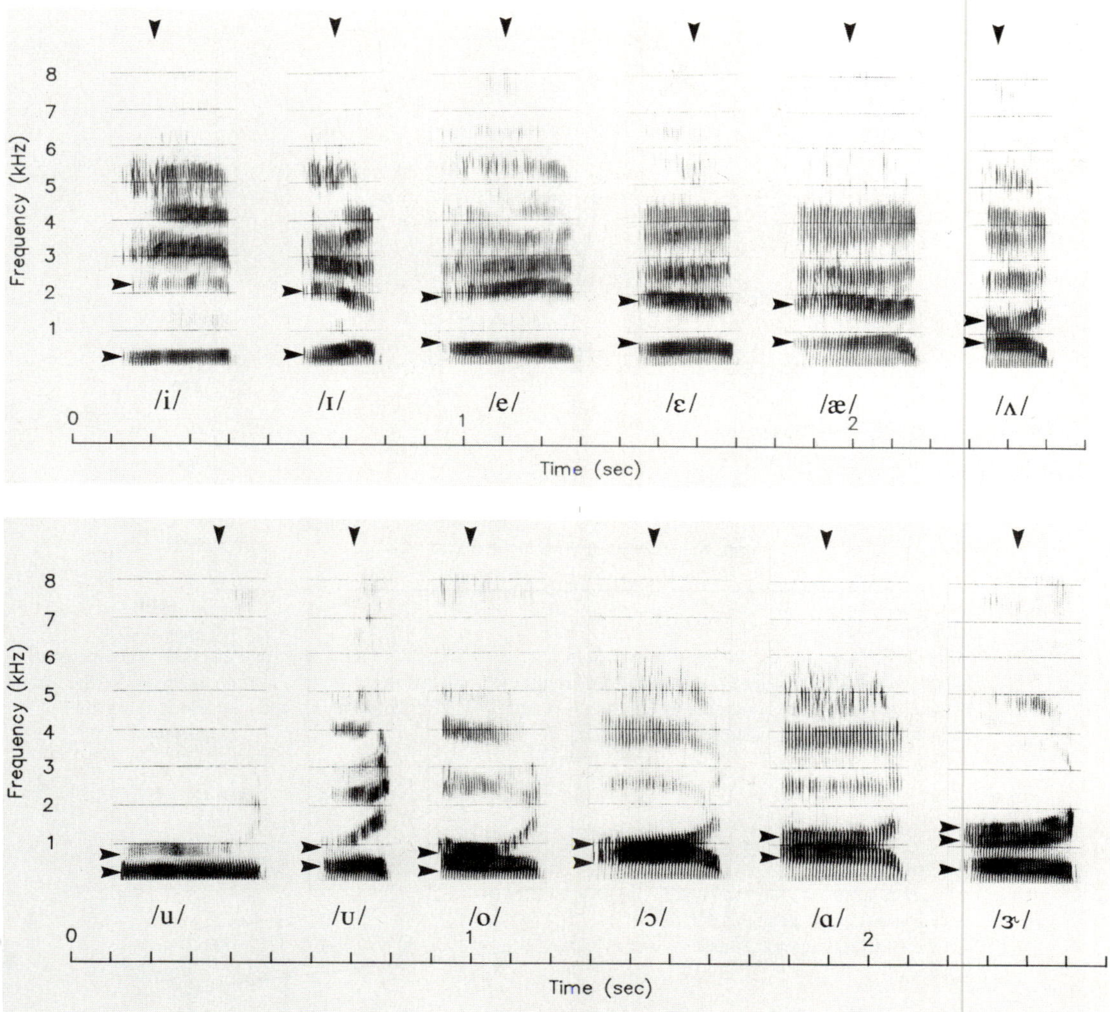

Figure 3–6
Spectrograms of front vowels and /ʌ/ (top panel) and back vowels and /ɝ/ (bottom panel) produced by an adult male in a /h Vd/ context. Approximate frequencies of F_1 and F_2 for each vowel, except /ɝ/, are indicated by the lowest and highest arrows on the *y* axis. These arrows reflect the different formant frequency patterns of the vowels plotted in Figure 3–7. For /ɝ/, F_3 is indicated by the highest arrow. Arrows along the upper *x* axis of each panel indicate approximate points in time for power spectrum analyses (amplitude sections) used to derive the formant frequencies.

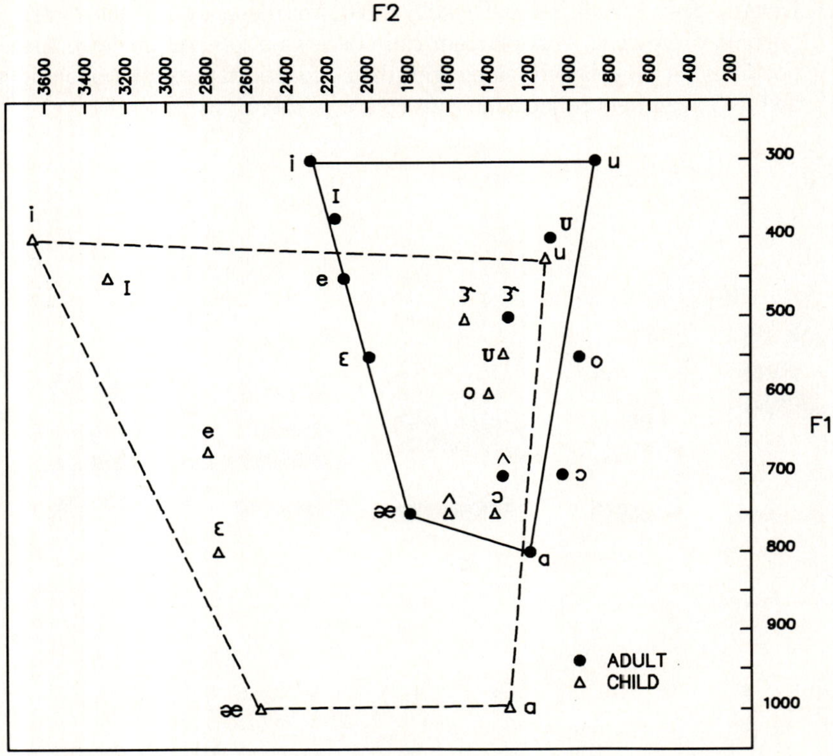

Figure 3–7
Plot of $F_1 \times F_2$ for the vowels illustrated in figures 3–5 and 3–6 for a child and an adult male speaker. Formant frequency values were calculated from power spectrums at a point in time indicated by the arrow at the top of the spectrograms in Figures 3–5 and 3–6. The plots for /ʌ / and /ɝ/ also indicate the approximate formant values for /ə / and /ɚ/.

Figure 3–8
Diagram illustrating vertical and horizontal tongue positions for the vowels of the General American dialect.

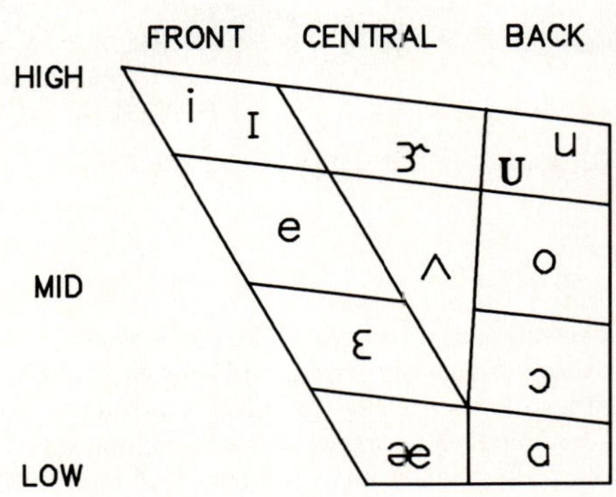

Since understanding the nature of the vowels of the General American dialect is so important, each will be considered with reference to its distinctiveness, as shown in Table 3–1, and its production, as shown in Figure 3–8. Tense vowels presumably are produced with greater tension of the tongue muscles than lax vowels. Rounded vowels are produced with a greater narrowing of the lip opening than unrounded vowels. High vowels are characterized by a slight drop of the lower jaw from its closed position, low vowels by a maximum opening of the lower jaw, and mid vowels by an intermediate jaw position.

/i/ High (Highest) Front Unrounded Tense Vowel

This vowel is produced with the tongue in the highest and most forward position of any vowel in English. It occurs in all positions, including the final position in monosyllables. Since it is tense, /i/ frequently is produced as a diphthong, which may be transcribed as [ɪi], particularly when there is no following consonant, as in 'see' [sɪi], or when the final consonant is voiced, as in 'seed' [sɪid] (Bronstein, 1960; Tiffany & Carrell, 1977).

/ɪ/ High Front Unrounded Lax Vowel

This vowel is produced with the tongue slightly lowered from the position for /i/. It does not occur in final position in monosyllabic words.

/e/ Mid (High-Mid) Front Unrounded Tense Vowel

This vowel is produced with the tongue lowered from the level for the high vowels. It occurs in all positions of words including the final position in monosyllables. Since it is tense, /e/ frequently is produced as a diphthong, particularly when there is no following consonant, as in 'say' [seɪ], or when the following consonant is voiced, as in 'same' [seɪm].

/ɛ/ Mid (Low-Mid) Front Unrounded Lax Vowel

This vowel is produced with the tongue slightly lowered from the position for /e/. It does not occur in word-final position.

/æ/ Low Front Unrounded Lax Vowel

This vowel is produced with the tongue lowered from the position for /ɛ/. It does not occur in word-final position. Some phoneticians classify this vowel as tense.

/u/ High (Highest) Back Rounded Tense Vowel

This vowel is produced with the tongue raised in the highest and most retracted position of any vowel in English. It occurs in all positions of words including the final position in monosyllables. Since it is tense, /u/ often is a diphthong, particularly when there is no consonant following, as in 'shoe' [ʃʊu], or when the final consonant is voiced, as in 'shoes' [ʃʊuz] (Bronstein, 1960; Tiffany & Carrell, 1977).

/ʊ/ High Back Rounded Lax Vowel

This vowel is produced with the tongue slightly lowered from the /u/ position, as in 'book' /bʊk/. It does not occur in word-initial or word-final positions.

/o/ Mid (High-Mid) Back Rounded Tense Vowel

This vowel is produced with the tongue slightly lowered from the position for /ʊ/. It occurs in all positions, including the final position of monosyllables. Since it is tense, /o/ often becomes a diphthong, particularly when there is no following consonant, as in 'sew' [soʊ], or when the final consonant is voiced, as in 'sewed' [soʊd].

/ɔ/ Mid (Low-Mid) Back Rounded Tense Vowel

This vowel is produced with the tongue slightly lowered from the position for /o/. It occurs in all positions, including word-final position in monosyllables like 'law' /lɔ/. Although it is tense, /ɔ/ does not become a diphthong.

/ɑ/ Low Back Unrounded Lax Vowel

This vowel is produced with the tongue at the lowest and most retracted position of any vowel. It occurs in all positions, though only occasionally in word-final position in monosyllabic words like 'pa,' 'ma,' and 'spa.' Some phoneticians classify /ɑ/ as tense.

/ɝ/ Mid to High Central Unrounded Tense Vowel

This vowel is usually produced with the tongue bunched and raised to about the same level as /e/ or /ɪ/ but with the tongue retracted toward /o/. It is much less likely to occur as a retroflex sound, at least in English. Some speakers produce this vowel with some lip rounding. It occurs in all positions including word-final position in monosyllables like 'sir' /sɝ/. Many phoneticians use this symbol to designate only the stressed syllables of words like 'perverse' and 'murder.'

/ɚ/ Mid to High Central Unrounded Lax Vowel

This vowel is produced from the same position as /ɝ/, and it may also be rounded by some speakers. It is used by many phoneticians to represent the equivalent of /ɝ/ in the unstressed syllables of words like 'perverse' and 'murder.'

/ə/ Mid (Low Mid) Central Unrounded Lax Vowel

This vowel, referred to as the schwa, is produced with the tongue lowered from the position for /ɝ/, in the unstressed syllables of words like 'subtract.' But its position shifts considerably when it occurs in the unstressed syllables of words like 'believe.' It does not occur in final position in monosyllabic words.

/ʌ/ Mid Back-Central Unrounded Lax Vowel

This vowel is produced from a position close to that of /ə/ in the first syllable of words like 'subtract,' but the tongue is slightly retracted toward /ɑ/. Many phoneticians use this symbol to represent the stressed syllables of words like 'substance,' but not the unstressed syllables of words like 'subtract.' Also, IPA uses this symbol to represent the unrounded equivalent of /ɔ/.

A number of vowels other than those shown in Figure 3–8 occur in other dialects of English and in foreign languages. Figure 3–9 includes two diagrams of IPA cardinal vowels, one for rounded vowels and one for unrounded vowels, with tongue positions represented for each vowel. The **cardinal vowels** constitute a system, devised by the phonetician Daniel Jones (Jones, 1940), for describing vowels in terms of the front, highest /i/ and lowest /a/ tongue positions and the back, highest /u/ and lowest /ɑ/ tongue positions from which vowels can be produced. Intermediate front /e, ɛ/ and back /o, ɔ/ vowels are located between these four corner vowels, supposedly on the basis of equal acoustic separation. It is generally acknowledged that the vowels can be learned only from an auditory model. Since the focus in this book is on clinical phonetics, these diagrams are covered only briefly. Basically, the diagrams show that any vowel can be produced with the lips rounded or unrounded. For example, you can put your tongue in

Figure 3–9
Diagrams illustrating vertical and horizontal tongue positions for rounded and unrounded vowels (IPA cardinal vowels). The relative positions for /ɚ/ also illustrate the approximate positions for /ɝ/.

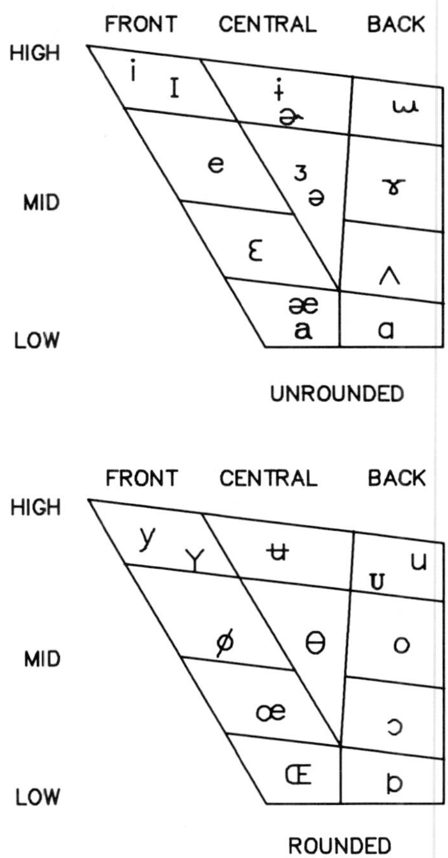

the position for /i/ as in 'heat,' round the lips while still maintaining the same tongue position, and produce the /y/ vowel. These two vowels, /i/ and /y/, are shown in the same positions in the unrounded and rounded diagrams in Figure 3–9. In addition, there are the following unrounded and rounded pairs: /ɪ/ and /ʏ/; /e/ and /ø/; /ɛ/ and /œ/. In each pair, the unrounded front vowel occurs in English as the standard.

In English, the standard back vowels /u, ʊ, o, ɔ/ are rounded, but /ɑ/ is not. You can produce the unrounded equivalents of these vowels by assuming their tongue positions and then unrounding the lips to produce the following pairs: /u/ and /ɯ/; /o/ and /ɤ/; /ɔ/ and /ʌ/. Just the opposite can be done to produce the /ɑ/ and /ɒ/ pair. As will be pointed out in Chapter 4 in discussing vowel allophones, the rounded vowels of English become somewhat unrounded when preceded by the glide sound /j/, as in 'you,' 'yolk,' and 'yawn.' Also, /ɑ/ may become rounded when preceded by the /w/ glide as in 'watch.' It should be noted that the /ʌ/ symbol is commonly used to represent the stressed equivalent of the /ə/ vowel rather than its IPA cardinal value.

In Figure 3–9, the /ɚ/ vowel is somewhat arbitrarily placed with the unrounded vowels. As noted earlier, phoneticians disagree as to the classification of this vowel; it may be rounded by some speakers of American English.

It is worthwhile specifically noting three of the vowels in Figure 3–9—/a/; /ɒ/; and /ɜ/—because they occur in New England and Southern dialects. The /a/ vowel occurs in New England in words like 'park,' 'card,' and 'sharp' in the speech of those who do not produce the /r/ sound in those words (Bronstein, 1960). The /ɒ/ vowel is used by New England speakers in some words produced with the /ɑ/ vowel by General American dialect speakers, like 'hot,' 'top,' and 'cod' (Bronstein, 1960). The /ɜ/ vowel is produced by speakers of Southern and New England dialects in words like 'bird,' 'first,' and 'work' instead of the /ɝ/ vowel (Bronstein, 1960). Also, as will be suggested in discussing deviant vowel and glide variants in Chapter 4, children who produce a distorted /r/ appear to start the sound from the /ɜ/ position. Note that the use of key words like 'hot' is not adequate for either the /ɑ/ or /ɒ/ vowels unless the dialect is specified, and 'bird' is not adequate for either /ɝ/ or /ɜ/ for the same reason.

There are gaps in the rounded vowel diagram for the equivalents of /æ/ and /ɝ/, not because they do not occur but merely because IPA does not provide symbols for them. There are, however, diacritic symbols, shown in Table 3–2, which can be used to indicate just about any type of vowel that might occur. The rounded equivalents of the vowels noted above can be indicated by using the symbol for lip rounding: /æ̹/. The

Table 3–2
Diacritics indicating modifications in lip rounding and tongue positions of vowels. Note that diacritics relating to the lips are placed above the vowel symbol. Those relating to the tongue follow the vowel symbol, according to the practice recommended by Shriberg & Kent (1982).

Symbol	Modification
[V̹]	Lips rounded
[V̜]	Lips unrounded
[V˔]	Tongue raised
[V˕]	Tongue lowered
[V˖]	Tongue moved forward
[V˗]	Tongue moved backward

modifiers can also be used to indicate various degrees of lip rounding. For example, [i˒] indicates some rounding toward /y/; [y˓] indicates some unrounding toward /i/.

In addition to lip rounding, the modifiers in Table 3–2 are useful for indicating degrees of modification in the tongue position of vowels. For example, General American dialect speakers who try to pronounce the /a / vowel tend to vacillate between /æ / and /ɑ / in their attempts. In doing so, they may produce: (1) a vowel between /æ / and /a / which can be indicated by using a diacritic for tongue lowering, [æ˕], or by using a diacritic for tongue raising, [a˔]; or (2) a vowel between /a / and /ɑ /, which can be indicated by using a tongue retraction diacritic, [a ˗], or by using a tongue advancement diacritic, [ɑ ˖].

RELATIONSHIPS AMONG VOWELS, GLIDES, AND LIQUIDS

Glides are sounds produced by shifting from the position for one vowel to the position for another within the same syllable. For example, you can shift from /i/ to /ɑ/ in one syllable and produce 'yon,' which begins with a glide, or you can shift between the same vowels in two syllables and produce 'eon,' which does not begin with a glide. Since a glide is contained within one syllable and a syllable has one peak of sound energy or sonority, one of the two vowels in a glide has greater energy or sonority than the other. Two types of glides, for example, can be formed from the /u/ and /ɑ/ vowels, one in which the second vowel is more prominent, as in /u ɑ t/ 'watt,' and another in which the first vowel is more prominent, as in /ɑ u t/ 'out.' The first type is a prevocalic glide, or **onglide,** and the second is a postvocalic glide, or **offglide.**

Four types of postvocalic glides or offglides can be produced: **fronting, retracting, centering,** and **lateralizing.** As the arrows in Figure 3–10 illustrate, these terms reflect shifts in tongue position from any vowel, such as /ɑ/, toward: (1) the highest front vowel /i/ for the fronting offglide, as in 'high' (*fronting* as used here to modify the postvocalic glide should not be confused with the *fronting* which denotes a phonological process, described in Chapter 6); (2) the highest back vowel /u/ for the retracting offglide, as in 'how'; (3) the mid central vowel /ɚ/ for the centering offglide, as in 'mar'; and (4) the lateral vowel /l/ for the lateralizing offglide, as in 'moll.'

The vowel target for each of these offglides has been described, except for the lateralizing one. Distribution of syllabic /l/ is limited in English, occurring only in the unstressed syllables of two-syllable words like 'cattle,' 'paddle,' 'tunnel,' and 'puzzle.' In these words the tongue apex contacts the alveolar ridge for the consonant that terminates the first syllable. In order to produce the following /l/, this apico-alveolar contact is maintained, but the rest of the tongue is lowered from its palatal contact, and no vowel intervenes between the preceding consonant and the /l/. In this position, /l/ acts as a vowel because it provides the peak of sound energy for the second syllable, and it is referred to as a syllabic consonant in such contexts. Unlike vowels, /l/ involves tongue contact, but air is free to flow over the sides of the tongue and out of the oral cavity.

Figure 3–11 shows the four types of prevocalic glides, or onglides: (1) /j/, which shifts from the /i/ vowel to the position for any other vowel, as in 'yacht'; (2) /w/, which

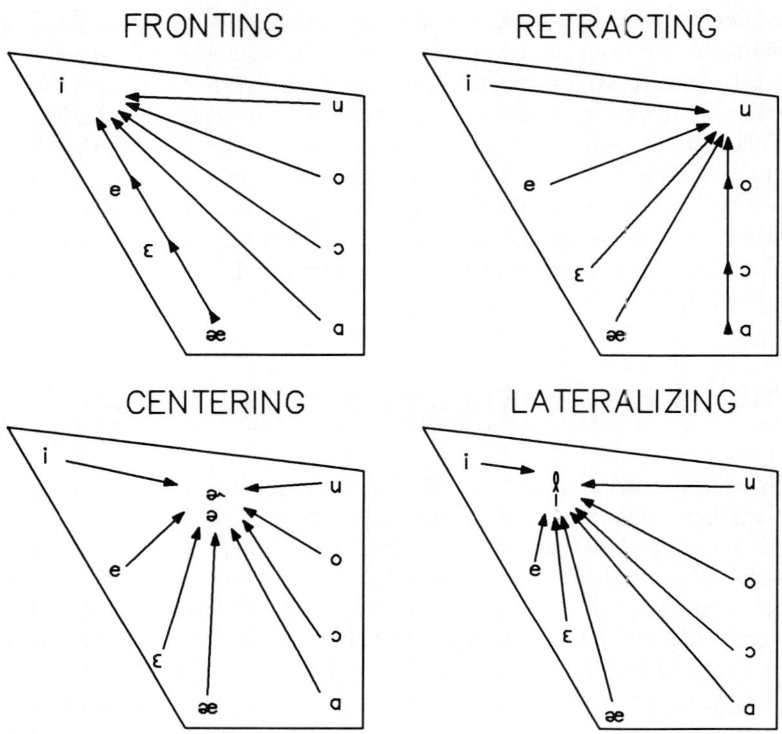

Figure 3–10
Schematic of fronting, retracting, centering, and lateralizing postvocalic glides or offglides.

shifts from the /u/ vowel to the position for any other vowel, as in 'watt'; (3) /r/, which shifts from the /ɚ/ vowel to the position for any other vowel, as in 'rot'; and (4) /l/, which shifts from the /l/ vowel to the position for any other vowel, as in 'lot.' These glides are generally classified as consonant sounds. In the interest of ease of transcription, this book follows the practice of others whose main concern is American English by using /r/ for the consonant in words like 'ray' rather than the upside down /ɹ/ recommended by IPA (Bronstein, 1960; Calvert, 1980; MacKay, 1987; Potter, Kopp, & Green, 1947; Shriberg & Kent, 1982; Singh & Singh, 1976; Tiffany & Carrell, 1977).

Although some phoneticians classify /l/ and /r/ as glides (Potter, Kopp, & Green, 1947; Bronstein, 1960; Calvert, 1980; Singh & Singh, 1976; Pickett, 1980), others either do not (Heffner, 1952; Jones, 1956; Shriberg & Kent, 1982) or include /r/ but not /l/ (Tiffany & Carrell, 1977). The /l/ and /r/ sounds are also referred to as liquids by some phoneticians (Heffner, 1952; Shriberg & Kent, 1982). **Liquid** is a cover term for /l/ and /r/, used to differentiate them from /w/ and /j/ in recognition of the distinctiveness of their articulatory configuration, which is lateral for /l/ and either retroflex or bunched for /r/. The distinction is particularly convenient when discussing the phonological process of gliding (see Chapter 4). Gliding is the substitution of /w/ for /r/ and

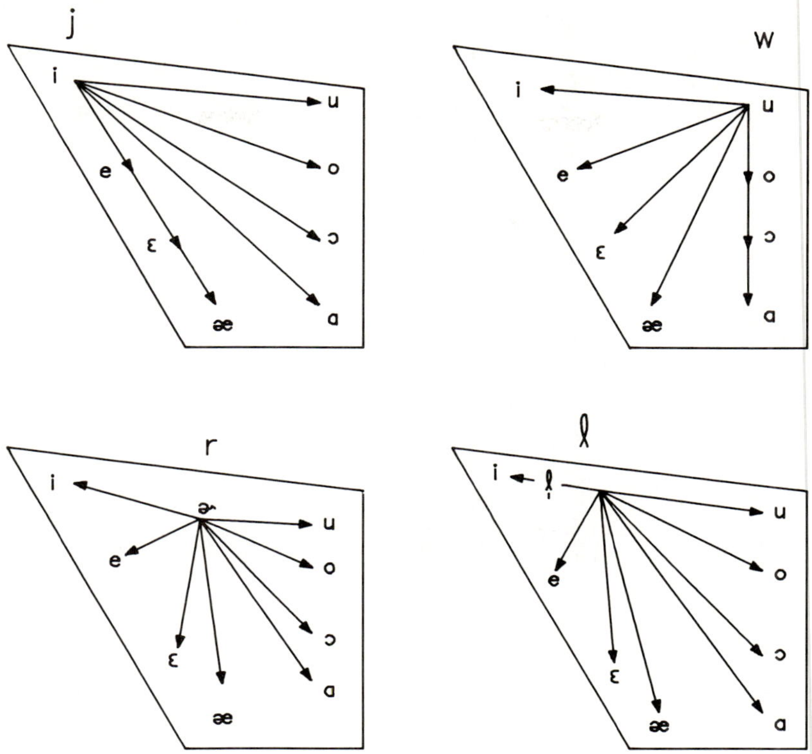

Figure 3–11
Schematic of /j/, /w/, /r/, and /l/ prevocalic glides, or onglides.

/l/, and is less confusing to think of as the substitution of a glide for a liquid than as the substitution of a glide for another glide.

The dynamic aspect of glides can be seen when one looks at the acoustic analyses of them in Figure 3–12, which shows shifts between /ɑ/ and following /ʊ/, /r/, /l/, /ɪ/. Each of these is paired with the analogous glide between /w/, /r/, /l/, /j/, and /ɑ/. Notice how F_1 and F_2 for the /j/ glide shift from the widely separated pattern characteristic of a front vowel to the close-knit pattern characteristic of a back vowel. For the /ɑɪ/ glide, the F_1 and F_2 pattern shows just the reverse. Similar comparisons can be made by examining the spectrograms for each of the other glide pairs. In making these comparisons, you should note that even though the /w/, /r/, /j/, and /l/ prevocalic glides are phonologically classified as consonants because 'watt,' 'rot,' 'yacht,' and 'lot' differ from words like 'cot,' the glides have formants just like the vowels.

Although only a few of them have been noted, many different glides are possible. The beginning and ending positions for the glides can vary. Most of the conceivable glides do not occur in any language, but some appear in English as phonemes or as dialectal variants. On the basis of minimal pair analysis, /ɑɪ/, /ɑʊ/, and /ɔɪ/ are identified as diphthong phonemes, /w/ and /j/ as glide phonemes, and /r/ and /l/ as liquid phonemes. Examples of minimal contrasts among these sounds are presented in Table 3–3. Even though only one way of transcribing the /ɔɪ/, /ɑɪ/, and /ɑʊ/ diphthongs is shown, there is a good deal of variation in the beginning and ending vowel positions as these sounds are produced. Phoneticians recognize that the representation of the start-

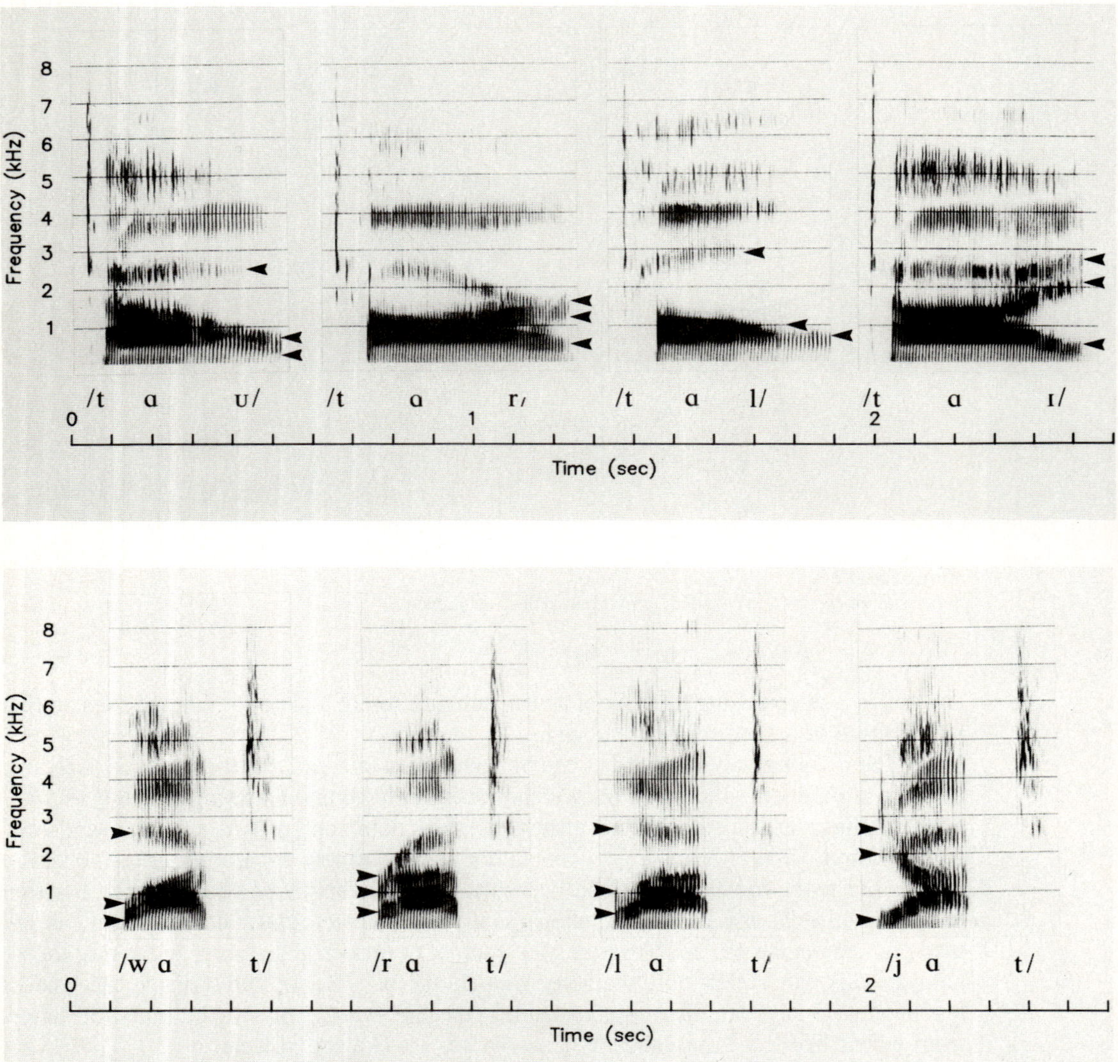

Figure 3–12
Spectrograms of an adult male's postvocalic glides, or offglides (top panel), and prevocalic glides, or onglides (bottom panel), produced in a /t ɑ / or an /ɑ t/ context. Glides in the top panel are between /ɑ / and /u/, /ɑ / and /ɚ/, /ɑ / and /l/, and /ɑ / and /i/. Glides in the bottom panel are between /u/ and /ɑ /, /ɚ/ and /ɑ /, /l/ and /ɑ /, and /i/ and /ɑ /. Formant onsets and offsets are indicated by arrows.

Table 3–3
Minimal pair contrasts of the glide-type phonemes of English, showing contrasts in CV and VC positions.

	Diphthongs			Glides		Liquids	
	/ɑɪ/	/ɑʊ/	/ɔɪ/	/w/	/j/	/r/	/l/
CV	buy	bow[a]	boy	watt	yacht	rot	lot
VC	aisle	owl	oil			bear	bell

[a]To bend forward at the waist.

Table 3–4
Examples of fronting, retracting, and centering glides in English.

Glide	Word	Usage
Fronting		
/eɪ/	say	General American dialect
[ɛɪ]	say	Variant of /e/
[æɪ]	can	Southern dialect
/ɑɪ/	rise	General American dialect
[aɪ]	rise	Variant of /ɑɪ/
[ʌɪ]	rice	Variant of /ɑɪ/ preceding voiceless consonants
/ɔɪ/	boy	General American dialect
[oɪ]	boy	Variant of /ɔɪ/
[ɜɪ]	bird	New York dialect
Retracting		
/ɑʊ/	how	General American dialect
[aʊ]	how	Variant of /ɑʊ/
[ɛʊ]	how	Canadian dialect
[æʊ]	how	Canadian dialect
/oʊ/	hoe	General American dialect
Centering		
/ɪɚ/	fear	General American dialect
[iə]	fear	Infrequent variant of /ɪɚ/
[ɪə]	fear	Southern and New England dialects
/ɛɚ/	pear	General American dialect
[ɛə]	pear	Southern and New England dialects
/ʊɚ/	poor	General American dialect
[uɚ]	poor	Infrequent variant of /ʊɚ/
[ʊə]	poor	Southern and New England dialects
/ɔɚ/	pour	General American dialect
[ɔə]	pour	New England dialect
[oə]	pour	Southern dialect
/ɑɚ/	par	General American dialect
[ɑə]	par	Southern and New England dialects

ing and ending points for these glides is only an approximation which serves the purpose of standardizing their phonetic transcription. The same can be said of the [eɪ] and [oʊ] diphthongs, described more fully in Chapter 4 as the allophonic variants of /e/ and /o/.

Table 3–4 includes examples of words in which fronting, retracting, and centering glide variants occur in various dialects of English. Some of these variants represent slight differences in the starting points for glides, as when [ɛɪ] and [eɪ] are used in a word like 'say.' In some cases variants indicate disagreement among phoneticians about the starting point for glides, as in the use of [ɑɪ] and [aɪ] for words like 'rise.' A number of dialectal variants are shown, including those for the starting points of the glides, for example, the Southern use of [æɪ] for words like 'can' and the Southern and New England use of [ɪə] in words like 'fear.'

The type of sounds identified as centering glides ending in /ɚ/ in Figure 3–10 are referred to by some phoneticians as r-colored vowels, or as diphthongs if they occur in English (Bronstein, 1960; Tiffany & Carrell, 1977). Examples of words in which such sounds occur are presented in Table 3–4. As indicated, r-coloring occurs in the General American dialect when the /ɪ/, /ɛ/, /ʊ/, /ɔ/, and /ɑ/ vowels are terminated by /ɚ/ as in 'fear,' 'pear,' 'poor,' 'pour,' and 'par,' respectively. In Southern and New England dialects, these same words terminate in /ə/, so that r-coloring does not occur.

GLOSSARY

Back vowel. A vowel made with the tongue retracted toward the back of the oral cavity.

Bunched. Raising and arching of the tongue as in the production of /ɝ/.

Cardinal vowels. A system for describing vowels in relation to the highest and lowest front and back vowels that can be produced.

Centering glide. A postvocalic glide, or offglide, that terminates in /ɚ/ or /ə/.

Central vowel. A vowel made with the tongue positioned midway between the most forward and the most retracted positions for vowels.

Diphthong. A sound made by shifting from the position for one vowel to another one within the same syllable.

Front vowel. A vowel made with the tongue advanced toward the front of the oral cavity.

Fronting glide. A postvocalic glide, or offglide, that terminates near the /i/ vowel. Not to be confused with the phonological process of the same name.

Glide. A sound made by shifting from one vowel position to another within the same syllable. May be an offglide or an onglide.

High vowel. A vowel made with the tongue raised toward the palate.

Lateralizing glide. A postvocalic glide, or offglide, that terminates in /l/.

Lax vowel. A vowel made with reduced tension in the tongue muscles.

Liquid. A cover term for /l/ and /r/ used to differentiate them from /w/ and /j/ in recognition of the distinctiveness of their articulatory configuration, that is, lateral for /l/ and either retroflex or bunched for /r/.

Low vowel. A vowel made with the tongue lowered toward the floor of the oral cavity.

Mid vowel. A vowel made with the tongue midway between the palate and the floor of the oral cavity.

Offglide. A postvocalic glide produced by shifting from a more prominent to a less prominent vowel within the same syllable.

Onglide. A prevocalic glide produced by shifting from a less prominent to a more prominent vowel within the same syllable. Also referred to as a glide and generally classified as a consonant.

Retracting glide. A postvocalic glide, or offglide, that terminates near /ʊ/.

Retroflex. Describes raising the body of the tongue toward the palate and arching the apex upward and backward in the production of certain sounds.

Rhoticized. Describes sounds with r-coloring. Commonly misspelled as *rhotacized.*

Rounded. Describes sounds made with a narrowing of the lip opening.

Schwa. A mid central vowel which includes a relatively wide range of variants in the unstressed syllables of words like 'above,' 'below,' 'today,' and 'conceive.'

Tense vowel. A vowel made with the tongue muscles relatively tense.

Unrounded. Describes sounds made with the lips with a relatively long horizontal opening.

Vowel. A speech sound that is produced with relatively open vocal tract resonance and functions as the nucleus of a syllable.

REVIEW QUESTIONS

A. Classify the vowels by checking the appropriate columns.

	Tense	*Lax*	*High*	*Low*	*Mid*	*Front*	*Central*	*Back*
1. /i/	____	____	____	____	____	____	____	____
2. /ɪ/	____	____	____	____	____	____	____	____
3. /e/	____	____	____	____	____	____	____	____
4. /o/	____	____	____	____	____	____	____	____
5. /ɔ/	____	____	____	____	____	____	____	____
6. /ə/	____	____	____	____	____	____	____	____

****

Key: 1. T,H,F; 2. L,H,F; 3. T,M,F; 4. T,M,B; 5. T,L,B; 6. L,M,C

B. Complete the minimal pair for each pair of vowels or glides. The word for the first vowel is given to you.

1. /i, e / bees ______________
2. /ɪ , o / hip ______________
3. /ɑ , æ / sock ______________
4. /ɛ , o / peck ______________

5. /l, w/ laced ____________ 7. /u, æ / food ____________

6. /r, l/ wrist ____________ 8. /j , w/ yolk ____________

****

Key: 1. bays; 2. hope; 3. sack; 4. poke; 5. waist or waste; 6. list; 7. fad; 8. woke

C. Note how F_1 reflects the tongue height of vowels by indicating whether the first vowel is higher (H) or lower (L) in frequency than the second vowel in each pair.

1. /i, e/ ________ 4. /u, o/ ________

2. /ɪ, ɛ/ ________ 5. /ɔ, o/ ________

3. /æ, ɛ/ ________ 6. /ɑ, o/ ________

****

Key: 1. L; 2. L; 3. H; 4. L; 5. H; 6. H

D. Note how F_2 reflects the horizontal position of the tongue by indicating whether the first vowel in each pair is higher (H) or lower (L) in frequency than the second vowel.

1. /i, o/ ________ 4. /e, o/ ________

2. /ɛ, ɔ/ ________ 5. /ɔ, i/ ________

3. /ʊ, ɪ/ ________ 6. /æ, ɑ/ ________

****

Key: 1. H; 2. L; 3. L; 4. H; 5. L; 6. H

E. Indicate the word in which each glide might occur by inserting the appropriate letter.

a. more b. gear c. say d. poor e. far f. nice g. sew h. doubt

i. bird j. coin

1. /ʊ ɚ/ ________ 6. [ʌ ɪ] ________

2. [ɜ ɪ] ________ 7. [o ʊ] ________

3. /ɔ ɪ/ ________ 8. [ɪ ɚ] ________

4. [ɛ ɪ] ________ 9. /ɑ ɚ/ ________

5. [æ ʊ] ________ 10. /ɔ ɚ/ ________

****

Key: 1. d; 2. i; 3. j; 4. c; 5. h; 6. f; 7. g; 8. b; 9. e; 10. a

LABORATORY ASSIGNMENT

Tape I, Side A
Sections 1–3: Vowels, Glides, and Liquids
IA1: Front Vowels (Tape running time 5:41; Elapsed time 00:00–05:41)

a. Front Vowel Models

Listen to the front vowels of the General American dialect as they are pronounced in the minimal contrast /h Vt/ context by an adult and a child. If necessary, stop the tape at any time, rewind, and listen again.

1. Adult: /h i t/; /h ɪ t/; /h e t/; /h ɛ t/; /h æ t/
2. Child repeats above.
3. Adult: /h i t/; /h ɪ t/. Child repeats.
4. Adult: /h ɪ t/; /h e t/. Child repeats.
5. Adult: /h e t/; /h ɛ t/. Child repeats.
6. Adult: /h ɛ t/; /h æ t/. Child repeats.
7. Child: /h i t/; /h ɪ t/; /h e t/; /h ɛ t/; /h æ t/
8. Adult repeats above.

In sections b through e, transcribe the vowels produced by an adult and a child. If necessary, stop the tape after each utterance, rewind, and listen again. After transcribing all the utterances in each section, check your answers with the key. Transcriptions for which there was majority agreement are identified as "Consensus" in the key. Other choices are identified as "Variants"; "None" indicates no variants. This procedure is used in all transcription exercises. If you make many errors, redo the section.

b. Transcription of Front Vowels in Minimal Pairs

1. ________ 2. ________ 3. ________ 4. ________ 5. ________

6. ________ 7. ________ 8. ________ 9. ________ 10. ________

****

Consensus: 1. /ɪ/ 2. /i/ 3. /æ/ 4. /e/ 5. /ɛ/ 6. /e/ 7. /ɪ/ 8. /æ/ 9. /i/ 10. /ɛ/

Variants: None.

c. Transcription of Front Vowels in Minimal Pairs in Context

1. ________ 2. ________ 3. ________ 4. ________ 5. ________

6. ________ 7. ________ 8. ________ 9. ________ 10. ________

****

Consensus: 1. /ɛ/ 2. /i/ 3. /e/ 4. /æ/ 5. /ɪ/ 6. /æ/ 7. /i/ 8. /ɛ/ 9. /ɪ/ 10. /e/

Variants: 1. /ɛ˔/ 4. /æ˕/

d. Transcription of Front Vowels in Words in Isolation

1. feet ________ 2. pin ________ 3. fat ________ 4. safe ________

5. pen ________ 6. bat ________ 7. gate ________ 8. itch ________

9. test ________ 10. gift ________

****

Consensus: 1. /i/ 2. /ɪ/ 3. /æ/ 4. /e/ 5. /ɛ/ 6. /æ/ 7. /e/ 8. /ɪ/ 9. /ɛ/ 10. /ɪ/

Variants: 6. /æ˔/

e. Transcription of Front Vowels in Words in Context

Transcribe the vowels in the following sentence types: 'I can say ________'; 'Say the word ________'; '________ is the word.'

1. cat ________ 2. late ________ 3. get ________ 4. ask ________

5. beat ________ 6. eight ________ 7. teach ________ 8. get ________

9. bed ________ 10. dip ________

****

Consensus: 1. /æ/ 2. /e/ 3. /ɛ/ 4. /æ/ 5. /i/ 6. /e/ 7. /i/ 8. /ɪ/ 9. /ɛ/ 10. /ɪ/

Variants: None.

If you continue to have trouble differentiating the /ɪ/ and /ɛ/ vowels, particularly on items 2 and 5 in section d and items 3 and 8 in section e, then you should complete the section 1 supplement (IA1S).

IA1S: Front Vowels: /ɪ –ɛ/ Discrimination
(Tape running time: 6:34; Elapsed time: 05:41–12:15)

a. /ɪ/ and /ɛ/ Models

Listen to the /ɪ/ and /ɛ/ vowels as they are pronounced in minimal contrast contexts by an adult and a child.

1. Adult: /gɛt/; /gɪt/; /gɪt/; /gɛt/
2. Child repeats above.
3. Adult: /tɪn/; /tɛn/; /tɛn/; /tɪn/
4. Child: /tɪn/; /tɛn/; /tɪn/; /tɛn/
5. Adult: /mɛni/; /mɪni/; /mɪni/; /mɛni/
6. Child repeats above.

b. Discrimination of /ɪ/ and /ɛ/

Listen to the following pairs of words and indicate if they are the same (S) or different (D). After responding to each item, check your answers with the key. If you get more than three wrong, redo this section.

1. ______	2. ______	3. ______	4. ______	5. ______
6. ______	7. ______	8. ______	9. ______	10. ______
11. ______	12. ______	13. ______	14. ______	15. ______
16. ______	17. ______	18. ______	19. ______	20. ______
21. ______	22. ______	23. ______	24. ______	25. ______
26. ______	27. ______	28. ______	29. ______	30. ______
31. ______	32. ______	33. ______	34. ______	35. ______
36. ______	37. ______	38. ______	39. ______	40. ______

41. ________ 42. ________ 43. ________ 44. ________ 45. ________

46. ________ 47. ________ 48.________

****

Key: 1. D; 2. S; 3. D; 4. S; 5. S; 6. D; 7. D; 8. S; 9. S; 10. D; 11. S; 12. D; 13. S; 14. S; 15. D; 16. S; 17. S; 18. D; 19. D; 20. S; 21. S; 22. D; 23. S; 24. D; 25. D; 26. D; 27. S; 28. D; 29. D; 30. S; 31. D; 32. S; 33. D; 34. S; 35. D; 36. S; 37. S; 38. D; 39. D; 40. S; 41. S; 42. D; 43. S; 44. D; 45. S; 46. D; 47. D; 48. S.

In sections c and d, transcribe the vowels in monosyllabic words or in the first syllable of polysyllabic words. If necessary, stop the tape after each utterance, rewind, and listen again. After transcribing all utterances in each section, check your answers with the key. If you make any errors, redo the section.

c. Transcription of /ɪ / and /ɛ / Vowels in Isolated Words

1. get ________ 2. ten ________ 3. many ________ 4. many ________

5. get ________ 6. ten ________ 7. pen ________ 8. tin ________

9. get ________ 10. get ________

****

Consensus: 1. /ɛ / 2. /ɪ / 3. /ɪ / 4. /ɛ / 5. /ɪ / 6. /ɛ / 7. /ɪ / 8. /ɪ / 9. /ɪ / 10. /ɛ /

Variants: 9. /ɪ˔/

d. Transcription of /ɪ / and /ɛ / in Words in Context

Transcribe the vowels in the following sentence types: 'I can say ________'; Say the word ________'; '________ is the word.'

1. penny ________ 2. get ________ 3. get ________ 4. penny ________

5. ten ________ 6. many ________ 7. hen ________ 8. ten ________

9. get ________ 10. many ________ 11. many ________ 12. tin ________

13. get ________ 14. get ________ 15. many ________ 16. ten ________

****

Consensus: 1. /ɪ / 2. /ɛ / 3. /ɪ / 4. /ɛ / 5. /ɪ / 6. /ɪ / 7. /ɪ / 8. /ɛ / 9. /ɪ / 10. /ɛ / 11. /ɪ / 12. /ɪ / 13. /ɪ / 14. /ɛ / 15. /ɛ / 16. /ɛ /

Variants: None.

IA2: Back Vowels (Tape running time: 5:28; Elapsed time: 12:15–17:43)

a. Back Vowel Models

Listen to the back vowels of the General American dialect as they are pronounced in the minimal contrast /h Vt/ context by an adult and a child. If necessary, stop the tape at any time, rewind, and listen again.

1. Adult: /h u t/; /h ʊ t/; /h o t/; /h ɔ t/; /h ɑ t/
2. Child repeats above.
3. Adult: /h u t/; /h ʊ t/. Child repeats.
4. Adult: /h ʊ t/; /h o t/. Child repeats.
5. Adult: /h o t/; /h ɔ t/. Child repeats.
6. Adult: /h ɔ t/; /h ɑ t/. Child repeats.

In sections b through e, transcribe the vowels produced by an adult and a child. If necessary, stop the tape after each item, rewind, and listen again. After transcribing all the items in each section, check your answers with the key. If you make any errors, redo the section.

b. Transcription of Back Vowels in Minimal Pairs

1. ________ 2. ________ 3. ________ 4. ________ 5. ________

6. ________ 7. ________ 8. ________ 9. ________ 10. ________

****

Consensus: 1. /ʊ/ 2. /u/ 3. /ɑ/ 4. /o/ 5. /ɔ/ 6. /o/ 7. /ʊ/ 8. /ɑ/ 9. /u/ 10. /ɔ/

Variants: 10. /ɔ˔/

c. Transcription of Back Vowels in Minimal Pairs in Context

1. ________ 2. ________ 3. ________ 4. ________ 5. ________

6. ________ 7. ________ 8. ________ 9. ________ 10. ________

****

Consensus: 1. /ɔ/ 2. /u/ 3. /o/ 4. /ɑ/ 5. /ʊ/ 6. /ɑ/ 7. /u/ 8. /ɔ/ 9. /ʊ/ 10. /o/

Variants: None.

d. Transcription of Back Vowels in Words in Isolation

1. boot ________ 2. could ________ 3. cot ________ 4. boat ________

5. got ________ 6. lots ________ 7. hope ________ 8. soup ________

9. caught ________ 10. foot ________

****

Consensus: 1. /u/ 2. /ʊ/ 3. /ɑ/ 4. /o/ 5. /ɑ/ 6. /ɑ/ 7. /o/ 8. /u/ 9. /ɔ/ 10. /ʊ/

Variants: None.

e. Transcription of Back Vowels in Words in Context

Transcribe the vowels in the following sentence types: 'I can say ________'; 'Say the word ________'; '________ is the word.'

1. wash ________ 2. rope ________ 3. wash ________ 4. top ________

5. two ________ 6. go ________ 7. book ________ 8. book ________

9. saw ________ 10. look ________

****

Consensus: 1. /ɑ/ 2. /o/ 3. /ɔ/ 4. /ɑ/ 5. /u/ 6. /o/ 7. /ʊ/ 8. /ʊ/ 9. /ɔ/ 10. /ʊ/

Variants: None.

If you continue to have trouble differentiating the /ɑ/ and /ɔ/ vowels, particularly on items 3 and 9 in section d and items 1 and 3 in section e, then you should complete the section 2 supplement (IA2S).

IA2S: Back Vowels: /ɑ –ɔ/ Discrimination (Tape running time: 7:05; Elapsed time: 17:43–24:48)

a. /ɑ/ and /ɔ/ Models

Listen to the /ɑ/ and /ɔ/ vowels as they are pronounced in minimal contrast contexts by an adult and a child.

1. Adult: /lɑg/; /lɔg/; /lɔg/; /lɑg/
2. Child repeats above.

3. Adult: /kɑt/; /kɔt/; /kɔt/; /kɑt/
4. Child repeats above.
5. Adult: /wɑʃ/; /wɔʃ/; /wɔʃ/; /wɑʃ/
6. Child repeats above.

b. Discrimination of /ɑ/ and /ɔ/

Listen to the following pairs of words and indicate if they are the same (S) or different (D). After responding to each item, check your answers with the key. If you get more than three wrong, redo this section.

1. ______	2. ______	3. ______	4. ______	5. ______
6. ______	7. ______	8. ______	9. ______	10. ______
11. ______	12. ______	13. ______	14. ______	15. ______
16. ______	17. ______	18. ______	19. ______	20. ______
21. ______	22. ______	23. ______	24. ______	25. ______
26. ______	27. ______	28. ______	29. ______	30. ______
31. ______	32. ______	33. ______	34. ______	35. ______
36. ______	37. ______	38. ______	39. ______	40. ______
41. ______	42. ______	43. ______	44. ______	45. ______
46. ______	47. ______	48. ______		

****

Key: 1. D; 2. S; 3. D; 4. S; 5. D; 6. S; 7. D; 8. S; 9. D; 10. S; 11. S; 12. D; 13. D; 14. S; 15. S; 16. D; 17. S; 18. D; 19. S; 20. D; 21. S; 22. D; 23. S; 24. D; 25. S; 26. D; 27. D; 28. S; 29. S; 30. D; 31. D; 32. S; 33. D; 34. D; 35. S; 36. S; 37. D; 38. S; 39. D; 40. S; 41. D; 42. S; 43. D; 44. S; 45. D; 46. S; 47. D; 48. S.

In sections c and d, transcribe the vowels in monosyllabic words or in the first syllable of polysyllabic words. If necessary, stop the tape after each utterance, rewind, and listen again. After transcribing all utterances in each section, check your answers with the key. If you make any errors, redo the section.

c. Transcription of /ɑ/ and /ɔ/ Vowels in Isolated Words

1. log ______	2. caught ______	3. wash ______	4. cot ______
5. log ______	6. wash ______	7. log ______	8. wash ______
9. caught ______	10. log ______		

****

Consensus: 1. /ɑ/ 2. /ɔ/ 3. /ɑ/ 4. /ɑ/ 5. /ɔ/ 6. /ɔ/ 7. /ɔ/ 8. /ɑ/ 9. /ɔ/ 10. /ɑ/

Variants: 10. /ɑ˔/

d. Transcription of /ɑ/ and /ɔ/ in Words in Context

Transcribe the vowels in the following sentence types: 'I can say ________'; 'Say the word ________'; '________ is the word.'

1. log ________	2. water ________	3. caught ________
4. waffle ________	5. wash ________	6. want ________
7. log ________	8. foreign ________	9. wash ________
10. foreign ________	11. log ________	12. water ________
13. wash ________	14. want ________	15. log ________
16. cot ________	17. caught ________	18. waffle ________

****

Consensus: 1. /ɔ/ 2. /ɔ/ 3. /ɔ/ 4. /ɔ/ 5. /ɑ/ 6. /ɔ/ 7. /ɔ/ 8. /ɔ/ 9. /ɔ/ 10. /ɑ/ 11. /ɑ/ 12. /ɑ/ 13. /ɑ/ 14. /ɑ/ 15. /ɔ/ 16. /ɑ/ 17. /ɔ/ 18. /ɑ/

Variants: 1. /ɑ/ 2. /ɑ/ 4. /ɑ/ 5. /ɔ/ 6. /ɑ/ 7. /ɑ/ 11. /ɔ˕/

IA3: Central Vowels (Tape running time: 5:20; Elapsed time: 24:48–30:08)

a. Central Vowel Models

Listen to the central vowels of the General American dialect as they are pronounced in the minimal contrast /h Vt/ context by an adult and a child. For contrast, two back vowels, /ʊ/ and /ɑ/, are included. If necessary, stop the tape at any time, rewind, and listen again.

1. Adult: /hɝt/; /hʌt/; /hʌt/; /hɝt/
2. Child repeats above.
3. Adult: /hɝt/; /hʌt/; /hʊt/; /hɑt/
4. Child repeats above.
5. Adult: /hɝt/; /hʌt/; /hʌt/; /hʊt/; /hɝt/; /hʊt/
6. Child repeats above.

In sections b through e, transcribe the vowels produced by an adult and a child. If necessary, stop the tape after each utterance, rewind, and listen again. After transcribing all the utterances in each section, check your answers with the key. If you make any errors, redo the section.

b. Transcription of Central Vowels in Minimal Pairs

1. ________ 2. ________ 3. ________ 4. ________ 5. ________

6. ________ 7. ________ 8. ________ 9. ________ 10. ________

****

Consensus: 1. /ɝ/ 2. /ʌ/ 3. /ʊ/ 4. /ɑ/ 5. /ɝ/ 6. /ɑ/ 7. /ɝ/ 8. /ɝ/ 9. /ʊ/ 10. /ʌ/

Variants: None.

c. Transcription of Central Vowels in Minimal Pairs in Context

1. ________ 2. ________ 3. ________ 4. ________ 5. ________

6. ________ 7. ________ 8. ________ 9. ________ 10. ________

****

Consensus: 1. /ʌ/ 2. /ʊ/ 3. /ɑ/ 4. /ɝ/ 5. /ɝ/ 6. /ʊ/ 7. /ʌ/ 8. /ɑ/ 9. /ɝ/ 10. /ʌ/

Variants: None.

d. Transcription of Central Vowels in Words in Isolation

1. third ________ 2. fussed ________ 3. could ________ 4. cot ________

5. first ________ 6. Turk ________ 7. took ________ 8. tuck ________

9. dock ________ 10. duck ________

****

Consensus: 1. /ɝ/ 2. /ʌ/ 3. /ʊ/ 4. /ɑ/ 5. /ɝ/ 6. /ɝ/ 7. /ʊ/ 8. /ʌ/ 9. /ɑ/ 10. /ʌ/

Variants: None.

e. Transcription of Central Vowels in Words in Context

Transcribe the vowels in the following sentence types: 'I can say ________'; 'Say the word ________'; '________ is the word.'

1. look ________ 2. lurk ________ 3. luck ________ 4. lock ________

5. pluck ________ 6. pa ________ 7. purr ________ 8. pull ________

9. pearl ________ 10. luck ________

****

Consensus: 1. /ʊ/ 2. /ɝ/ 3. /ʌ/ 4. /ɑ/ 5. /ʌ/ 6. /ɑ/ 7. /ɝ/ 8. /ʊ/ 9. /ɝ/ 10. /ʌ/

Variants: None.

IB1: Offglides (Tape running time: 6:23; Elapsed time: 00:00–06:23)

a. Offglide Models

Listen to the offglides of the General American dialect as they are pronounced for you in a minimal contrast /h Vd / context by an adult and a child. If necessary, stop the tape, rewind, and listen again.

1. Adult: /hɑɪd/; /hɑʊd/; /hɔɪd/; /hɑɚd /; /hɑld/
2. Child repeats above.
3. Adult: /hɑɪd/; /hɑʊd /; /hɑʊd /; /hɔɪd /; /hɑɪd/; /hɔɪd/; /hɑɚd/; /hɑld/; /hɑɚd/; /hɑʊd/;
4. Child repeats above.
5. Adult: /hɑɪd/; /hɑd/; /hɑʊd/; /hɑd/; /hɔɪd/; /hɔd/; /hɑɚd/; /hɑd/; /hɑld/; /hɑd/
6. Child repeats above.

In sections b through e, transcribe the offglides produced by an adult and a child. If necessary, stop the tape after an utterance, rewind, and listen again. After transcribing all the utterances in each section, check your answers with the key. If you make an error, redo the section.

b. Transcription of Offglides in Minimal Pairs

1. ________ 2. ________ 3. ________ 4. ________ 5. ________

6. ________ 7. ________ 8. ________ 9. ________ 10. ________

****

Consensus: 1. /ɑʊ/ 2. /ɑɚ/ 3. /ɑɪ/ 4. /ɑl/ 5. /ɔɪ/ 6. /ɑl/ 7. /ɑʊ/ 8. /ɔɪ/ 9. /ɑɚ/ 10. /ɑɪ/

Variants: 1. /aʊ/ 3. /aɪ/ 4. /ɔl/ 6. /ɔl/ 7. /aʊ/ 10. /aɪ/

c. Transcription of Offglides in Minimal Pairs in Context

1. ________ 2. ________ 3. ________ 4. ________ 5. ________

6. ________ 7. ________ 8. ________ 9. ________ 10. ________

****

Consensus: 1. /ɑʊ/ 2. /ɑɚ/ 3. /ɑɪ/ 4. /ɑl/ 5. /ɔɪ/ 6. /ɔl/ 7. /ɑʊ/ 8. /ɔɪ/ 9. /ɑɚ/ 10. /ɑɪ/

Variants: 1. /aʊ/ 3. /aɪ/ 4. /ɔl/ 6. /ɑl/ 7. /aʊ/ 10. /aɪ/

d. Transcription of Offglides in Words in Isolation

1. size ________ 2. boys ________ 3. cart ________ 4. mouse ________

5. cold ________ 6. cows ________ 7. finds ________ 8. cars ________

9. noise ________ 10. balls ________

****

Consensus: 1. /ɑɪ/ 2. /ɔɪ/ 3. /ɑɚ/ 4. /ɑʊ/ 5. /ol/ 6. /ɑʊ/ 7. /ɑɪ/ 8. /ɑɚ/ 9. /ɔɪ/ 10. /ɔl/

Variants: 1. /aɪ/ 4. /aʊ/ 6. /aʊ/ 7. /aɪ/ 10. /ɑl/

e. Transcription of Offglides in Words in Context

Transcribe the glides in the following sentence types: 'I can say ________'; 'Say the word ________'; '________ is the word.'

1. lies ________ 2. mice ________ 3. calls ________ 4. bounce ________

5. boards ________ 6. coins ________ 7. course ________ 8. toys ________

9. rolls ________ 10. towns ________

****

Consensus: 1. /ɑɪ/ 2. /ɑɪ/ 3. /ɔl/ 4. /ɑʊ/ 5. /ɔɚ/ 6. /ɔɪ/ 7. /ɔɚ/ 8. /ɔɪ/ 9. /ol/ 10. /ɑʊ/

Variants: 1. /aɪ/ 2. /aɪ/ 3. /ɑl/ 4. /aʊ/ 5. /oɚ/ 7. /oɚ/ 10. /aʊ/

IB2: Onglides (Tape running time: 5:20; Elapsed time: 06:23–11:43)

a. Onglide Models

Listen to the General American onglides pronounced in the minimal contrast /Cɑt/ context by an adult and a child speaker. If necessary, stop the tape at any time, rewind, and listen again.

1. Adult: /wɑt/; /rɑt/; /jɑt/; /lɑt/
2. Child repeats above.

3. Adult: /wɑ t/; /rɑ t/. Child repeats.
4. Adult: /rɑ t/; /jɑ t/. Child repeats.
5. Adult: /jɑ t/; /lɑ t/. Child repeats.
6. Adult: /lɑ t/; /wɑ t/. Child repeats.

In sections b through e, transcribe the onglides produced by an adult and a child. If necessary, stop the tape after each utterance, rewind, and listen again. After transcribing all the utterances in each section, check your answers with the key. If you make an error, redo the section.

b. Transcription of Onglides in Minimal Pairs

1. ________ 2. ________ 3. ________ 4. ________ 5. ________

6. ________ 7. ________ 8. ________ 9. ________ 10. ________

****

Consensus: 1. /w/ 2. /w/ 3. /r/ 4. /j / 5. /w/ 6. /w/ 7. /r/ 8. /l/ 9. /j / 10. /l/

Variants: None.

c. Transcription of Onglides in Minimal Pairs in Context

1. ________ 2. ________ 3. ________ 4. ________ 5. ________

6. ________ 7. ________ 8. ________ 9. ________ 10. ________

****

Consensus: 1. /r/ 2. /l/ 3. /j / 4. /w/ 5. /r/ 6. /r/ 7. /l/ 8. /r/ 9. /w/ 10. /j /

Variants: None.

d. Transcription of Onglides in Words in Isolation

1. twist ________ 2. praise ________ 3. cube ________ 4. fleas ________

5. plays ________ 6. sweeps ________ 7. sleeps ________ 8. trips ________

9. fumes ________ 10. freeze ________

****

Consensus: 1. /w/ 2. /r/ 3. /j / 4. /l/ 5. /l/ 6. /w/ 7. /l/ 8. /r/ 9. /j / 10. /r/

Variants: None.

e. Transcription of Onglides in Words in Context

Transcribe the onglides in the following sentence types: 'I can say ________'; 'Say the word ________'; '________ is the word.'

1. trees ________ 2. please ________ 3. bruise ________ 4. blues ________
5. tweeze ________ 6. quits ________ 7. slaps ________ 8. straps ________
9. cute ________ 10. slave ________

****

Consensus: 1. /r/ 2. /l/ 3. /r/ 4. /l/ 5. /w/ 6. /w/ 7. /l/ 8. /r/ 9. /j/ 10. /l/

Variants: None.

CHAPTER 4

Vowel, Glide, and Liquid Variants

Variants in the production of vowels, glides, and liquids can be allophonic or abnormal. Allophonic variants are attributable to contextual changes in sound production which are consistent with adult speech patterns. Abnormal variants are attributable to an articulatory or phonological problem. Table 4–1 includes descriptions of the vowel, glide, and liquid variants covered in this chapter.

ALLOPHONIC VOWEL, GLIDE, AND LIQUID VARIATIONS

Vowel Lengthening

In discussing diphthongizing and lengthening of tense vowels, allusion was made to the influence of the openness of the syllable, that is, the difference between the /i/ of the open syllable 'see' and the closed syllable 'seed.' The evidence supporting the existence of this distinction is mixed. One study has shown that adults produce longer vowels in open syllables than in closed syllables (Rositzke, 1939); another has shown a nonsignificant tendency in this direction for adults, but no such tendency for children (Lehman, 1988); a third has shown a difference in vowel length for normal and deaf adolescents (Monsen, 1974).

Although the evidence about vowel length in open syllables is mixed, the influence of the voicing of a postvocalic consonant on vowel length is unequivocal. Pronounce the following minimal pairs. You will hear that the vowel is longer in the second word of each pair, the word ending in a voiced consonant: 'heat' versus 'heed,' 'cap' versus 'cab,' 'buck' versus 'bug,' and 'race' versus 'rays.' Figures 4–1 and 4–2 are spectrograms of child and adult speech illustrating the lengthening influence of a final voiced consonant.

Table 4–1
Allophonic and misarticulated vowel (V), glide (G), and liquid (L) variants with diacritics and symbols for indicating them.

Variation	Diacritic	Nature of Variation
Allophonic[a]		
Lengthening	[V:]	Vowels lengthen before voiced consonants
Rounding	[V͗], [G͗]	Vowels and glides round after and before /w/
Nasalizing	[Ṽ], [G̃]	Vowels and glides nasalize, before or after nasals
Devoicing	[G̥]	Glides lose voicing after voiceless consonants
Dentalizing	[l̪]	Tongue tip/teeth contact, before or after *th*
Palatalizing	[lʲ]	/l/ assumes high front vowel position before /j/
Velarizing	[lʷ]	/l/ assumes high back vowel position before back vowels or after any vowel
Syllabicizing	[l̩]	/l/ acts as vowel in unstressed syllables
Abnormal[b]		
Gliding	–	/w/ replaces prevocalic /r/; /w/ or /j/ replaces /l/
Distorting /r/ or derhoticizing	[r˕]	Prevocalic /r/ loses r-coloring
Delateralizing	[l˕]	Prevocalic /l/ loses lateral quality
Vocalization	–	/u/ and /o/ replace [l̩] and postvocalic /l/; /ʊ/ and /ə/ replace /ɝ/ and /ɚ/
Dentalizing	[l̪]	Linguadental contact is made for /l/ in all contexts
Neutralizing	–	Vowels are replaced by /ʌ/ or /ɑ/
Lengthening	[V:]	Vowels lengthen before deleted or devoiced final consonants[c]
Nasalizing	[Ṽ], [G̃]	Vowels and glides are nasalized in all contexts
	[Ṽ]	Vowels are nasalized before deleted final consonant[c]
Denasalizing	[V͊]	Vowels lose normal allophonic nasal quality due to nasal cavity blockage

[a]See tables 4–2 and 4–4 for examples.
[b]See tables 4–5 and 4–6 for examples.
[c]Compensation for phonological process affecting consonants.

The beginning and end of the vowels in the figures are marked by the onset and offset of formants (shown by arrows). The /i/ vowel is shorter when followed by /t/ than by /d/, and the /e/ vowel is shorter when followed by /s/ than by /z/.

The difference in vowel duration preceding voiced and voiceless consonants is a robust distinction observed in acoustic studies both of adults (House & Fairbanks, 1953; Peterson & Lehiste, 1960; House, 1961) and of children (Naeser, 1970a; DiSimoni, 1974; Krause, 1982a; Lehman, 1988). Vowel duration is a sufficient perceptual cue for adults (Raphael, 1972) and children (Krause, 1982b; Lehman, 1988) to differentiate voiced and voiceless consonants. The absolute vowel durations and differences vary with the age of the speaker, the vowel, and the phonetic context, but the ratio of the prevoiceless vowel to the prevoiced vowel duration stays about the same, around 0.65. When it is necessary to indicate such variations, a colon is used for long duration, as in [hi:d] 'heed' versus [hit] 'heat.'

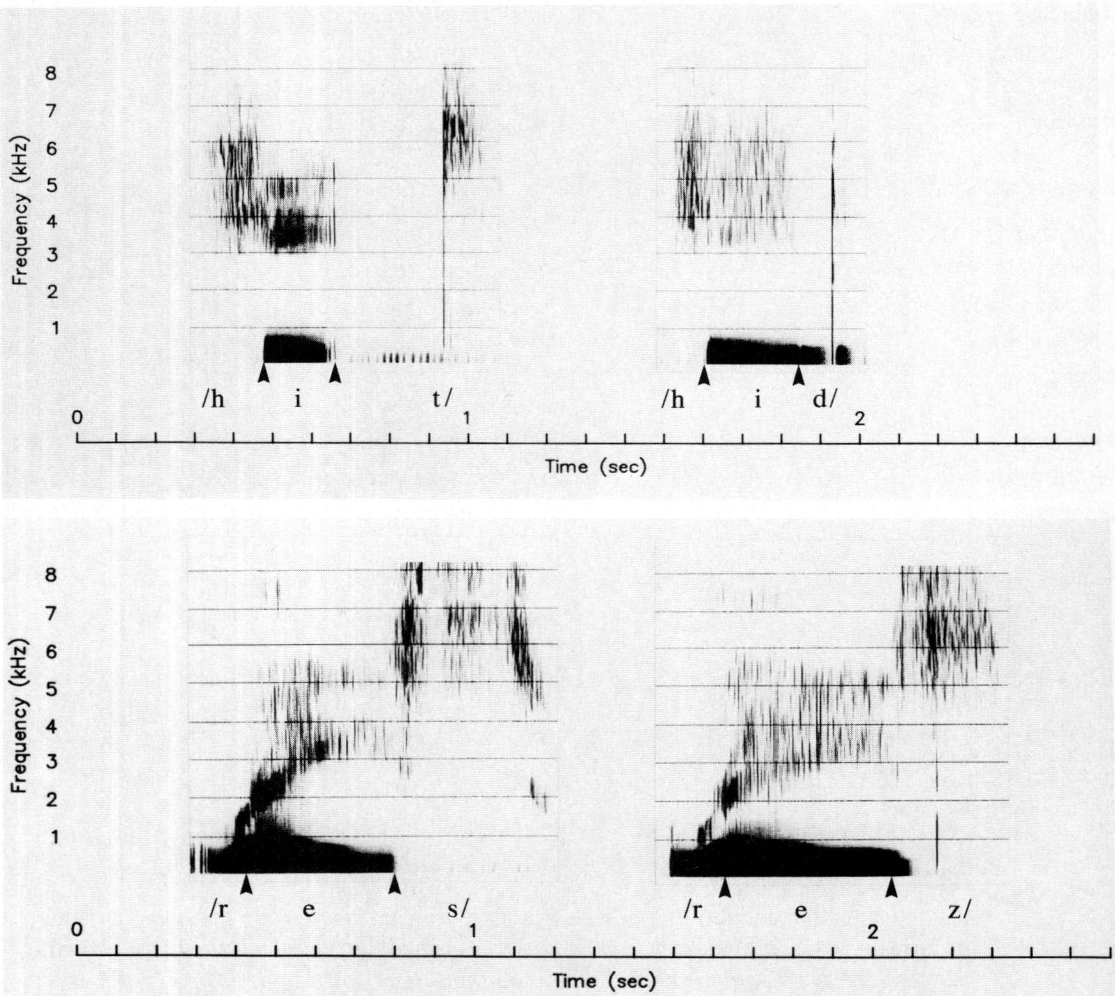

Figure 4–1
Spectrograms illustrating vowel durations for /hit/ (184 msec) versus /hid/ (239 msec) and /res/ (359 msec) versus /rez/ (415 msec) for a child. Arrows along the *x* axis (abscissa) indicate the onset and offset of each vowel.

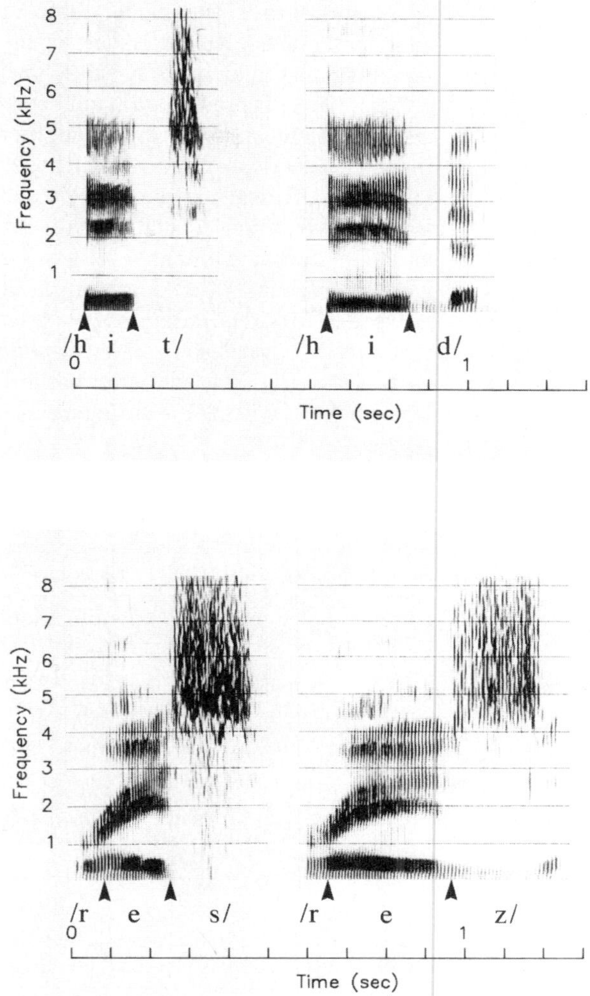

Figure 4–2
Spectrograms illustrating vowel durations for /h i t/ (128 msec) versus /h i d/ (215 msec) and /r e s/ (160 msec) versus /r e z/ (279 msec) for an adult male. Arrows along the *x* axis indicate the onset and offset of each vowel.

In order to explain the difference in vowel duration associated with postvocalic voiced and voiceless consonants, the concept of the allophone must be introduced. Earlier the phoneme was identified as a sound which makes a meaningful distinction between words. For example, 'heat' and 'hit' are distinguished by the /i/ and /ɪ/ vowels. The difference between the long /i/ of 'heed' and the short /i/ of 'heat' was also noted. Are the long and short /i/ vowels also different phonemes? The answer is no, because the difference between /i/ and /ɪ/ makes for meaningful distinctions between words, but the difference between [i:] and [i] does not. The /t/ and the /d/ of 'heat' and 'heed' differentiate these words, not their vowels. Therefore, [i:] and [i] are classified as allophones of the /i/ phoneme. Table 4–2 shows the allophones for a sampling of vowels and diphthongs. The vowels and diphthongs not included in Table 4–2 also have durational variants influenced by the following consonant.

Table 4–3 presents a number of rules and examples of the influence of phonetic and structural context on vowel duration. The rules have been limited to those for which there is objective evidence and those that serve a practical purpose in analyzing the variations in vowel duration associated with misarticulated speech. There may be cases in which you want to differentiate three degrees of duration, as in the case of the variation according to number of syllables shown in Table 4–3. The duration of the stem word decreases as the length of the utterance increases (House, 1961). According to Lehiste (1970), this variation is a rule-governed phonological behavior. It is worth noting that such behavior has been observed in apraxics, adults with motor speech disorders, as well as in normal adults in words like 'please,' 'pleasing,' and 'pleasingly' (Collins, Rosenbek, & Wertz, 1983). Figures 4–3 and 4–4 show spectrograms of a child and an

Table 4–2
Allophones (in brackets) of some vowels and diphthong phonemes (between slant lines) of the General American dialect, with diacritics for indicating them.

Phoneme	Lengthening		Rounding	Nasalizing
/i/	[i] beat	[ɪ i:] bead; bee	[iᵓ] weep	[ĩ:] bean; knee
/u/	[u] suit	[ʊ u:] sued; sue	–	[ũ:] soon; new
/e/	[e] ate	[e ɪ:] aid; hay	[eᵓ] wait	[ẽɪ̃:] aim; may
/o/	[o] boat	[o ʊ:] bode; beaux	–	[o͠ʊ:] bone; no
/aɪ/	[aɪ] sight	[a ɪ:] side; sigh	[aᵓɪ] wipe	[ãɪ̃:] sign; nigh

Table 4–3
Rules and examples of the influence of postvocalic consonant context and structural context on vowel duration. (Contexts preceding > produce longer vowels than those following it.)

Rule	Example
Postvocalic Consonant Context	
Voiced > voiceless	heed, heat
Fricative > stop	hiss, hit
Voiced stop > nasal	dab, dam
Structural Context	
Monosyllabic > polysyllabic	please, pleasing, pleasingly
Stressed syllable > unstressed syllable	seam, inseam
Phrase stress > phrase unstress	I did, I did not

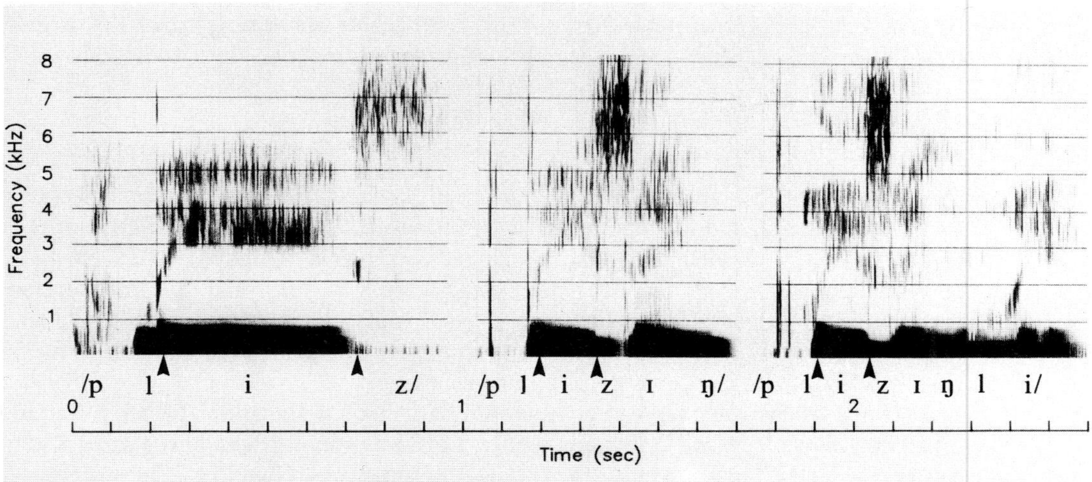

Figure 4–3
Spectrograms of a child illustrating the effects of increasing the number of syllables on the duration of /i/ in 'please' (447 msec), 'pleasing' (148 msec), and 'pleasingly' (104 msec). Arrows along the *x* axis indicate the onset and offset of each vowel.

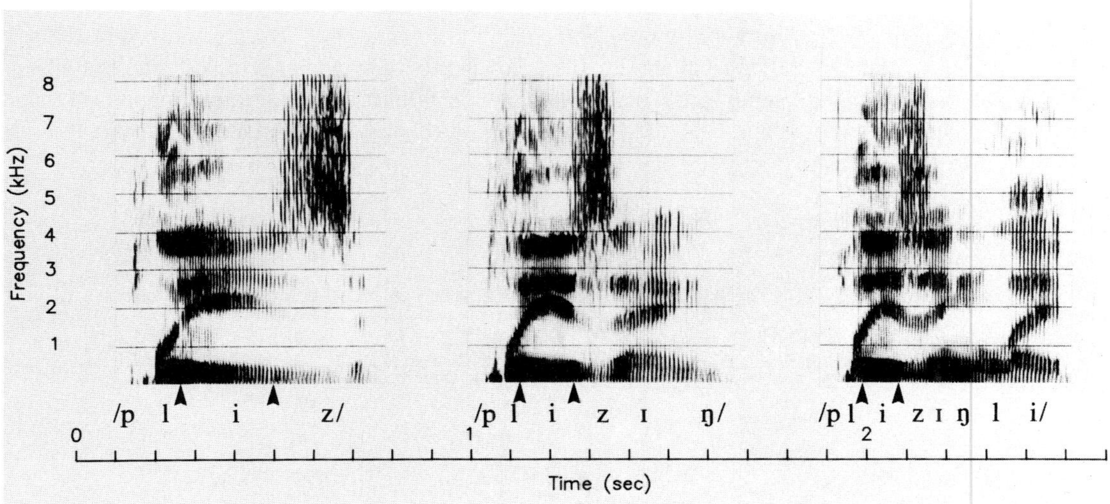

Figure 4–4
Spectrograms of an adult male illustrating the effects of increasing the number of syllables on the duration of /i/ in 'please' (271 msec), 'pleasing' (160 msec), and 'pleasingly' (96 msec). Arrows along the *x* axis indicate the onset and offset of each vowel.

adult producing these words. You can observe the variation in vowel duration. Since decreasing vowel duration in words as a function of the number of syllables that follow is allophonic in English speech, it is not necessary to transcribe these variations.

Vowel, Glide, and Liquid Rounding

The /u/, /ʊ/, /o/, and /ɔ/ vowels are rounded in English. This is an intrinsic difference from other vowels, and it occurs even when the vowels are spoken in isolation or in a context like /h Vt/, which has a minimal influence on vowels. As indicated in Table 4–1, however, the unrounded vowels, /i/, /ɪ/, /e/, /ɛ/, /æ/, /ɑ/, /ʌ/, and /ɝ/, may become rounded when preceded by /w/ in 'weep,' 'wit,' 'wait,' 'wet,' 'wag,' 'watt,' 'what,' and 'word,' respectively. The rounding of the lips for the /w/ carries over into the following vowel so that it too has some degree of lip rounding.

If necessary, rounding can be indicated by using the rounding symbol, as in the transcription of 'weep' as [w i̹p]. For speakers of American English, however, rounding can be assumed when a vowel follows /w/, so the diacritic is redundant. The occurrence of rounded vowels following /w/ is another example of an allophonic variation. In no case in American English does the distinction between rounded and unrounded vowels following /w/ differentiate words. Therefore, [i̹] and [i] are allophones of the /i/ phoneme, as indicated in Table 4–2. The same is true of each of the other unrounded vowels in this context.

The /r/, /l/, and /j/ sounds are also subject to a rounding influence when they precede the /u/ vowel in words like 'rude,' 'loot,' and 'you.' During the production of these sounds, the lip rounding for the following /u/ vowel is anticipated, and the glides are uttered with some lip rounding. Rounded onglides are considered allophones of their phonemes (see Table 4–4): [j] in 'yet' and [j̹] in 'you' are classified as two allophones of /j/.

Table 4–4
Allophones of glide and liquid phonemes of the General American dialect and diacritics for indicating them.

Variation	/w/	/j/	/r/	/l/
Rounding	–	[j̹] you	[r̹] root	[l̹] loot
Nasalizing	–	[j̃] new[a]	[r̃] arm[b]	[l̃] elm
Devoicing	[w̥] twin	/j̥/ few	[r̥] tree	[l̥] fly
Dentalizing	–	–	–	[l̪] health
Palatalizing	–	–	–	[lʲ] million
Velarizing	–	–	–	[lʷ] pill; pull
Syllabicizing	–	–	–	[l̩] pedal; panel

[a]Pronounced [n j u :].
[b]May be transcribed with [ɚ] instead of [r].

Vowel and Liquid Nasalizing

Normally the vowels of American English are not nasalized, that is, the velopharyngeal port is closed so that no nasality occurs. However, as indicated in Table 4–1, in the context of the nasal consonants, /m/ in 'beam,' /n/ in 'bin,' and /ŋ/ in 'bing,' for example, all vowels are nasalized to some extent. (Nasal consonants are covered more thoroughly in Chapter 9.) For now, it is sufficient for you to know that, in the production of nasal consonants, the velopharyngeal port is open so that nasality is produced. During the production of the /i/ vowel in words like 'bean,' the articulatory system responsible for opening up the nasal cavity anticipates the production of the nasal so that some nasalization occurs for the vowel. Nasalization may also occur on /l/ in words like 'elm,' 'calm,' and 'film,' and on /ɚ/ in words like 'arm,' 'form,' and 'barn.' Note that the offglide in the *r* words can be transcribed as /ɚ/ or /r/.

Nasalization of vowels can also occur when they are preceded by nasal consonants, as in the case of the /ɪ/ vowel in 'mitt' and 'knit,' and the /ɚ/ vowel in 'singer.' In this case, the nasalization of the consonant carries over to the vowel. Nasalization may also occur on the /j/ glide in words like 'music,' which all speakers produce with the glide following /m/, and words like 'new' and 'nuisance,' which only some speakers produce with the glide following /n/.

Nasalization can be indicated by placing the nasal modifier over the vowel, but nasalization of vowels and glides is predictable in English due to the influence of the nasal consonants. Nasal and nonnasal vowel and glide variants, therefore, are considered allophones of the same phoneme, as indicated in Tables 4–2 and 4–4. English does not distinguish words because of nasal and nonnasal vowels.

Glide and Liquid Devoicing

Glide and liquid **devoicing** is described in Table 4–1. Frequently /w/, /j/, /r/, and /l/ occur in consonant clusters in which they are preceded by a voiceless consonant, as in the /w/ of 'sweet,' 'twist,' and 'quick'; the /j/ of 'pure,' 'tune,' 'cube,' and 'few'; the /r/ of 'proof,' 'true,' 'crew,' 'free,' and 'shrew'; and the /l/ of 'please,' 'club,' 'fly,' and 'slow.' In each case the absence of vocal fold vibration during the voiceless consonant carries over to the following glide or liquid, which becomes partially devoiced. Such devoicing can be indicated by using the appropriate diacritic below the glide or liquid symbol, as shown in Table 4–4. Note that while all speakers pronounce 'pure,' 'cube,' and 'few' with /j/, only a small percentage do the same for 'tune.' In each case, the devoiced sound is an allophone.

/l/ Dentalizing

In words like 'health,' 'wealth,' and 'athlete,' the /l/ is **dentalized,** that is, the usual alveolar ridge contact of the tongue tip for /l/ changes to either an apicodental (tongue tip contacting back of upper teeth) or interdental (tongue tip protruded between upper and lower teeth) position under the influence of the interdental *th* sound (see

Table 4–1). Dentalization may be noted by using the appropriate IPA diacritic just below the /l/, as shown in Table 4–4. Because this variation is determined by context, the interdental and the alveolar /l/ are treated as allophones of one phoneme.

Glide and Liquid Palatalizing, Velarizing, and Syllabicizing

The **palatalizing, velarizing,** and **syllabicizing** of /l/ are briefly described in Table 4–1. In words like 'million,' 'milieu,' and 'bullion,' in which the /lj/ sequence occurs, the tongue tip and blade contact the alveolar ridge and anterior hard palate to produce a palatalized /l/. The effect is as though you are trying to produce /l/ and /j/ simultaneously. If the tongue tip continues to be close to the alveolar ridge, the /l/-quality is maintained, and the word can be transcribed as /mɪljən/ 'million.' If not, only the /j/ quality survives, and the word is transcribed as /mɪjən/. Palatalized /l/, transcribed as [lʲ], is another allophone of the /l/ phoneme.

When /l/ precedes front vowels, as in 'leap,' 'lip,' and 'lap,' the back part of the tongue does not approximate the palate. This sound has been referred to as clear or **light** /l/; it shares the concentration of energy at the higher resonance frequencies with the front vowels. But when /l/ precedes back vowels, as in 'loop,' 'loan,' and 'lot,' when it is in postvocalic position, following front or back vowels, as in 'pill' or 'pull,' or when it is in unstressed syllables, as in 'noodle' and 'panel,' the back of the tongue is raised to approximate the palate. This velarized sound is commonly known as **dark** /l/, and it shares a concentration of energy at the lower resonance frequencies with the back vowels. Velarized /l/ can be transcribed as [lʷ] and is classified as an allophone of /l/.

In words like 'cattle,' 'noodle,' and 'tunnel,' where /l/ appears in an unstressed syllable and is preceded by /t/, /d/, or /n/, a special type of velarized /l/ occurs. As you can see from the palatograms in Figure 4–5 and feel by producing 'toe,' 'doe,' and 'low,' each of the initial sounds is produced with apico-alveolar contact, that is, with the tongue tip touching the alveolar ridge. But in the production of /l/ the rest of the tongue does not contact the palate, and for /t/, /d/, and /n/ it does. In saying 'cattle,' 'noodle,' and 'tunnel,' the transition from /t/, /d/, or /n/ to /l/ is made by lowering the back of the tongue. In this transition, no vowel is produced, so that only the velarized /l/ occurs in the second syllable. Since /l/ acts in the place of a vowel by being the peak of sonority

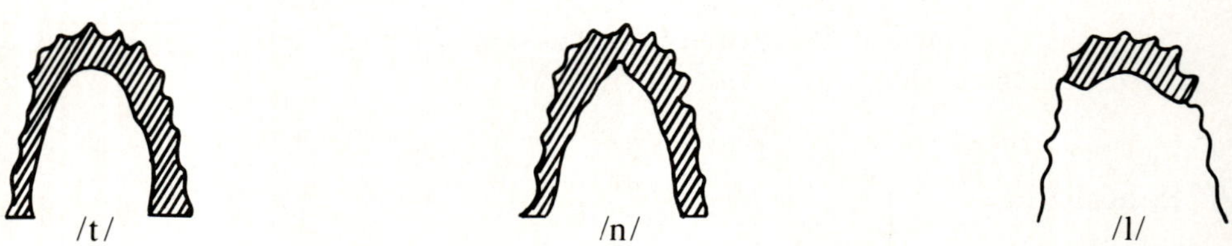

Figure 4–5
Palatograms of an adult, showing tongue contact for /t/, /n/, and /l/. Palatal contact for /d/ is nearly identical to the positions for /t/ and /n/.

for a syllable, it is called a **syllabic consonant** and is transcribed with a diacritic, as in [nudl̩] 'noodle.' This variant is considered another allophone of /l/, as shown in Table 4–4.

ABNORMAL VOWEL AND LIQUID VARIATIONS

Before dealing specifically with the various vowel and liquid misarticulations listed in Tables 4–1, 4–5, and 4–6, the types of errors covered in this book should be described. Allophonic variations in the production of vowels and liquids have already been dealt with. Since these are normal modifications due to changes in phonetic context, they should not be confused with misarticulations. For example, dentalized /l/ occurs consistently in the General American dialect adjacent to the *th* sounds. But some

Table 4–5
Examples of misarticulations of /r/, /ɚ/, /ɝ/, /l/, and [l̩], with symbols and diacritics for indicating them.

		Misarticulation			
	Context	Gliding	Derhoticizing[a]	Delateralizing	Vocalization
/r/	run	/w/	[r˔]	–	–
/ɚ/	car	–	–	–	/ə/
/ɝ/	bird	–	–	–	/ʊ/
/l/	leave	/j/ or /w/	–	[l˔]	–
/l/	bell	–	–	–	/o, u/
[l̩]	noodle	–	–	–	/o, u/

[a]Commonly known as distorted /r/.

Table 4–6
Examples of misarticulations and phonological processes that involve all vowels.

Variation	Example
Neutralizing	/ʌ/ for /u/ in 'tooth' and /ɑ/ for /o/ in 'boat'; phonological process
Lengthening	[bæ:t] for 'bad'; accommodation to process of final consonant devoicing [bæ:] for 'bad'; accommodation to process of final consonant deletion
Nasalizing	[læ̃p] for 'lap'; misarticulation [læ̃p] for 'lamp'; accommodation to process of cluster reduction

speakers dentalize /l/ in all contexts, and such sounds are classified as **misarticulations,** since they are clearly not due to context.

Another useful distinction has recently been elaborated between phonological and phonetic errors. For example, the substitution of /w/ for /r/ by children is described as a **phonological disorder** called gliding (Ingram, 1976; Hodson & Paden, 1983). The production of a distorted /r/ by children, however, is described as a **phonetic disorder.** For many years, no distinction was made between them, except calling one a substitution and the other a distortion. With the development of phonological process analysis, a basic distinction has been drawn between the two. Presumably, the gliding error results from a cognitive process: The child is not aware of the phonemic importance of the distinction between /w/ and /r/. Such a child is not assumed to have a phonetic problem achieving the articulatory adjustment required to produce /r/. But a child who distorts /r/ has a phonetic problem, not a cognitive one. Since this distinction has implications for therapy planning, it is worthwhile stressing it in the phonetic analysis of misarticulated speech.

The third important distinction is between primary and secondary vowel variations. For example, the incorrect production of /r/ and /ɝ/ by children may be characterized as a **primary variation,** since it is the direct consequence of a phonological or phonetic problem. Some children who delete or devoice final consonants tend to lengthen the preceding vowel. For example, they may delete or devoice the final consonant in 'bird' and abnormally lengthen the /ɝ/ vowel. This is a **secondary variation,** an accommodation or compensation for either the devoiced or deleted final consonant.

Gliding

Gliding applies to /l/ and /r/ (see Table 4–1). In the case of /r/, gliding involves the substitution of /w/ for /r/ in words like 'round' and 'around.' For /l/, substitution may involve /w/ or /j/. Although the process is not completely predictable, /w/ may more often replace /l/ when it precedes back vowels, as in 'low' and 'below,' and /j/ may more often replace /l/ when it precedes front vowels, as in 'leave,' 'lip,' and 'believe.' In earlier terminology, these errors were described as substitutions, but they are currently characterized as gliding errors.

Distorting, Derhoticizing, and Vocalization of /r/

Distorting, derhoticizing, and vocalization all apply to /r/, which is described by Ladefoged (1975) as rhoticized when produced normally. This term refers to the r-coloring that is characteristic of the auditory quality of /r/, and it covers both the retroflex and the bunched productions used to achieve it. **Derhoticized** /r/ is a sound which has lost its r-quality as a result of deviation from the positions necessary for normal production. The term refers to the misarticulation in which a **distorted** /r/ substitutes for normal /r/. The spelling error mentioned in Chapter 3 has persisted, so that you will see *derhotacized* used for this misarticulation (Shriberg & Kent, 1982).

There is considerable difference of opinion and lack of clarity as to the characteristics of distorted /r/. It has been variously described as being produced with too much lip rounding (Van Riper & Irwin, 1958; Tiffany & Carrell, 1977), without the necessary bunching and retroflexing of the tongue (Van Riper & Irwin, 1958), with the tongue in position as though you were about to say 'shoe' (Shriberg & Kent, 1982), with the tongue too far forward (Van Riper & Irwin, 1958), and with the tongue too far back (Tiffany & Carrell, 1977).

There is little physiological or acoustic evidence for the articulation of distorted /r/. In studies of synthesized child speech (Sharf & Ohde, 1983), an acoustic and perceptual study of a child before and after successful therapy for distorted /r/ (Sharf, Ohde, & Lehman, 1986), and an acoustic and perceptual study of children reliably identified as producing distorted /r/ (Ohde, McCarver, & Sharf, 1989), it was found that F_3 for one variant of this sound is higher than for normal /r/. This difference may be observed in Figure 4–6 by comparing the real child distorted /r/ and normal /r/ patterns. For another variant of [r˔], F_3 is too high and F_2 too low. This difference may be observed by comparing the synthesized child distorted /r/ and normal /r/ patterns in Figure 4–6. Both of these variants will be perceived predominantly as distorted /r/, but alternatively as /r/ or /w/, depending on how closely their F_2 and F_3 values approximate those for /r/ or /w/.

On the basis of the results of these studies and of observations of children, some inferences can be made about an idealized model of distorted /r/. In normal speech, prevocalic /r/ starts from a mid central tongue position /ɚ/ and moves to the position for the following vowel. The relatively small difference in F_2 between normal and

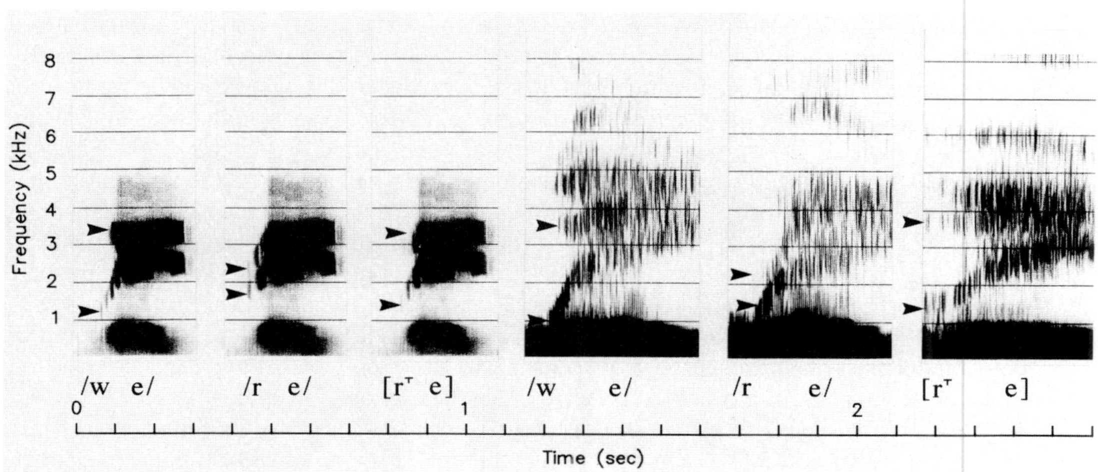

Figure 4–6
Spectrograms of synthesized child (three left panels) and natural child (three right panels) productions of /we/, /re/, and distorted /re/ or [r˔e]. Arrows along the *y* axis indicate the approximate locations of F_2 (lower arrow) and F_3 (upper arrow).

distorted /r/ shown in Figure 4–6 plus our own observations suggests that distorted /r/ also starts from a mid central vowel position. But the initiation of the glide is from the /ɜ/ rather than the /ɚ/ position. The /ɜ/ vowel occurs in New England and Southern dialects in words like 'bird' and 'sir.' Its production requires a slight lowering of the tongue from the position for /ɚ/ without moving the tongue forward or backward and without changing the lip position. If you vocalize with the tongue in the /ɝ/ position and then in the /ɜ/ position, you will hear the loss of r-coloring occur, but each vowel will still sound like a central one. If you glide from the /ɜ/ vowel to any other vowel, for example, /e/ or /o/, you will produce the derhoticized versions of the words 'ray' and 'row.'

You may hear children whose distorted /r/ sounds vary from this idealized model. The most common variation is a slight shifting of the tongue toward the back vowel /ʊ/. Too much backing will result in a /w/ for /r/ substitution. Children who distort prevocalic /r/ or substitute /w/ for it tend to substitute a vowel like /ə/ for /ɚ/ in 'father' and in 'car,' which can be transcribed as /kɑɚ/ or /kɑr/ as normally pronounced. Unfortunately, the objective evidence for these variants is considerably less than that for prevocalic /r/. In the misarticulations in 'car' and 'father,' children substitute a vowel like /ə/. In the case of the /ɝ/ vowel in 'bird,' children substitute a vowel like /ʊ/. The substitution of a vowel for a postvocalic or syllabic liquid is a phonological process called **vocalization.**

Delateralizing and Vocalization of /l/

Like derhoticizing, **delateralizing** applies to prevocalic glides. Recall that in the gliding error, /w/ or /j/ substitutes for /l/, just as /w/ substitutes for /r/. Some children, however, produce prevocalic /l/ without tongue tip contact by starting from a position close to the /ɪ/ or /ʊ/ vowel. The resulting sounds differ from /w/ in not having rounded lips or high back vowel quality and from /j/ in not having high front vowel quality. By analogy with the misarticulation of prevocalic /r/, delateralizing /l/ could be referred to as distorted /l/. Some phoneticians describe an /l/ that appears to be missing (Tiffany & Carrell, 1977) or produced without apico-alveolar contact (Bronstein, 1960; Shriberg & Kent, 1982). Although the description of delateralizing may give the impression that no sound replaces /l/, you can reassure yourself that this is not the case by comparing words like 'ate' and 'late' produced by a child. If the child delateralizes, the /l/ will sound like an unrounded glide from a high back vowel position. If delateralizing is not present, and the child is omitting /l/, then these words should sound identical. If the child says 'wait' for 'late,' then the problem is gliding rather than delateralizing. This is an important distinction for the purpose of deciding whether therapy procedures can be based on the assumption of a cognitive rather than an articulatory problem.

With regard to the postvocalic and vowel /l/, apico-alveolar contact does not occur, and a vowel like /o/ or /u/ is substituted. This type of substitution is described as the phonological process of vocalization or vowelization (see tables 4–1 and 4–6). Children who use this process substitute /u/ or /o/ for [l̩] as in /nudo/ or /nudu/ for 'noodle.'

Dentalizing

As was noted previously, the /l/ of words like 'health' is a dentalized allophone of the /l/ phoneme. Some speakers dentalize /l/ no matter where it occurs, which is abnormal. The difference between alveolar and dental /l/ is not always easy to hear, but it is easy to see if the tongue tip protrudes between the teeth. If, instead, the tongue tip contacts the inner surface of the upper teeth, several repetitions of an utterance may be necessary to perceive the misarticulation. The dentalization of /l/ is easier to identify if it is part of a pattern that includes dentalization of all of the apico-alveolar consonants, /t, d, n, s, z/.

Neutralization

Although correct production of vowels is not usually a problem for native speakers of English, during early speech development children often neutralize vowels, substituting /ɑ/ and /ʌ/ for the target vowels, as in /bɑt/ for 'boat' and 'boot' and /tʌf/ for 'teeth.' This phonological process is called **neutralization.** Because data are lacking on the normal development of vowels, it is not clear when this phenomenon disappears. Some children apparently continue to neutralize beyond the age when most children are producing vowels correctly (Ingram, 1976), but neutralization is not often a problem in children with even the most severe articulation disorders (Hodson & Paden, 1981).

Lengthening

Lengthening of vowels preceding voiced consonants is not usually transcribed in normal speech because it is allophonic. But it should be noted if lengthened vowels occur in the speech of children who delete or devoice final consonants. Final consonant deletion and devoicing of final consonants are phonological processes which neutralize the distinction between voiced and voiceless consonants (Ingram, 1976). Some children may only partially neutralize the distinction by maintaining the difference in vowel duration even when they delete or devoice final consonants, as in [bæː] or [bæːt] for 'bad' (see Table 4–6). Acoustic measures have shown that four of five children who deleted final stops differentiated long and short vowels preceding voiced and voiceless consonants (Weismer, Dinnsen, & Elbert, 1981; Weismer, 1984). But acoustic analysis is not always needed to detect vowel duration differences in such cases. The acoustic data indicate that the vowel duration distinctions maintained by children in the Weismer et al. (1981) and Weismer (1984) studies are of the same order of magnitude as those produced by normal speakers. These distinctions should be perceptible to the careful listener.

Nasalizing and Denasalizing

Allophones and misarticulations involving **nasalizing** and **denasalizing** are shown in Table 4–1. In normal speech production, vowels and glides are not nasalized except in the context of nasal consonants. The difference in velopharyngeal port opening for normal and nasalized /ɛ/ is shown in Figure 4–7. Deviations from the normal pattern should be noted. Some speakers, for example, those with cleft palates, nasalize all vowels no matter what the context. This type of nasalization generally involves a large opening of the velopharyngeal port during most, if not all, of the vowel. The spectrograms in Figure 4–8 show that nasality has a considerable effect on the acoustic correlates of vowels. The following acoustic characteristics of nasalized vowels can be observed in Figure 4–8: (1) Some formants are lower in intensity than those in nonnasal vowels, as can be observed by comparing F_1 of [ĩ] and /i/ and F_2 of [ɑ̃] and /ɑ/; (2) a very low nasal formant is added, as can be observed by comparing the lowest formant in [ɑ̃] and its absence in /ɑ/; and (3) a formant is missing, as can be observed by comparing F_3 of /ɑ/ and its absence in [ɑ̃]. In addition, the overall intensity of nasalized vowels is generally lower than that for nonnasal vowels. Some higher formants are weaker in intensity or missing in the production of both [ĩ] and [ɑ̃], and the overall intensity of the vowel is less than for a nonnasal vowel. The acoustic cues to nasalization of vowels vary greatly depending on the vowel, the speaker, and the degree of opening of the velopharyngeal port. As indicated in Table 4–6, nasalization of vowels and glides in all contexts is considered a misarticulation.

Nasalized vowels occur in the speech of children with the phonological disorder of cluster reduction when they simplify nasal consonant plus stop clusters that occur in

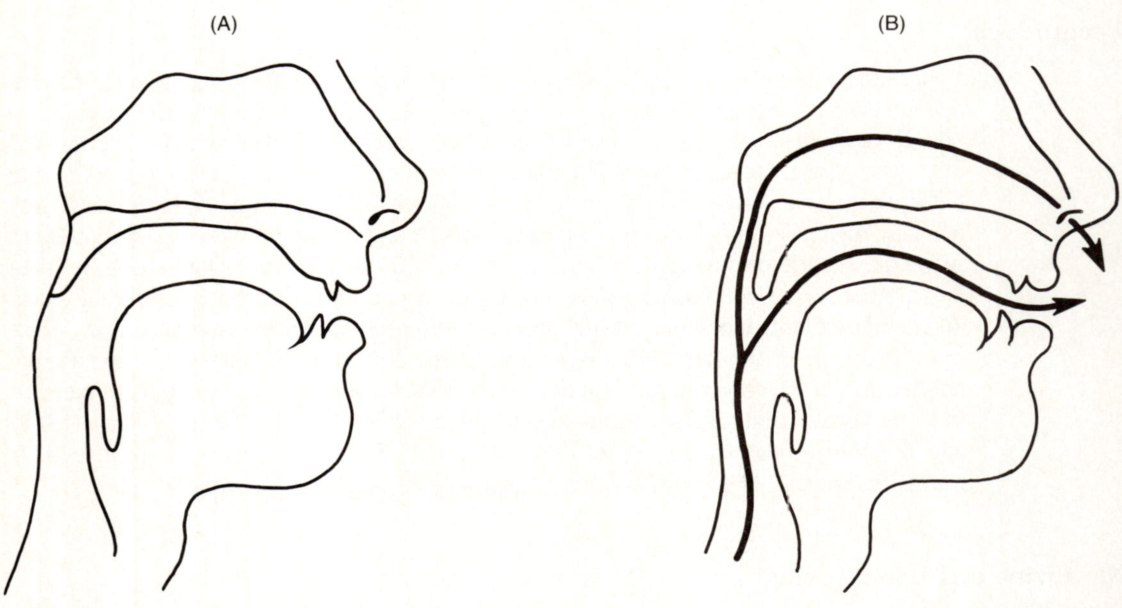

Figure 4–7
Schematized midsagittal sections illustrating velopharyngeal opening and closing during the production of normal /ɛ/ (A) and nasalized /ɛ/ (B). Arrows in (B) indicate airflow from both the oral and nasal cavities.

words like 'lamp' and 'plant' by deleting the nasal consonant. These children may nasalize the preceding vowel, as in [læ̃p] for 'lamp' (Compton & Hutton, 1980). Such nasalization should be noted, because it provides evidence that the child is aware of the need for a nasal consonant following the vowel. Nasalization of vowels due to the

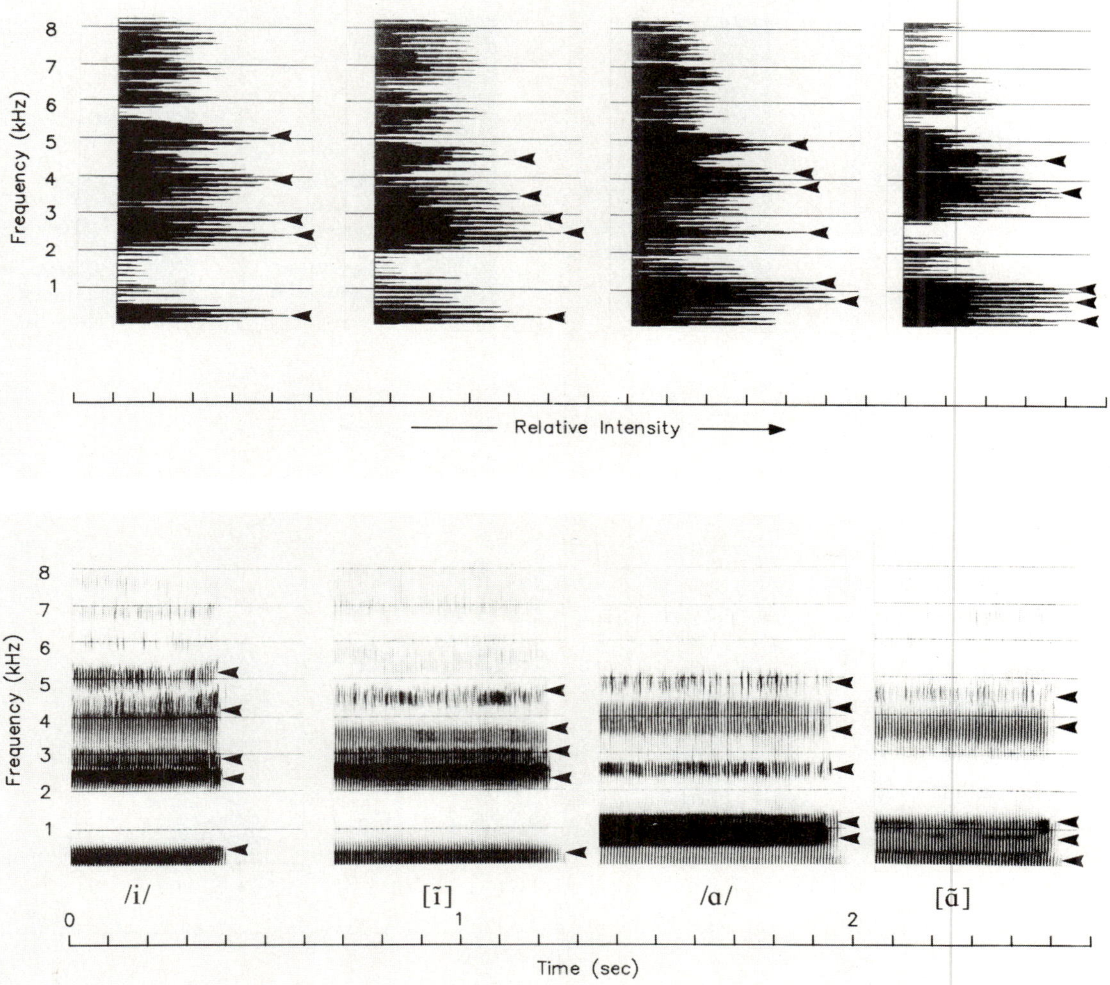

Figure 4–8
Spectrograms of an adult male's productions of normal /i/, nasalized /i/, or [ĩ], normal /ɑ/, and nasalized /ɑ/, or [ɑ̃]. Narrow band power spectrums (amplitude sections) above the wide band patterns show the amplitudes of formants and harmonics and the variations in them between normal and nasalized vowels. Alignment of these power spectrums along the *x* axis shows the approximate location of the analysis. Arrows along the *y* axis of both wide band and narrow band analyses indicate the approximate location of formants. The lowest arrow is F_1 except for [ɑ̃].

influence of nasal consonants is less noticeable than the effects of abnormal nasality. Figure 4–9 shows spectrograms of an adult producing /æ/ in nonnasal and nasal contexts: 'add' versus 'mad' and 'lap' versus 'lamp.' Most evident is the lower intensity level of F_1 for the nasal as compared with the nonnasal vowels, but there also appears to be a low nasal formant below F_1 in [æ̃], but not in /æ/.

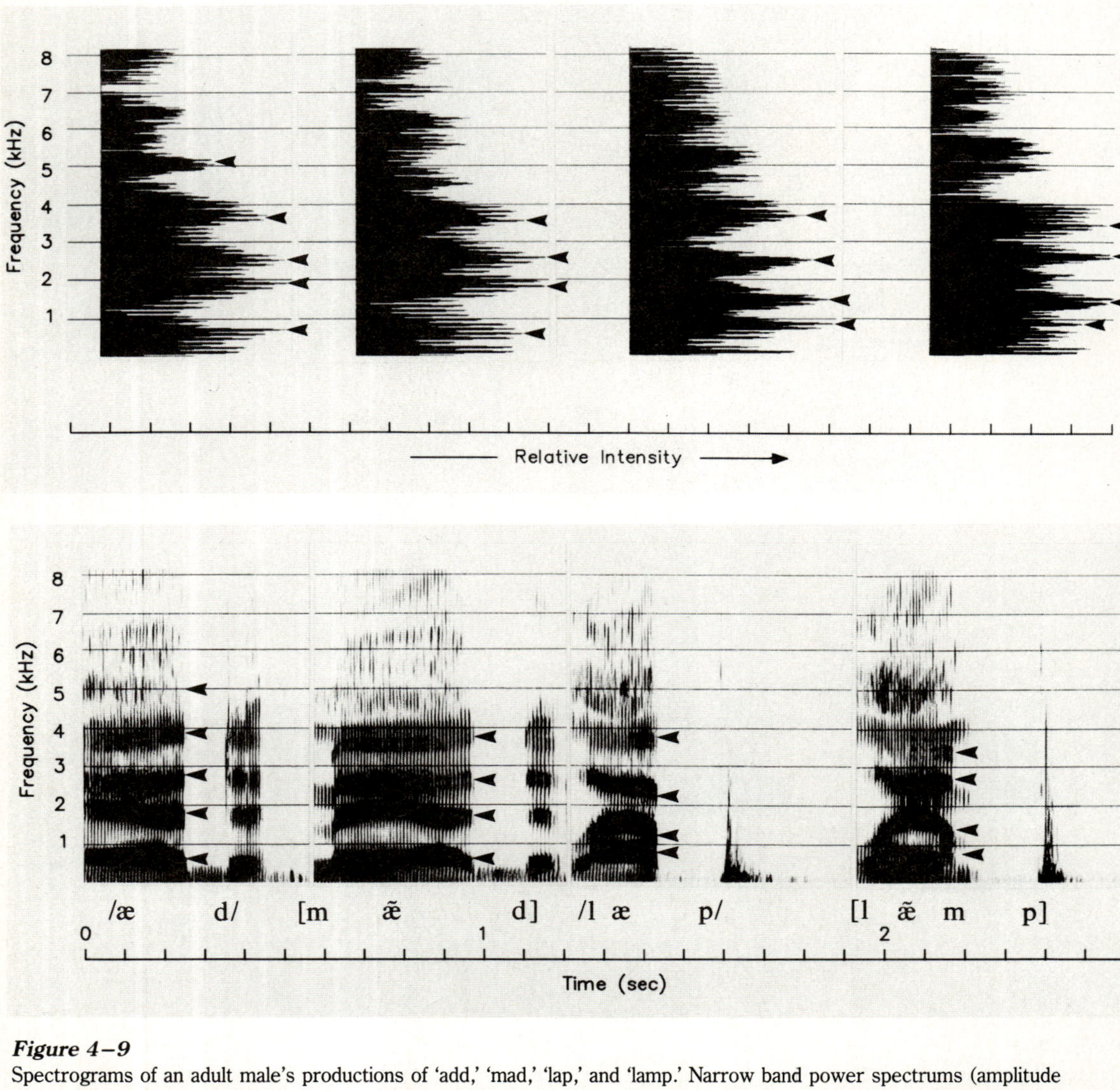

Figure 4–9
Spectrograms of an adult male's productions of 'add,' 'mad,' 'lap,' and 'lamp.' Narrow band power spectrums (amplitude sections) above the wide band spectrograms show the amplitudes of formants and harmonics and their variations between contextually nonnasal and nasal environments. Alignment of these power spectrums along the *x* axis shows the approximate location of the analysis. Arrows along the *y* axis of both wide band and narrow band analyses indicate the approximate location of formants. The lowest arrow is F_1.

Denasalization of vowels (and consonants) may result if there is blockage of the nasal cavity, as when a speaker has a bad cold. The speaker's velopharyngeal port may be open, but the blockage in the nasal cavity alters the normal resonance. The result will be denasalization of the vowel, as in [kæ̃n] for 'can.' Because denasalization of vowels is not allophonic, it should be noted if heard. It is an unusual phenomenon, however, extremely difficult to perceive, and clinically of little importance (Compton & Hutton, 1980). Nasalization and denasalization are also called **hypernasality** and **hyponasality,** respectively.

GLOSSARY

Dark /l/. A variant of /l/ produced with considerable raising of the tongue dorsum; generally occurs in the context of back vowels.

Delateralized. Having some /l/ coloring but not enough for a normal /l/.

Denasalizing. The production of nasal consonants with a blockage in the nasal cavity. Results in a replacement of nasal quality by stop quality, or hyponasality.

Dentalizing. The production of apico-alveolar consonants as apicodentals.

Derhoticized. Having some /r/ coloring but not enough for a normal /r/.

Devoicing. The production of voiced consonants with partial or complete loss of vocal fold vibration.

Distorted /r/. A sound used for normal /r/ that shares some features of /r/ and /w/.

Gliding. A phonological process which results in the substitution of the glides /w/ and /j/ for the liquids /r/ and /l/.

Hypernasality. Excessive nasal quality in the production of nonnasal consonants or vowels, or the nasalizing of such sounds.

Hyponasality. Loss of nasal quality in the production of nasal consonants, or the denasalizing of such sounds.

Light /l/. A variant of /l/ produced with little or no raising of the tongue dorsum; generally occurs in the context of front vowels.

Misarticulation. An error in speech production. May result in the replacement, deletion, distortion, or addition of sounds or the deletion of syllables.

Nasalization. The production of nonnasal consonants or vowels with excessive nasal quality, or hypernasality; also called nasalizing.

Neutralization. A phonological process involving the substitution of /ɑ/ or /ʌ/ for vowels so that the contrast between them is decreased.

Palatalizing. The production of an alveolar sound with approximation of the tongue dorsum to the hard palate.

Phonetic disorder. A misarticulation or pattern of misarticulations due to an articulatory problem.

Phonological disorder. A pattern of misarticulations due to phonological processes.

Primary variation. A misarticulation that is the direct consequence of a phonological or phonetic problem.

Secondary variation. A compensation for a primary variation, for example, lengthening of a vowel when a final voiced consonant is devoiced.

Syllabic consonant. A consonant that functions as the nucleus, or peak of sonority, of a syllable.

Syllabicizing. The production of a consonant as the nucleus, or peak of sonority, of a syllable.

Velarizing. The production of an alveolar sound with approximation of the tongue dorsum to the velum, or soft palate.

Vocalization. A phonological process which results in the substitution of a vowel for a postvocalic or syllabic liquid; also called vowelization.

REVIEW QUESTIONS

A. Indicate which diacritic represents each sound feature by inserting the correct letter.

(a) [l̪] (b) [æ̃] (c) [æ̹] (d) [æ˗] (e) [æ˔] (f) [æ˖] (g) [æ˕] (h) [æ̥]

1. Rounded ________ 5. Dentalized ________

2. Tongue raised ________ 6. Tongue retracted ________

3. Tongue lowered ________ 7. Tongue advanced ________

4. Nasalized ________ 8. Devoiced ________

****

Key: 1. c; 2. e; 3. g; 4. b; 5. a; 6. d; 7. f; 8. h

B. Indicate the context in which gliding and vocalization occur by inserting the correct letter.

(a) Gliding (b) Vocalization

1. red ________ 5. mother ________

2. below ________ 6. around ________

3. medal ________ 7. fill ________

4. car ________ 8. lamp ________

****

Key: 1. a; 2. a; 3. b; 4. b; 5. b; 6. a; 7. b; 8. a

C. Indicate whether the pronunciations would be considered allophonic or a misarticulation by inserting the correct letter.

(a) Allophonic (b) Misarticulation

1. [l̪] in 'wealth' ________
2. [æ̃] in 'lap' ________
3. [w̥] in 'twirl' ________
4. [iː] in 'key' ________
5. [iː] in 'we' ________
6. [ʊː] in 'bird' ________
7. [l̩] in 'model' ________

****

Key: 1. a; 2. b; 3. a; 4. a; 5. a; 6. b; 7. a

LABORATORY ASSIGNMENT

Tape I, Side B
Sections 3–4: Consonantal /r/
IB3: Prevocalic /r/ (Tape running time: 13:43; Elapsed time: 11:43–25:26)

a. Synthetic Speech Models

Listen to synthetic versions of /w/, /r/, and [r̞] produced in a consonant-vowel (CV) context by an adult and a child. If necessary, stop the tape at any time, rewind, and listen again.

1. Adult: /re/; /we/; [r̞e]
2. Child repeats above.
3. Adult: /rɑ/; /wɑ/; [r̞ɑ]
4. Child repeats above.

b. Discrimination of Synthetic /w/, /r/, and [r̞] Sounds

Listen to the following pairs of CV synthetic syllables of a child and indicate if they are the same (S) or different (D).

1. ______ 2. ______ 3. ______ 4. ______ 5. ______
6. ______ 7. ______ 8. ______ 9. ______ 10. ______
11. ______ 12. ______ 13. ______ 14. ______ 15. ______

16. ________ 17. ________ 18. ________ 19. ________ 20. ________

21. ________ 22. ________ 23. ________ 24. ________ 25. ________

26. ________ 27. ________ 28. ________ 29. ________ 30. ________

31. ________ 32. ________ 33. ________ 34. ________ 35. ________

36. ________ 37. ________ 38. ________ 39. ________ 40. ________

41. ________ 42. ________ 43. ________ 44. ________ 45. ________

46. ________ 47. ________ 48. ________ 49. ________ 50. ________

51. ________ 52. ________ 53. ________ 54. ________

****

Key: 1. D; 2. S; 3. D; 4. S; 5. D; 6. S; 7. S; 8. S; 9. S; 10. D; 11. D; 12. D; 13. S; 14. S; 15. S; 16. D; 17. D; 18. D; 19. D; 20. D; 21. S; 22. D; 23. S; 24. D; 25. S; 26. D; 27. D; 28. D; 29. S; 30. S; 31. D; 32. S; 33. D; 34. D; 35. D; 36. S; 37. S; 38. D; 39. D; 40. D; 41. D; 42. D; 43. S; 44. S; 45. S; 46. D; 47. D; 48. S; 49. D; 50. S; 51. D; 52. S; 53. S; 54. D.

c. Transcription of Synthetic /w/, /r/, and [r˔] Sounds

Transcribe the initial consonants produced in a CV context.

1. ________ 2. ________ 3. ________ 4. ________ 5. ________

6. ________ 7. ________ 8. ________ 9. ________ 10. ________

11. ________ 12. ________

****

Consensus: 1. /r/ 2. /w/ 3. [r˔] 4. /w/ 5. [r˔] 6. /r/ 7. /r/ 8. [r˔] 9. /w/ 10. [r˔] 11. /w/ 12. /r/

Variants: 1. [r˔] 3. /w/ 10. /r/ 11. [r˔]

d. Natural Speech Models

Listen to /w/, /r/, and [r˔] as they are produced by an adult and a child.

1. Adult: /we d/; /re d/; [r˔e d]
2. Child repeats above.
3. Adult: /wɑ t/; /rɑ t/; [r˔ɑ t]
4. Child repeats above.

e. Discrimination of Natural /w/, /r/, and [r˕] Sounds

Listen to the following pairs of natural syllables produced by a child and indicate if they are the same (S) or different (D).

1. ________ 2. ________ 3. ________ 4. ________ 5. ________
6. ________ 7. ________ 8. ________ 9. ________ 10. ________
11. ________ 12. ________ 13. ________ 14. ________ 15. ________
16. ________ 17. ________ 18. ________ 19. ________ 20. ________
21. ________ 22. ________ 23. ________ 24. ________ 25. ________
26. ________ 27. ________ 28. ________ 29. ________ 30. ________
31. ________ 32. ________ 33. ________ 34. ________ 35. ________
36. ________ 37. ________ 38. ________ 39. ________ 40. ________
41. ________ 42. ________ 43. ________ 44. ________ 45. ________
46. ________ 47. ________ 48. ________ 49. ________ 50. ________
51. ________ 52. ________ 53. ________ 54. ________

****

Key: 1. D; 2. S; 3. D; 4. S; 5. D; 6. S; 7. S; 8. S; 9. S; 10. D; 11. D; 12. D; 13. S; 14. S; 15. S; 16. D; 17. D; 18. D; 19. D; 20. D; 21. S; 22. D; 23. S; 24. D; 25. S; 26. D; 27. D; 28. D; 29. S; 30. S; 31. D; 32. S; 33. D; 34. D; 35. D; 36. S; 37. S; 38. D; 39. D; 40. D; 41. D; 42. D; 43. S; 44. S; 45. S; 46. D; 47. D; 48. S; 49. D; 50. S; 51. D; 52. S; 53. S; 54. D.

f. Transcription of Natural /w/, /r/, and [r˕] in Minimal Contrast Context

Transcribe the initial consonant as it is pronounced by an adult and a child in a minimal contrast context, /Ce d/ or /Ca t/, in which C represents contrast among /w/, /r/, and [r˕].

1. ________ 2. ________ 3. ________ 4. ________ 5. ________
6. ________ 7. ________ 8. ________ 9. ________ 10. ________
11. ________ 12. ________

****

Consensus: 1. [r˕] 2. /w/ 3. /r/ 4. /r/ 5. /w/ 6. [r˕] 7. /w/ 8. /r/ 9. [r˕] 10. /r/ 11. [r˕] 12. /w/

Variants: None.

g. Transcription of Natural /w/, /r/, and [r^ᵀ] in Minimal Contrast Context in a Sentence

Transcribe the initial consonant as it is pronounced by an adult and a child in syllables in the sentence 'Say ________ again.'

1. ________ 2. ________ 3. ________ 4. ________ 5. ________

6. ________

****

Consensus: 1. [rᵀ] 2. /w/ 3. /r/ 4. /w/ 5. [rᵀ] 6. /r/

Variants: None.

h. Transcription of Natural /w/, /r/, and [rᵀ] in Words in Isolation

Transcribe the initial consonants in the words pronounced by an adult and a child.

1. rude ________ 2. rock ________ 3. reed ________ 4. white ________

5. wake ________ 6. red ________

****

Consensus: 1. /r/ 2. [rᵀ] 3. [rᵀ] 4. /w/ 5. /w/ 6. /r/

Variants: None.

i. Transcription of Natural /w/, /r/, and [rᵀ] in Words in Sentences

Transcribe the initial consonants as they are pronounced by an adult and a child in words in the following sentences: 'I can say ________'; 'Say the name ________'; '________ is the name.'

1. rake ________ 2. witch ________ 3. rope ________ 4. rat ________

5. web ________ 6. ride ________

****

Consensus: 1. [rᵀ] 2. /w/ 3. /r/ 4. /r/ 5. /w/ 6. [rᵀ]

Variants: None.

IB4: Intervocalic /r/ (Tape running time: 3:59; Elapsed time: 25:26–29:25)

a. Intervocalic /r/ Models

Listen to /w/, /r/, and [rᵀ] produced in the intervocalic position by an adult and a child. If necessary, stop the tape at any time, rewind, and listen again. If you have difficulty hearing the differences among these sounds in any part of this section, complete the discrimination exercises on Tape II, Section IIA1.

1. Adult: /d ɛ r i/; /d ɛ w i/; [d ɛ rᵀi]
2. Child repeats above.
3. Adult: /pə re d/; /pə we d/; [pə rᵀe d]
4. Child repeats above.

b. Transcription of Intervocalic /w/, /r/, and [rᵀ] in Minimal Contrast Context

Transcribe the intervocalic consonants as they are pronounced by an adult and a child.

1. ________ 2. ________ 3. ________ 4. ________ 5. ________

6. ________ 7. ________ 8. ________ 9. ________ 10. ________

11. ________ 12. ________

****

Consensus: 1. /r/ 2. /w/ 3. [rᵀ] 4. /w/ 5 [rᵀ] 6. /r/ 7. [rᵀ] 8. /w/ 9. /r/ 10. /w/ 11. /r/ 12. [rᵀ]

Variants: None.

c. Transcription of Intervocalic /w/, /r/, and [rᵀ] in Minimal Contrast Context in a Sentence

Transcribe the intervocalic consonants as they are pronounced by an adult and a child in syllables in the sentence 'Say ________ again.'

1. ________ 2. ________ 3. ________ 4. ________ 5. ________

6. ________

****

Consensus: 1. /r/ 2. [rᵀ] 3. /w/ 4. [rᵀ] 5. /r/ 6. /w/

Variants: None.

d. Transcription of Intervocalic /w/, /r/, and [rᵀ] in Words

Transcribe the intervocalic consonants as they are pronounced in words by an adult and a child.

1. erase ________ 2. berry ________ 3. garage ________ 4. parrot ________

5. Harry ________ 6. very ________

****

Consensus: 1. /r/ 2. /w/ 3. /w/ 4. [r˕] 5. [r˕] 6. /r/

Variants: None.

e. Transcription of Intervocalic /w/, /r/, and [r˕] in Words in Sentences

Transcribe the intervocalic consonants as they are pronounced by an adult and a child in the following sentences: 'I can say ________'; 'Say the name ________'; '________ is the name.'

1. carrot ________ 2. sorrow ________ 3. merry ________ 4. around ________

5. borrow ________ 6. merry ________

****

Consensus: 1. [r˕] 2. /w/ 3. /w/ 4. [r˕] 5. /r/ 6. /r/

Variants: None.

Tape II, Side A
Sections 1–5: Consonantal and Vocalic /r/ and /l/
IIA1: Intervocalic /r/ Discrimination (Tape running time: 4:25; Elapsed time: 00:00–4:25)

The purpose of this section is to train students to discriminate the difference between normal and abnormal /r/ variants in intervocalic position.

a. Discrimination Training

Listen to the following pairs of syllables produced by a child and indicate if they are the same (S) or different (D).

1. ________ 2. ________ 3. ________ 4. ________ 5. ________

6. ________ 7. ________ 8. ________ 9. ________ 10. ________

11. ________ 12. ________ 13. ________ 14. ________ 15. ________

16. ________ 17. ________ 18. ________ 19. ________ 20. ________

21. ________ 22. ________ 23. ________ 24. ________ 25. ________

26. ________ 27. ________ 28. ________ 29. ________ 30. ________

31. ________ 32. ________ 33. ________ 34. ________ 35. ________

36. ________ 37. ________ 38. ________ 39. ________ 40. ________

41. ________ 42. ________ 43. ________ 44. ________ 45. ________

46. ________ 47. ________ 48. ________ 49. ________ 50. ________

51. ________ 52. ________ 53. ________ 54. ________

****

Key: 1. D; 2. S; 3. D; 4. S; 5. D; 6. S; 7. S; 8. S; 9. S; 10. D; 11. D; 12. D; 13. S; 14. S; 15. S; 16. D; 17. D; 18. D; 19. D; 20. S; 21. S; 22. D; 23. S; 24. D; 25. S; 26. D; 27. D; 28. D; 29. S; 30. S; 31. D; 32. S; 33. D; 34. D; 35. D; 36. S; 37. S; 38. D; 39. D; 40. D; 41. D; 42. D; 43. S; 44. S; 45. S; 46. D; 47. D; 48. S; 49. D; 50. S; 51. D; 52. S; 53. S; 54. D.

IIA2: Vocalic /r/ (Tape running time: 3:58; Elapsed time: 04:25– 08:23)

a. Vocalic /r/ Variant Models

Listen to models of vocalic /r/ variants produced in /b Vd / and /f ɑ ð V/ contexts by an adult and a child. If necessary, stop the tape at any time, rewind, and listen again.

1. Adult: /b ɝ d /; /b ʊ d /
2. Child repeats above.
3. Adult: /f ɑ ð ɚ/; /f ɑ ð ə /
4. Child repeats above.

b. Transcription of Vocalic /r/ Variants in Minimal Contrast Context

Transcribe the vocalic /r/ variants as they are pronounced in /b Vd / and /f ɑ ð V/ contexts by an adult and a child.

1. ________ 2. ________ 3. ________ 4. ________ 5. ________

6. ________ 7. ________ 8. ________

****

Consensus: 1. /ɝ/ 2. /ʊ/ 3. /ə/ 4. /ɚ/ 5. /o/ 6. /ɚ/ 7. /ɝ/ 8. /ʊ/

Variants: 5. /ə/

c. Transcription of Vocalic /r/ Variants in Sentence Context

Transcribe the vocalic /r/ variants as they are pronounced by an adult and a child in /b Vd / and /f ɑ ð V/ contexts in the sentence 'Say ________ again.'

1. ________ 2. ________ 3. ________ 4. ________ 5. ________

6. ________ 7. ________ 8. ________

****

Consensus: 1. /ə/ 2. /ɚ/ 3. /ɝ/ 4. /ʊ/ 5. /ɝ/ 6. /ʊ/ 7. /ə/ 8. /ɚ/

Variants: None.

d. Transcription of Vocalic /r/ Variants in Words in Isolation

Transcribe the vocalic /r/ variants as they are pronounced in words by an adult and a child.

1. burn ________ 2. Bert ________ 3. dirt ________ 4. fern ________

5. honor ________ 6. mother ________ 7. holler ________ 8. sister ________

****

Consensus: 1. /ɝ/ 2. /ʊ/ 3. /ʊ/ 4. /ɝ/ 5. /ə/ 6. /o/ 7. /ɚ/ 8. /ɚ/

Variants: 6. /ə/

e. Transcription of Vocalic /r/ Variants in Words in Sentences

Transcribe the vocalic /r/ variants as they are pronounced by an adult and a child in words in the following sentences: 'I can say ________'; 'Say the name ________'; '________ is the name.'

1. curve ________ 2. burst ________ 3. curb ________ 4. verb ________

5. sugar ________ 6. victor ________ 7. doctor ________ 8. actor ________

****

Consensus: 1. /ɝ/ 2. /ʊ/ 3. /ʊ/ 4. /ɝ/ 5. /ə/ 6. /ɚ/ 7. /ɚ/ 8. /ə/

Variants: 3. /ʌ/ 5. /ʊ/

IIA3: Prevocalic /l/ (Tape running time: 10:02; Elapsed time: 08:23–18:25)

a. Models of Prevocalic /l/ Variants

Listen to /w/, /l/, /j /, and [l˔] produced in CVC syllables by an adult and, all except [l˔], by a child. If necessary, stop the tape at any time, rewind, and listen again.

1. Adult: /wɛ t/; /lɛ t/; /j ɛ t/; [l˔ɛ t]
2. Child: /wɛ t/; /lɛ t/; /j ɛ t/
3. Adult: /wɑ t/; /lɑ t/; /j ɑ t/; [l˔ɑ t]
4. Child: /wɑ t/; /lɑ t/; /j ɑ t/

b. Discrimination of Prevocalic /l/ Variants

Listen to the following pairs of syllables produced by an adult and a child and indicate if they are the same (S) or different (D).

1. ________ 2. ________ 3. ________ 4. ________ 5. ________
6. ________ 7. ________ 8. ________ 9. ________ 10. ________
11. ________ 12. ________ 13. ________ 14. ________ 15. ________
16. ________ 17. ________ 18. ________ 19. ________ 20. ________
21. ________ 22. ________ 23. ________ 24. ________ 25. ________
26. ________ 27. ________ 28. ________ 29. ________ 30. ________
31. ________ 32. ________ 33. ________ 34. ________ 35. ________
36. ________ 37. ________ 38. ________ 39. ________ 40. ________
41. ________ 42. ________ 43. ________ 44. ________ 45. ________
46. ________ 47. ________ 48. ________ 49. ________ 50. ________
51. ________ 52. ________ 53. ________ 54. ________ 55. ________
56. ________ 57. ________ 58. ________ 59. ________ 60. ________
61. ________ 62. ________ 63. ________ 64. ________ 65. ________
66. ________

****

Key: 1. D; 2. S; 3. D; 4. S; 5. S; 6. S; 7. S; 8. S; 9. D; 10. D; 11. D; 12. D; 13. S; 14. S; 15. D; 16. D; 17. D; 18. D; 19. D; 20. D; 21. D; 22. S; 23. S; 24. D; 25. S; 26. S; 27. S; 28. D; 29. D; 30. D; 31. D; 32. D; 33. S; 34. D; 35. D; 36. S; 37. S; 38. D; 39. D; 40. D; 41. S; 42. S; 43. D; 44. S; 45. S; 46. D; 47. S; 48. D; 49. S; 50. D; 51. D; 52. S; 53. S; 54. D; 55. D; 56. S; 57. S; 58. D; 59. S; 60. S; 61. D; 62. D; 63. S; 64. D; 65. S; 66. D.

c. Transcription of Prevocalic /l/ in a Minimal Contrast Context

Transcribe the initial consonant as it is produced by an adult and a child in a CVC context.

1. ________ 2. ________ 3. ________ 4. ________ 5. ________
6. ________ 7. ________ 8. ________ 9. ________ 10. ________
11. ________ 12. ________ 13. ________ 14. ________

****

Consensus: 1. [l˔] 2. /w/ 3. /l/ 4. /j/ 5. /l/ 6. /w/ 7. [l˔] 8. /j/ 9. /w/ 10. /l/ 11. /j/ 12. /l/ 13. /w/ 14. /j/

Variants: None.

d. Transcription of Prevocalic /l/ in Sentences

Transcribe the initial consonant in the CVC utterances as they are pronounced by an adult and a child in the sentence 'Say ________ again.'

1. ________ 2. ________ 3. ________ 4. ________ 5. ________

6. ________ 7. ________

****

Consensus: 1. [lʳ] 2. /w/ 3. /l/ 4. /j/ 5. /w/ 6. /l/ 7. /j/

Variants: None.

e. Transcription of Prevocalic /l/ Variants in Words in Isolation

Transcribe the initial consonant in the words pronounced by an adult and a child.

1. loose ________ 2. lead ________ 3. week ________ 4. lane ________

5. leaf ________ 6. least ________ 7. yawn ________

****

Consensus: 1. /l/ 2. [lʳ] 3. /w/ 4. /w/ 5. /l/ 6. /j/ 7. /j/

Variants: None.

f. Transcription of Prevocalic /l/ Variants in Words in Sentences

Transcribe the initial consonants in the words pronounced by an adult and a child in the following sentences: 'I can say ________'; 'Say the name ________'; '________ is the name.'

1. lip ________ 2. leg ________ 3. limb ________ 4. wag ________

5. late ________ 6. yes ________ 7. lamb ________

****

Consensus: 1. /w/ 2. /l/ 3. /l/ 4. /w/ 5. [lʳ] 6. /j/ 7. /j/

Variants: None.

IIA4: Intervocalic /l/ (Tape running time: 4:39; Elapsed time: 18:25–23:04)

a. Intervocalic /l/ Variant Models

Listen to /w/, /l/, /j/, and [lʳ] as they are produced in intervocalic position by an adult and, all except [lʳ], by a child. If necessary, stop the tape at any time, rewind, and listen again.

1. Adult: /bɪli/; /bɪwi/; /bɪji/; [bɪlʳi]
2. Child: /bɪli/; /bɪwi/; /bɪji/
3. Adult: /jɛlo/; /jɛwo/; /jɛjo/; [jɛlʳo]
4. Child: /jɛlo/; /jɛwo/; /jɛjo/

b. Transcription of Intervocalic /l/ in Minimal Contrast Context

Transcribe the intervocalic consonants as they are pronounced by an adult and a child.

1. ________ 2. ________ 3. ________ 4. ________ 5. ________

6. ________ 7. ________ 8. ________ 9. ________ 10. ________

11. ________ 12. ________ 13. ________ 14. ________

****

Consensus: 1. /l/ 2. /w/ 3. /j/ 4. [lʳ] 5. /w/ 6. [lʳ] 7. /j/ 8. /l/ 9. /w/ 10. /j/ 11. /l/ 12. /w/ 13. /l/ 14. /j/

Variants: None.

c. Transcription of Intervocalic /l/ in a Sentence

Transcribe the intervocalic consonants as they are pronounced by an adult and a child in syllables in the sentence 'Say ________ again.'

1. ________ 2. ________ 3. ________ 4. ________ 5. ________

6. ________ 7. ________

****

Consensus: 1. /j/ 2. /l/ 3. /w/ 4. [lʳ] 5. /w/ 6. /j/ 7. /l/

Variants: None.

d. Transcription of Intervocalic /l/ Variants in Words in Isolation

Transcribe the intervocalic consonants as they are pronounced in words by an adult and a child.

1. willow ________ 2. alive ________ 3. hilly ________ 4. follow ________

5. calling ________ 6. believe ________ 7. Millie ________

****

Consensus: 1. /l/ 2. /w/ 3. /w/ 4. /j/ 5. /l/ 6. [lʳ] 7. /j/

Variants: None.

e. Transcription of Intervocalic /l/ Variants in Words in Sentences

Transcribe the intervocalic consonants pronounced by an adult and a child in the following sentences: 'I can say ________'; 'Say the name ________'; '________ is the name.'

1. fellow ________ 2. hello ________ 3. pilot ________ 4. belly ________

5. tally ________ 6. sally ________ 7. mellow ______

****

Consensus: 1. /j/ 2. /j/ 3. /w/ 4. /w/ 5. /l/ 6. /l/ 7. [l˔]

Variants: None.

IIA5: Syllabic and Dark /l/ (Tape running time: 4:02; Elapsed time: 23:04–27:06)

a. Syllabic and Dark /l/ Variant Models

Listen to models of syllabic and dark /l/ variants produced in /f i C or V/ and /k æ t V/ contexts by adult and child speakers. If necessary, stop the tape at any time, rewind, and listen again.

1. Adult: /f i l/; /f i o/
2. Child repeats above.
3. Adult: [k æ t l̩]; /k æ t o/
4. Child repeats above.

b. Transcription of Syllabic and Dark /l/ in Minimal Contrast Context

Transcribe the syllabic and dark /l/ variants pronounced in /f i l/ and [k æ t l̩] contexts by an adult and a child.

1. ________ 2. ________ 3. ________ 4. ________ 5. ________

6. ________ 7. ________ 8. ________

****

Consensus: 1. /l/ 2. /o/ 3. /o/ 4. [l̩] 5. [l̩] 6. /o/ 7. /l/ 8. /o/

Variants: None.

c. Transcription of Syllabic and Dark /l/ Variants in a Sentence

Transcribe the syllabic and dark /l/ variants pronounced by an adult and a child in /f i l/ and [k æ t l̩] contexts in the sentence 'Say ________ again.'

1. ________ 2. ________ 3. ________ 4. ________ 5. ________

6. ________ 7. ________ 8. ________

****

Consensus: 1. [l̩] 2. /o / 3. /o / 4. /l/ 5. /o / 6. /l/ 7. /o / 8. [l̩]

Variants: None.

d. Transcription of Syllabic and Dark /l/ Variants in Words

Transcribe the syllabic and dark /l/ variants pronounced in words by an adult and a child.

1. eel ________ 2. wheel ________ 3. kneel ________ 4. sail ________

5. idle ________ 6. kettle ________ 7. settle ________ 8. noodle ________

****

Consensus: 1. /l/ 2. /o / 3. /o / 4. /l/ 5. /o / 6. [l̩] 7. [l̩] 8. /o /

Variants: 8. [l̩]

e. Transcription of /l/ Variants in Words in Sentences

Transcribe the syllabic and dark /l/ variants pronounced by an adult and a child in words in the following sentences: 'I can say ________'; 'Say the name ________'; '________ is the name.'

1. tail ________ 2. steal ________ 3. nail ________ 4. pool ________

5. metal ________ 6. turtle ________ 7. saddle ________ 8. pedal ________

****

Consensus: 1. /o / 2. /l/ 3. /l/ 4. /o / 5. /o / 6. [l̩] 7. [l̩] 8. /o /

Variants: None.

CHAPTER 5

Articulatory Potential for Consonants

MECHANISMS OF PRODUCTION

Consonants are sounds produced by restricting or blocking airflow out of the oral cavity, or, as in some African languages, blocking the airflow into the oral cavity. In this regard consonants differ from vowels and glides, which require minimal interference with airflow. There are borderline sounds like /l/, which are classified as a glide consonant in 'low' but as a vowel in 'noodle.' The oral cavity is blocked at the alveolar ridge by the tongue tip for /l/, as it is for a number of consonants we will describe, but the margins of the tongue are lowered so that air continues to flow over its sides and out of the oral cavity. Consonants are distinctive; they involve a complete stoppage of airflow for stop consonants, a constriction that produces frication noise for fricative consonants, and a complete stoppage of the oral cavity with air shunted into the nasal cavity for nasal consonants.

Consonants are described in terms of at least five features: (1) **place of articulation,** or where the blockage or restriction of airflow occurs; (2) **manner of articulation,** or the nature of the interference with the airflow; (3) voicing, or what is happening at the vocal folds or glottal source; (4) type of resonance, or whether airflow is through the oral or the nasal cavity; and (5) airflow direction, or whether airflow is out of or into the oral cavity. Each of these features is considered primarily as it relates to normal and misarticulated consonants in English.

Place of Articulation

The articulatory system can be divided into lower jaw and upper jaw articulators. These structures, shown in Figure 5–1, were described briefly in Chapter 1. Here the ter-

Figure 5–1
Midsagittal sections of the vocal tract illustrating upper jaw (A) and lower jaw (B) articulators.

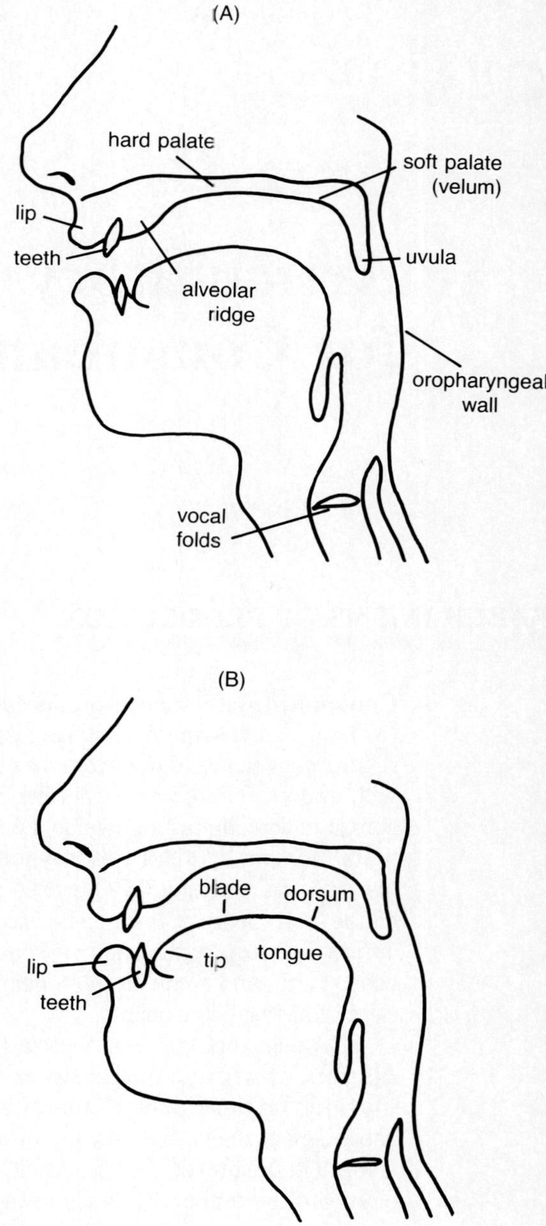

minology for the articulatory configurations of a large variety of consonants that occur in normal, misarticulated, or foreign speech is reviewed.

Table 5–1 lists articulatory structures as lower jaw or upper jaw with regard to their function in consonant production (Catford, 1977). In speech production, lower jaw structures usually move to contact upper jaw structures. The lower jaw structures are (1) the lower lip; (2) the lower front teeth; (3) the tongue tip, or apex, which can make contact with the margins of the tongue raised or lowered and can make anterior or posterior (retroflex) palatal contact; (4) the tongue blade; and (5) the tongue dorsum. The upper jaw structures are: (1) the upper lip; (2) the upper front teeth; (3) the alveolar ridge; (4) the hard palate; (5) the soft palate, or velum; and (6) the uvula. The pharyngeal wall and the vocal folds are articulatory structures outside the oral cavity. The pharyngeal wall functions as a contact location for the tongue for sounds that are not normally produced in English, and the vocal folds make contact with each other.

Table 5–1
Terminology of articulatory structures and positions for consonant production.

Term	Structure
Lower Jaw	
1. Labial (**labio-**)	Lower lip
2. **Dental (dento-)**	Lower front teeth
3. Apical (**apico-**)[a]	Tongue tip or apex
a. Lateral	Margins of tongue lowered
b. Retroflex	Tongue tip bent backward
4. Laminal (**lamino-**)[a]	Tongue blade
5. Dorsal (**dorso-**)[a]	Tongue dorsum
Upper Jaw	
1. **Labial**	Upper lip
2. Interdental	Between upper and lower teeth
3. Dental	Upper front teeth
4. Alveolar	Ridge posterior to upper/lower front teeth
5. Prepalatal	Palate just posterior to alveolar ridge
6. Palatal	Hard palate, posterior part
7. Velar	Soft palate, extending from the hard palate to the uvula
8. Uvular	Most posterior part of the velum
9. Pharyngeal	Wall of oropharynx
10. Glottal	Vocal folds

[a]In some systems, all tongue contacts are described as *lingua-*.

In compound words used to describe the place of articulation, the first element refers to the lower jaw structure and the second to the upper jaw structure. For example, *labiodental* sounds have contact between the upper teeth, which are approximated by the lower lip in saying the initial and final consonants of 'five.' Tongue, teeth, and lip are assisted in their function by the movement of the lower jaw.

It is theoretically possible to produce a consonant at any point in the vocal tract where airflow can be stopped or restricted, but only a small number of those sounds occur in any language. For example, the initial sound of 'face' is labiodental because the lower lip contacts the upper teeth. Labiodental articulation is used commonly in other languages. It is also possible to produce a dentolabial sound by having the lower teeth contact the upper lip. This sound does not normally occur in any language, but it has been used by at least one individual with abnormal jaw structure (Bloomer, 1971). As far as we know, no language has an apicolabial consonant in which the tongue tip contacts the upper lip, but this type of sound was used by an individual with radical loss of lower lip structure. Since he was unable to produce sounds that required involvement of the lower lip, like the bilabials that occur as the initial consonants of 'pet' and 'bet' and the labiodentals that occur as initial consonants in 'fine' and 'vine,' this individual was forced to improvise by using apicolabial sounds instead. A speech and language pathologist should be prepared to suggest alternative articulations for individuals whose articulatory structures do not permit normal ones. The clinician must have a basic knowledge of the sound-producing potential of the articulatory system. In the chapters that deal specifically with stops, fricatives, and nasals, variations in consonant productions are covered in greater detail.

Manner of Articulation

Consonants can be grouped into two categories on the basis of the degree of vocal tract constriction, the obstruent and the sonorant. An **obstruent** is a consonant made with a complete closure or narrow constriction in the oral cavity so that the airstream is stopped or frication noise is produced. A **sonorant** is a consonant made with a relatively open vocal tract so that cavity resonance occurs. Obstruents include stops, fricatives, affricates, and trills. Sonorants include nasals, glides, and liquids. The glides and liquids are sometimes categorized as **approximants.** This term refers to sounds produced by approximating two articulators, but not quite as closely as for fricatives (Ladefoged, 1975; Catford, 1977).

In the production of **fricatives,** a constriction is created in the oral cavity to produce frication noise. This constriction can be produced by using the soft tissue articulators, such as the tongue, lips, and palate, or by using the hard tissue articulators, the teeth. When the teeth are involved, air is directed between them by articulators behind them to produce a sibilant type of frication. For example, in the production of /s/ and /z/, the tongue is raised so that its margins make contact with the palate, but the tongue tip only approaches the upper or lower alveolar ridge. The channel formed between the hard palate and the upper surface of the tongue directs the airstream against the front teeth so that turbulence is produced. Sibilants are generally characterized by greater intensity noise than other fricatives, as you can hear if you compare the initial sibilants of 'so' and 'shin' with the nonsibilants of 'foe' and 'thin.'

There is general agreement that sibilants include the /s, z, ʃ, ʒ/ fricatives (Bronstein, 1960; Singh & Singh, 1976; Tiffany & Carrell, 1977; Shriberg & Kent, 1982), except for Malmberg (1963), who refers to /ʃ, ʒ/ as *shibilants,* a term that is not generally recognized. **Sibilants** are defined as "sounds with higher frequency than any other sounds in our language" by Bronstein (1962), as sounds that "have energy components in the high frequencies and also have longer duration than any other consonant category" by Singh and Singh (1976), as "sounds of more strident quality than other fricatives" by Tiffany and Carrell (1977), and as "sounds characterized by intense, high-pitched noise" by Shriberg and Kent (1982). Phoneticians who describe the mechanism for achieving the high frequency levels for sibilants implicate the teeth. Potter, Kopp, and Green (1947) describe sibilants as being produced by "directing the breath stream against the cutting edges of the teeth," and Tiffany and Carrell (1977) suggest that the strident quality of sibilants is achieved by "directing a more concentrated jet of air against the hard palate and dental surfaces."

As their name implies, **stop** consonants are produced by closing off the oral cavity at some point so that the flow of air is stopped. In postvocalic position, this is the only articulatory gesture needed to represent the stop. In prevocalic and intervocalic positions, however, air pressure builds up behind the closure until it is released by the action of the articulatory muscles. With the release, the air bursts out of the oral cavity. Contextual and deviant stop variants are covered in greater detail in Chapter 6.

Nasal consonants are produced by closing off the oral cavity at some point and opening the velopharyngeal port so that air flows out through the nasal cavity. The open nasal cavity and closed oral cavity result in the nasal resonance quality characteristic of nasal consonants. Because the oral cavity is closed completely, there is some logic to classifying nasal consonants as stops (Ladefoged, 1975). Many phoneticians, however, continue to classify them as sonorants or some other category distinct from stops (Bronstein, 1960; Singh & Singh, 1976; Tiffany & Carrell, 1977; Calvert, 1980; Pickett, 1980; Shriberg & Kent, 1982).

Affricates are produced by releasing a stop into a fricative. Some phoneticians limit affricates to combinations of stops and fricatives that are **homorganic,** that is, made from the same place of articulation (Heffner, 1952; Ladefoged, 1975; Calvert, 1980; MacKay, 1987). Acoustic evidence, however, indicates that nonhomorganic consonants like /ps/ and /ks/ also produce affricate-like spectrographic patterns (Potter et al., 1947). Some phoneticians limit affricates to stop and fricative combinations within the same syllable (Catford, 1977; Calvert, 1980), but others have recognized exceptions to syllabic limitations in such words as 'pizza' and 'outside' (Bronstein, 1960; Tiffany & Carrell, 1977).

Trills are produced by rapid and repetitive contacts and separations of articulators caused by an appropriate adjustment of muscle tension and air pressure buildup. Like stops, trills involve a closure at some point in the oral cavity and an increase in air pressure posterior to it. For stops, the articulators are separated by muscle action, but for trills the air pressure overcomes the resistance of the articulators and blows them apart. Then the articulators are brought together again as a result of their elasticity and the Bernoulli effect. The Bernoulli effect, which is produced by the air passing between the articulators, lowers the air pressure between them, creating a suction effect that draws the articulators together. This cycle repeats itself as long as the speaker maintains the proper muscle tension and air pressure.

Try the trill mechanism by bringing the lips together, blowing air out as you protrude the lips slightly and keeping the lips closed until the air pressure starts them vibrating. Even with rather sluggish articulators like the lips, trills can be produced at vibratory rates of about 30 per second. The vocal folds are the most versatile mechanism for producing vibratory sounds. They are capable of being vibrated slowly (25 or 30 vibrations per second) to produce a glottal or laryngeal trill (Heffner, 1952). This mechanism can be substituted for the normal voice in speech production. When used in this way, the glottal trill is known as **glottal fry,** creaky voice, or laryngealization. When the rate is increased to about 100 vibrations per second, the sound becomes a continuous glottal tone.

Glides are produced by shifting from one vowel to another within the same syllable. The potential for a large number of such sounds was described in Chapter 3. Postvocalic glides are commonly called diphthongs and fall into the vowel category. Prevocalic glides are commonly called glide consonants. There are two prevocalic glides in English that most phoneticians agree are consonants: /w/ and /j/, the former involving a rapid transition between the /u/ vowel and a following vowel within the same syllable, as in 'win,' and the latter involving a rapid transition between the /i/ vowel and a following vowel within the same syllable, as in 'yet.' There is less agreement about the classification of /r/ and /l/ in the glide or liquid category. Since these sounds appear to have unique articulatory configurations, they are discussed under liquids below.

Liquids are vowellike sounds. They are produced with the vocal cavity constricted less than for other consonants but more than for vowels. Like glides, liquids are the starting points for transitions to following vowels within the same syllable. Unlike glides, liquids are produced with unique articulatory tongue configurations, lateral in the case of /l/ and bunched or retroflex in the case of /r/. There is some confusion regarding the status of the postvocalic sound that occurs in words like 'bar,' which some phoneticians transcribe with /r/, implying that it is a liquid or glide, and others with /ɚ/, implying that it is a vowel.

Type of Voicing

Type of voicing refers to what is occurring at the vocal folds during the consonant closure or restriction. Most consonants in English are classified as voiced or voiceless. In voiceless sounds the air flows through the glottis unimpeded, and the only sound is the noise at the point of constriction. In voiced sounds the vocal folds are approximated so that air coming through the trachea from the lungs vibrates them. In the case of voiced consonants, this means that two sounds are being produced at the same time: glottal tone at the vocal folds, and frication noise at the point of constriction.

A number of modifications of the basic adjustments of the vocal folds for voiced and voiceless sounds are possible; three are of particular interest. One possibility is the glottal trill. This type of voice production, described earlier, is called glottalized or creaky voice, and it occurs in English particularly at the ends of utterances. A second possibility is adjusting the vocal folds so that they vibrate to produce a glottal tone, but with a gap between them that lets air escape. This type of voicing, called a breathy or murmured voice, may occur when /h/ occurs intervocalically in words like 'ahead.' The third modification, the whisper, results when the vocal folds are separated so that they are not set into vibration but constrict the airflow, producing frication noise.

Resonance Type

Resonance may be oral, nasal, or denasal. For all consonants except nasals, the normal resonance for English is **oral.** The nasal cavity is closed off, and the oral cavity serves as the resonator. In the production of **nasal** consonants, the channel between the oral and nasal cavities is opened so that both cavities act as resonators. When a consonant is **denasal,** there is some blockage in the nasal cavity that modifies the resonance usually present for nasal consonants, and 'tam,' 'tan,' and 'tang' tend to sound like 'tab,' 'tad,' and 'tag.'

Airflow Direction

The normal airflow pattern for English is **egressive,** or out of the oral cavity. Although egressive stops are normal in English, there are other possible mechanisms which are of interest because they are used by hearing-impaired speakers. In Figure 5–2, mechanisms for stop variants are shown schematically. In each drawing, the vocal tract is closed in front; the point of closure could be bilabial, alveolar, or palatal. In the normal stop production mechanism for English, shown in Figure 5–2(a), compression of the lungs, as indicated by the dashed line, increases pressure in the vocal tract so that it becomes greater than the outside pressure. When the anterior closure is released, air bursts out of the vocal tract. These sounds are **pulmonic pressure** stops because they are produced with egressive airflow from the lungs. Frequently they are called **explosives,** or just **plosives.** This mechanism is the one normally used for English stops.

In Figure 5–2(b), the lungs are expanded following an anterior stop closure, as indicated by the dashed line. Expansion of the vocal tract decreases the air pressure so that it is less than the outside air pressure. When the anterior closure is released, air bursts into the vocal tract. These sounds are pulmonic **suction** stops, and are rarely used in speech (Catford, 1977).

In Figure 5–2(c), a back closure is formed by the vocal folds (solid line). Pressure is increased within the vocal tract by raising the level of the larynx (dashed line), decreasing the size of the vocal tract from the vocal folds to the anterior stop closure. When the front closure is released, air bursts from the vocal tract. Compared to pulmonic stops, the amount of air is small, since it is only what can be trapped between the laryngeal closure and the anterior closure. These sounds are **glottalic** pressure stops. They are frequently called **ejectives.** Normally this mechanism is not used in English, but some hearing-impaired speakers use it to produce stops (see Chapter 6).

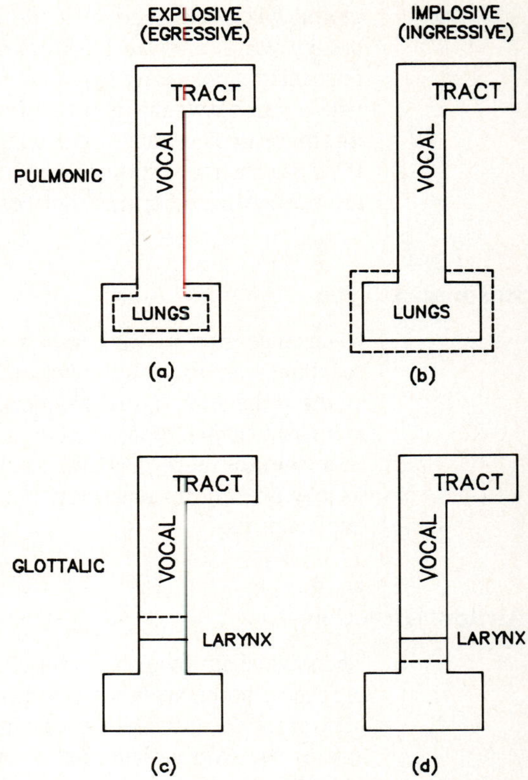

Figure 5–2
Diagram of the mechanism for achieving pressure adjustments for the production of (a) pulmonic pressure stops (explosives) involving compression of the lungs; (b) pulmonic suction stops (implosives) involving expansion of the lungs; (c) glottalic pressure stops (ejectives) involving a raised larynx; and (d) glottalic suction stops involving a lowered larynx. Dashed lines indicate the mechanisms involved.

These sounds can be transcribed by using an apostrophe following the stop symbol to denote the place of articulation.

In Figure 5–2(d), a back closure is produced at the larynx, which is then lowered to the level shown by the dashed line. This increases the size of the vocal tract so that the air pressure within it decreases. When the anterior closure is released, air bursts into the vocal tract. These sounds are glottalic suction stops, which are very rare if they are unvoiced (Catford, 1977). Voiced glottalic suction stops are commonly called voiced **implosives,** or **ingressives,** and are represented by the bilabial, alveolar, and velar voiced stop symbols with superior right-pointing hooks.

It is possible to produce stop sounds using just the air trapped between a dorsovelar closure and bilabial or alveolar anterior closures. This is the mechanism for click sounds used in some African languages (Catford, 1977). Since this mechanism is not used in normal, misarticulated, or dialectal variants of English, it is not covered in detail.

A unique method of producing phonation can be used by an individual whose larynx has been surgically removed, usually as a treatment for cancer. The sound-producing mechanism involves a process of injecting or swallowing air into the upper esophagus, then forcing it out to produce vibration while the individual articulates speech sounds. This practice is referred to as alaryngeal or esophageal speech.

SPECTROGRAPHIC CUES TO PHYSIOLOGIC EVENTS IN CONSONANTS

The cues that differentiate consonants with regard to manner, voicing, and resonance are discussed in this chapter. Details of contextual and misarticulated variations in place of articulation are covered with stops, nasals, and fricatives in later chapters. The following connects sound production to its reflection in acoustic cues, particularly those in sound spectrograms. Such spectrographic cues to the physiologic events of consonant production are listed in Table 5–2.

Fricative Consonants

In the production of fricatives, a constriction is produced at any point in the vocal tract where articulators can be approximated. The approximation must be closer than it is for any vowel, yet not so close that contact is made which stops airflow. The constriction limits the passage of air out of the oral cavity, and frication noise results. Unlike vowels,

Table 5–2
Spectrographic cues to physiologic events in consonant production (see also Figures 5–1, 5–2, 5–3, and 5–4).

Event	Cue
Fricatives	
Frication	Fill (vertical lines) with no pattern
Voicing/oral cavity constricted	Voice bar (lowest formant) with some higher formants
Stops	
Pressure buildup	Blank space, if CV; gap in other positions or preceded by /s/
Closure release	Spike following blank or gap
Frication	Fill following spike
Aspiration	Fill following frication
Voicing/closed oral cavity	Relatively short VOT, with voice bar sometimes preceding spike
Nasals	
Resonance change	Discontinuity between nasal and vowel formants
Constant nasal resonance	Relatively level formants
Voicing/open nasal cavity	Formant patterns
Trills	
Vibration of articulators	Series of spikes

which are characterized by resonance frequency patterns, or formants, fricatives are distinguished primarily by random frequency patterns, or fill. As indicated in figures 5–3 and 5–4, the random frequency distribution in the initial voiceless fricative of 'sip' shows up as random vertical lines on the spectrograms for both adult and child speakers. This fill represents sound energy that is distributed across a range of frequencies with no formant-like concentration at any level. When voicing is added to the frication noise of 'sip' /s ɪ p/, the result is the voiced analog, 'zip' /z ɪ p/. If you alternate voiceless and

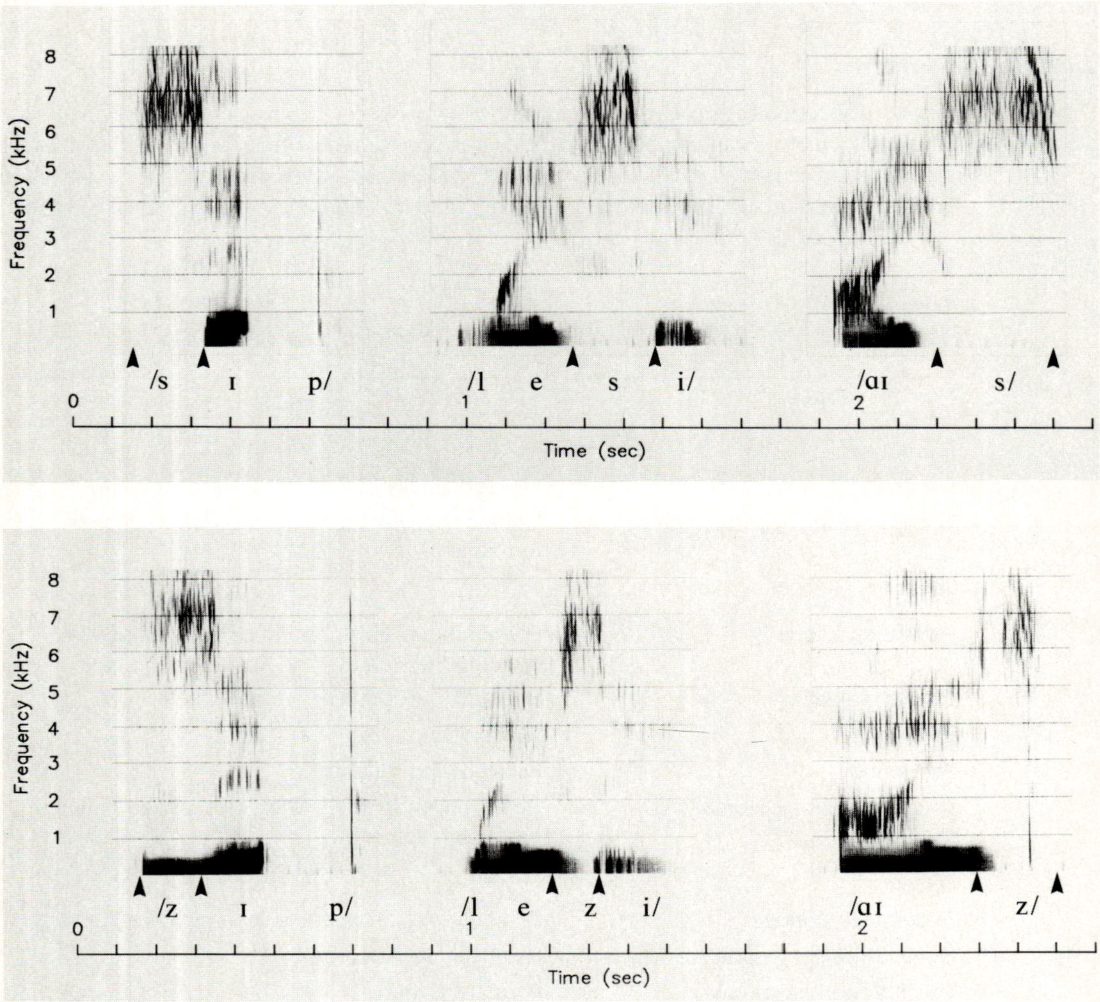

Figure 5–3
Spectrograms of a child's productions of 'sip,' 'lacy,' and 'ice' (top panel), and 'zip,' 'lazy,' and 'eyes' (bottom panel). Arrows along the *x* axis (abscissa) mark the beginning and ending of frication noise.

voiced words, you will hear the difference as the glottal tone is added to and subtracted from the frication noise. The glottal tone tends to energize the resonances of the vocal tract in the articulatory positions for fricatives. Spectrograms (Figures 5–3 and 5–4) reflect this by recording some resonance bars, or formants, in the patterns for 'zip' /zɪp/, 'lazy' /lezi/, and 'eyes' /ɑɪz/. These formants show that the fricatives are voiced. Fill represents the frication noise produced in the anterior part of the vocal

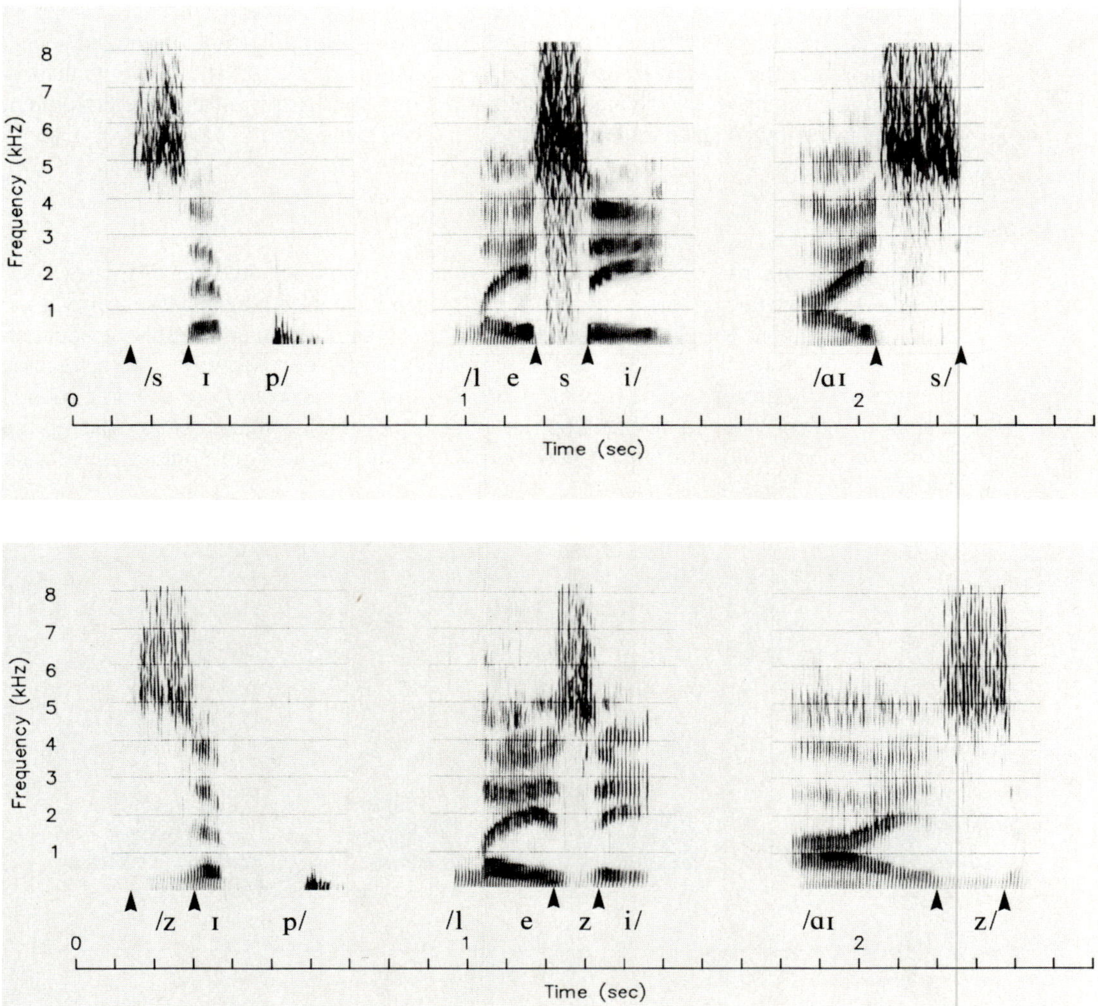

Figure 5–4
Spectrograms of an adult male's productions of 'sip,' 'lacy,' and 'ice' (top panel), and 'zip,' 'lazy,' and 'eyes' (bottom panel). Arrows along the *x* axis mark the beginning and ending of frication noise.

tract; formants represent resonances of the vocal tract. The relative strength or intensity of the glottal tone and frication noise components of each voiced fricative depends on the energy in the two sound sources. Darkness of formants and fill varies depending on the fricative produced and the pronunciation of the speaker. Table 5–2 summarizes the spectrographic cues which signal the physiologic events of fricative production.

Fricatives look much the same in prevocalic, postvocalic, and intervocalic positions. Their dynamics do not change greatly with context. Once the position for a fricative is assumed, the fricative can be prolonged as long as there is breath to support it. This is one difference from stops, which can be repeated but not prolonged, but it does not mean that fricatives are easier to produce than stops. The fine articulatory adjustments required to produce the constrictions for fricatives and their frequent misarticulation by children and adults attest to their difficulty.

Stop Consonants

Spectrograms are presented for a child in Figure 5–5 and for an adult in Figure 5–6, who are each producing 'pie,' 'spy,' and 'buy,' which have stop consonants in prevocalic position. Beginning with the voiceless stop in 'pie,' what happens during the production of each of the stops can be described. Physiologic events represented by the schematic diagram of stop production phases in Figure 5–7 can be related to the acoustic cues in the spectrogram. For the bilabial stop that begins 'pie,' the lips make contact to stop the flow of air. Since no utterance precedes it, this prevocalic stop contact movement

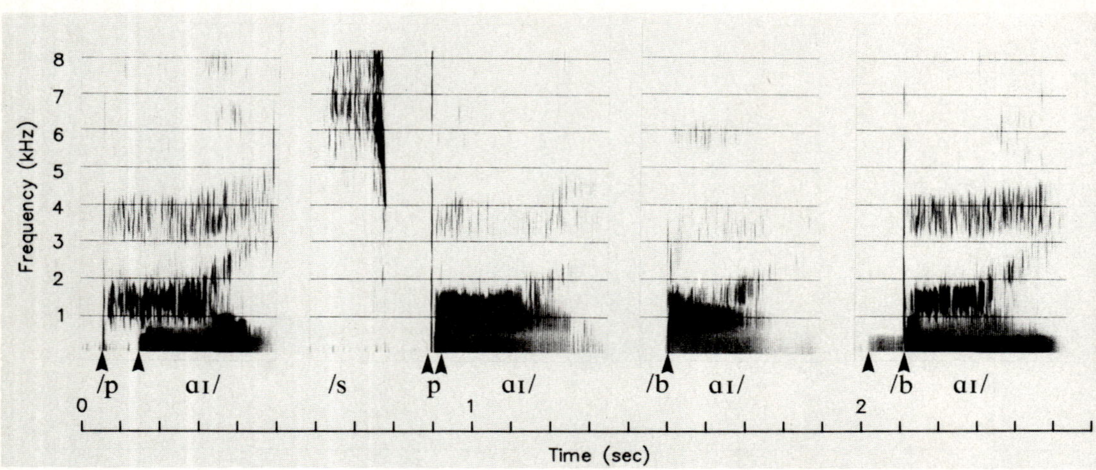

Figure 5–5
Spectrograms of voice onset time (VOT) for a child's productions of 'pie,' 'spy,' 'buy' (without prevoicing) and 'buy' (with prevoicing). VOT, identified for each utterance by arrows on the *x* axis, is 72 msec for 'pie,' 15 msec for 'spy,' 0 msec for 'buy' without prevoicing, and −76 msec for 'buy' with prevoicing. A single arrow indicates simultaneous stop consonant release and vocal fold vibration so that VOT is 0 msec. Due to space limitations, arrows for 'spy' are slightly misaligned.

produces no sound, and no physiologic event is represented in the spectrograms in figures 5–5 and 5–6. After bilabial contact is made, air flows out of the lungs into the vocal tract, where it is blocked by the bilabial closure. Because this is a voiceless stop, no sound accompanies this physiologic event either, and no representation appears in

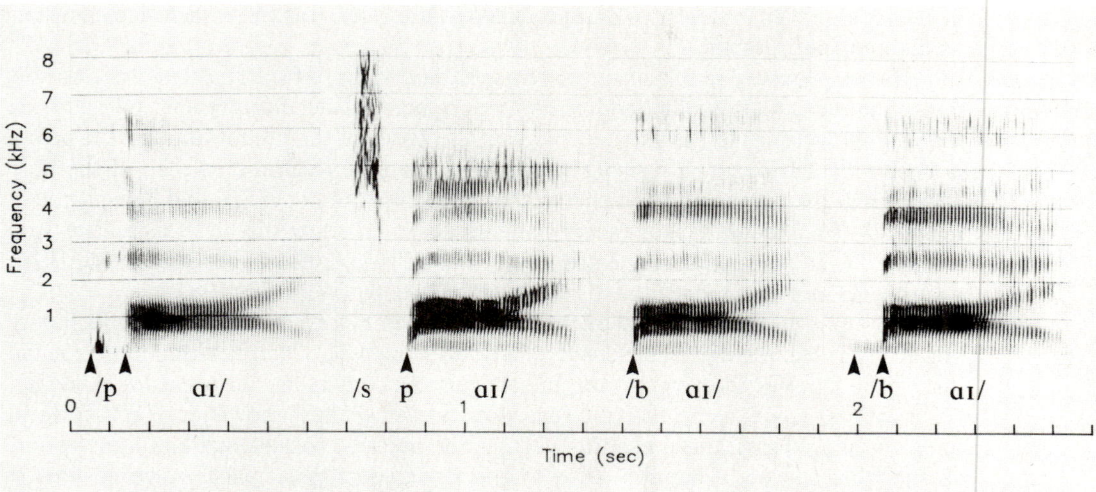

Figure 5–6
Spectrograms of VOT for an adult male's productions of 'pie,' 'spy,' 'buy' (without prevoicing) and 'buy' (with prevoicing). VOT, identified for each utterance by arrows on the x axis, is 72 msec for 'pie,' 0 msec for 'spy,' 0 msec for 'buy' without prevoicing, and −60 msec for 'buy' with prevoicing. A single arrow indicates simultaneous stop consonant release and vocal fold vibration so that VOT is 0 msec.

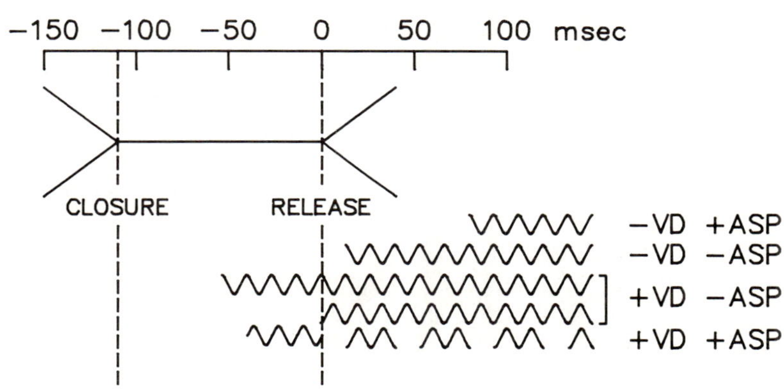

Figure 5–7
Schematic diagram of stop consonant production phases and of VOT, with vocal fold vibration indicated by the wavy line (−VD +ASP = voiceless aspirated stop; −VD −ASP = voiceless unaspirated stop; +VD −ASP = voiced unaspirated stop; +VD +ASP = voiced aspirated stop).

the spectrogram. For a brief period, air pressure builds up behind the closure, until it is released by the separation of the lips and the air rushes out of the oral cavity. The pulse of air that marks this release produces the initial stop noise and the first marking on the spectrogram, the long vertical line, or spike. As the lips begin to separate, the air passing out of the mouth produces frication noise, which shows up as a series of vertical lines, or fill, immediately after the spike. After the lips separate, aspiration noise occurs. This is similar to that produced at the glottis for /h/, which also shows up as fill on spectrograms.

Stops produced in this manner are **aspirated** stops. After the release of this flow of air, the vocal folds contact and begin to vibrate as the articulators shift into position for the following vowel. In the spectrogram the onset of the glottal tone for the vowel is shown by the onset of formant energy. The gap between the release of the stop closure and the beginning of voicing is the voice onset time (VOT), and is indicated in figures 5–5 and 5–6. This measure has been used to study the development of stop production and perception in children (Wolf, 1973; Zlatin & Koenigsknecht, 1975, 1976) and as evidence to support prevocalic voicing of stops (Weismer, 1984).

The physiologic events shown schematically in Figure 5–7 for the production of voiced stops like the initial consonant in 'buy' are somewhat different from those for the voiceless stop. For the voiced stop, the articulators contact and air pressure builds up, often with no sound, as for the voiceless stop. Some speakers, however, start the vocal folds vibrating during the pressure buildup. The acoustic representation of this event, as shown in figures 5–5 and 5–6, is a very low frequency formant, or **voice bar.** It reflects the glottal tone produced with the oral cavity closed off so that no higher frequency resonance occurs, and is referred to as **prevoicing.** For comparison, figures 5–5 and 5–6 include spectrograms of speakers who did not phonate during the pressure buildup. You can see the absence of any acoustic cue.

After the pressure buildup, the closure is released, producing a spike on the spectrogram. In figures 5–5 and 5–6, voicing during the buildup leads right into the vowel formants following the spike. When the speakers did not phonate during pressure buildup, voicing onset, marked by formants, begins shortly after the spike. Note that VOT is much shorter for voiced than for voiceless stops. When a speaker prevoices, voicing leads the stop release so that VOT is a negative value.

Figures 5–5 and 5–6 include spectrograms of 'spy' /spɑɪ/ in which the stop is preceded by /s/. In the spectrograms there is little or no aspiration for 'spy' as compared with 'pie.' Since the utterances differ only in the presence or absence of /s/ before the stop, the loss of aspiration in 'spy' is attributed to the /s/. Note that in the spectrogram for 'spy' a blank space follows the fill for /s/, corresponding to the buildup phase of the stop. Even though this event is silent, it shows up on the spectrogram as a gap between the end of the fricative and the release of the stop. The aspiration in 'spy' is more like that seen in 'buy' than that seen in 'pie.' These variations are shown schematically in Figure 5–7; the stop in 'pie' is voiceless aspirated, the stop in 'spy' is voiceless **unaspirated,** and the stop in 'buy' is voiced unaspirated. Analogous stops made from other positions are 'tie,' 'sty,' and 'die,' which are apico-alveolar, and 'cool,' 'school,' and 'ghoul,' which are dorsovelar. Research shows that VOT increases as the place of articulation changes from bilabial to apico-alveolar to dorsovelar (Klatt, 1975;

Zue, 1976; Kewley-Port, 1982), and that this property is a perceptual cue to place of articulation (Kewley-Port, 1983).

In Figure 5–7, a voiced aspirated stop is shown schematically by intermittent vocal fold vibration starting with the release. This is a simplification of the pressure buildup, glottal tone, and aspiration that characterize these stops (Catford, 1977). Although voiced aspirated stops do not occur in English, they occur in some Indian languages, as reflected by the spelling of words like 'bhakti,' 'ghee,' and 'dharma.' The spelling of English words like 'ghost' indicates that voiced aspirated stops may have been used in English at one time. When necessary, aspiration is indicated by using a superscript /h/ as in the pronunciation of 'pie' [p^{h}ɑɪ]. Table 5–2 summarizes the spectrographic cues to the physiologic events in the production of stops.

Nasal Consonants

For nasals, a closure is produced at some point along the vocal tract anterior to the velopharyngeal area. At the same time, the channel between the nasal and oral cavities is opened so that the nasal cavity becomes the main resonator and the oral cavity becomes the secondary resonator. The vocal folds contact so that air flowing out of the lungs produces a glottal tone. Figures 5–8 and 5–9 show child and adult spectrograms of initial and final nasals in 'man,' 'Nan,' and 'sang.' Unlike stops and fricatives, the nasals have formants with no fill, since they are produced with voicing, an open resonating system, and no frication or aspiration noise. In figures 5–8 and 5–9, note that the formants for the initial and final nasal consonants are level compared to

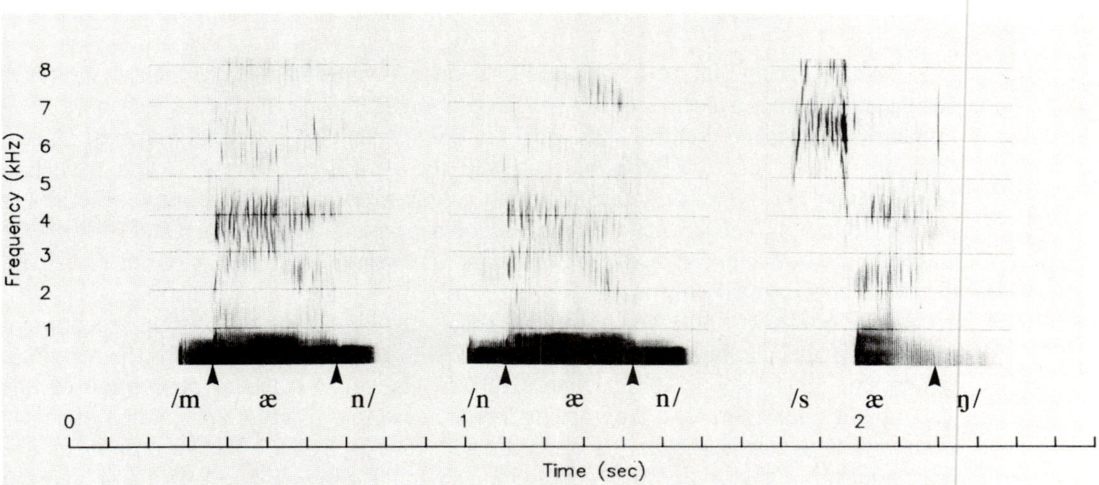

Figure 5–8
Spectrograms of a child's productions of 'man,' 'Nan,' and 'sang.' Arrows on the *x* axis indicate the point of discontinuity between the nasal consonant and the vowel.

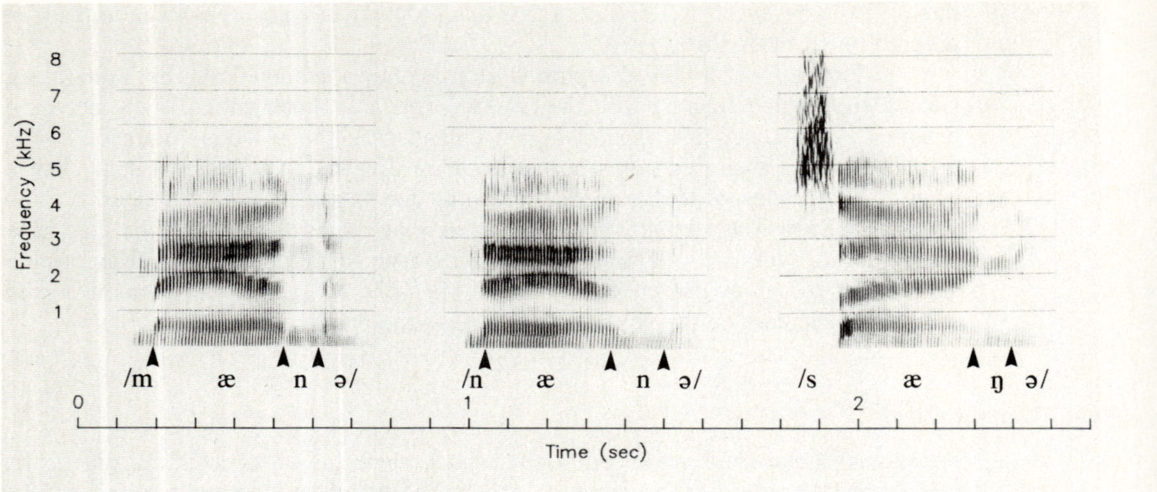

Figure 5–9
Spectrograms of an adult male's productions of 'man,' 'Nan,' and 'sang.' Arrows on the *x* axis indicate the point of discontinuity between the nasal consonant and the vowel. (This adult speaker released the final nasal into a schwa, shown by an additional arrow).

those for the vowel. The formants reflect the configuration of the articulators in the resonating system, which is stable for nasal consonants but dynamic for vowels as the tongue shifts between vowel and consonant positions. There are no articulators which can change the configuration of the nasal cavity during nasal consonant production.

In the production of a CV or VC sequence with nasal consonants, a radical change in resonance occurs between the vowel and the nasal. During the nasal, the oral cavity is blocked and the nasal cavity is open, resulting in a nasal murmur. During the vowel, the nasal cavity is blocked and the oral cavity is open. The transition between the two types of sound generally involves an abrupt shift between oral and nasal resonators. This is reflected in the spectrograms in Figures 5–8 and 5–9 by the discontinuity between the vowel and nasal (at arrows). F_1, F_2, and F_3 of the vowel and the nasal consonant do not match.

Discontinuity between vowel and nasal is an important cue to the perception of the place of articulation of nasal consonants in both adult and child speech (Kurowski & Blumstein, 1984; Repp, 1986; Ohde, 1988a). The importance to perception of this discontinuity has been tested by having listeners identify place of articulation of nasals from various acoustic properties of nasals and vowels. Some of these properties are illustrated for a child in Figure 5–10 and for an adult in Figure 5–11. In these figures, the shorter segments (50M, MT, 50T) have been removed from the full syllable using a computer software editing program. The 50M segment is the nasal murmur just

Figure 5–10
Spectrograms of a child's production of /n ɑ /. The segments shown are the full syllable (FS), 50-msec murmur preceding the discontinuity (50M), 25-msec murmur preceding the discontinuity plus 25-msec vowel transition following the discontinuity (MT), and 50-msec vowel transition following the discontinuity (50T).

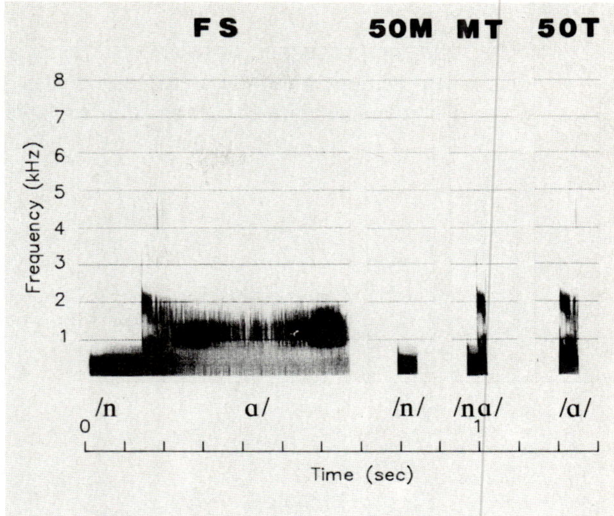

Figure 5–11
Spectrograms of a male adult's production of /n ɑ /. The segments shown are the same as in Figure 5–10.

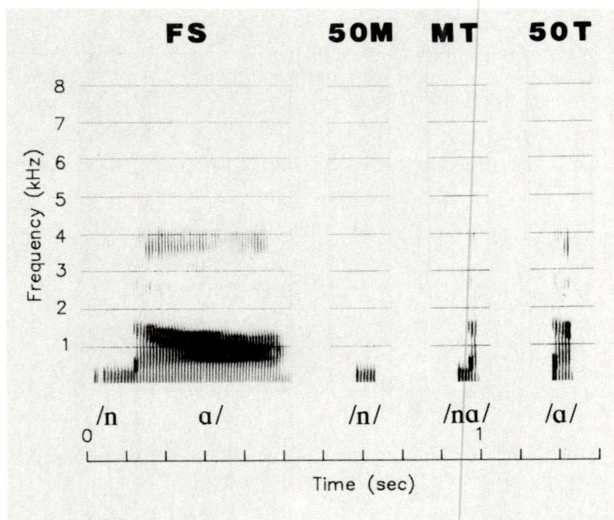

preceding the vowel. The MT segment is the end of the nasal murmur and the beginning of the vowel, the period of discontinuity. The 50T segment represents the initial portion of the vowel immediately following the discontinuity. It has been found that listeners given stimuli including the discontinuity (MT) achieved about 90% correct identification of the place of articulation of nasal consonants. The preceding murmur stimuli (50M) and following vowel stimuli (50T) resulted in about 80% correct identification (Kurowski & Blumstein, 1984; Repp, 1986; Ohde, 1988a).

Trills

In the production of trills, a series of air pressure pulses is produced as the vibratory movement of the articulators occurs. A child's bilabial, alveolar, and uvular trills are shown in Figure 5–12; an adult's bilabial, alveolar, uvular, and glottal trills are shown in

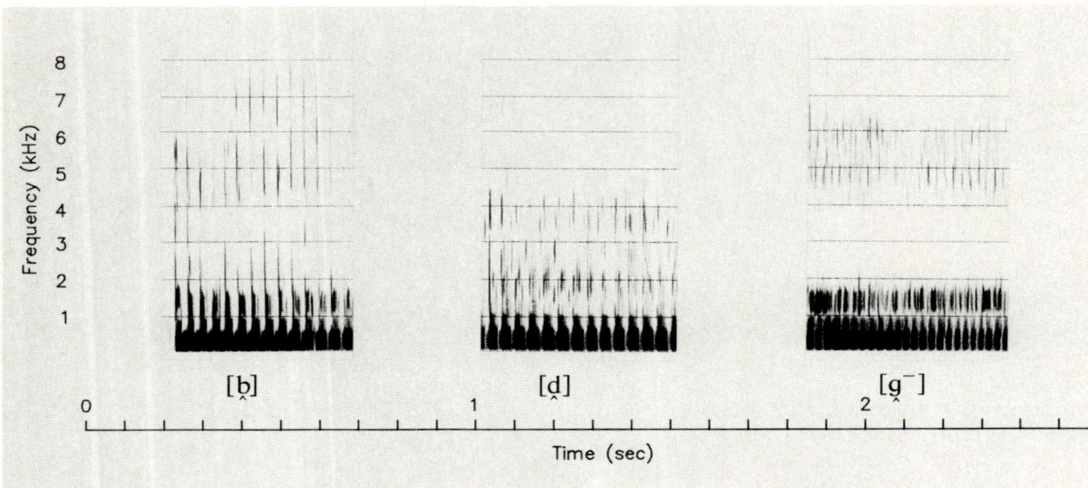

Figure 5–12
Left to right: Spectrograms of a child's productions of bilabial, alveolar, and uvular trills.

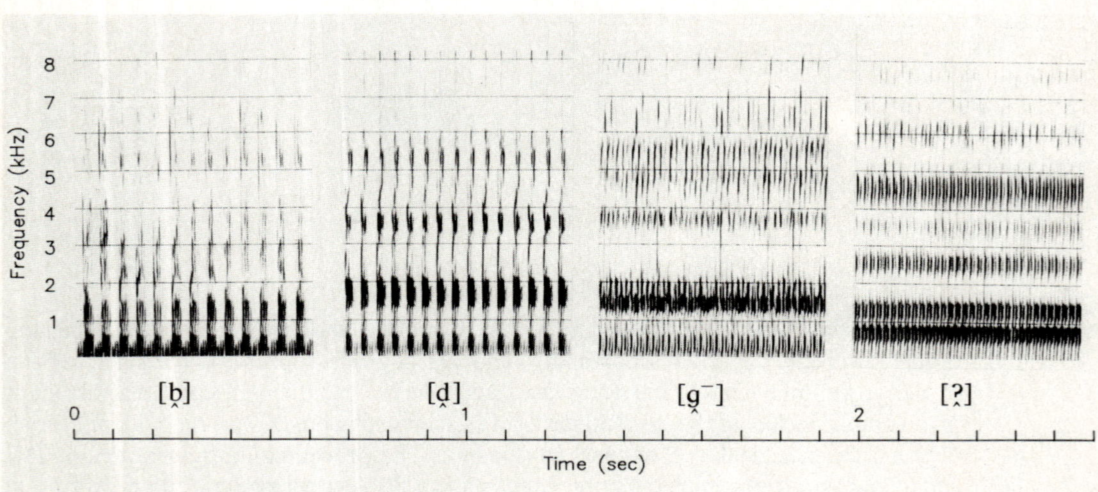

Figure 5–13
Left to right: Spectrograms of an adult male's productions of bilabial, alveolar, uvular and glottal trills.

Figure 5–13. Each trill shows a series of spikes, which represents the slow pulsing of the vibratory system.

POTENTIAL FOR CONSONANT ARTICULATORY POSITIONS

In this section, descriptions of places of articulation and symbols to represent them for stops, fricatives, nasals, and trills are presented. Some of the sounds described occur in English as phonemes, allophones, or misarticulated sounds; others occur in foreign languages, and still others may not occur in any language. The articulatory positions considered are limited to those where at least one type of sound is produced that occurs in normal or misarticulated English or may be substituted for an English sound by a foreign speaker or one with abnormal articulatory structures. The entire system is presented as an indication of the sound-producing capabilities of the speech mechanism. Some sound descriptions and symbols may be more useful to you than others, depending on your particular interest. From among the various sounds described in tables 5–3 and 5–4, those that may be especially useful for the analysis of articulatory and pho-

Table 5–3
Potential articulatory positions for consonant production.

Term	Nature of Occurrence
Bilabial	Stops and nasals in English; also fricatives in Spanish
Labiodental	Fricatives in English and other languages
Dentolabial	No language occurrence; compensatory use for abnormal jaw structure
Apicolabial	No language occurrence; compensatory use for abnormal lower lip structure
Apicodental[a]	Fricatives in English; allophonic or abnormal substitution for apico-alveolar stops and fricatives in English
Apico-alveolar[b]	Stops, fricatives, and nasals in English
Apicopalatal[c]	Retroflex sibilants in Indian languages but not in English
Lamino-prepalatal	Fricatives in English; nasals in other languages
Dorsovelar	Stops and nasal in English; fricatives in German
Dorsopharyngeal	Not in English except as used for stops and fricatives by cleft-palate speakers
Glottal	Fricative phoneme in English; stop used in Brooklyn dialect and by other speakers intervocalically as /t/ substitute

[a]May also be interdental.
[b]Upper alveolar ridge is usual for stops and nasals, but lower alveolar ridge can be used for /s/ and /z/ in English.
[c]Also called *retroflex.*

Table 5–4
Place of articulation for consonants. The first symbol in each pair is for a voiceless consonant, the second for a voiced one. Voiceless nasals are not shown.

Place	Nasal	Stop		Fricative		Trill	
Labial Sounds							
Bilabial	m	p	b	ɸ	β	p̭	b̭
Apicolabial	M	P	B	Ᵽ	Ƀ	P̭	B̭
Labiodental	ɱ	p̪	b̪	f	v	—	—
Tongue Tip/Blade Sounds							
Apico-interdental	n̪͇	t̪͇	d̪͇	θ	ð	—	—
Apicodental	n̪	t̪	d̪	s̪	z̪	—	—
Apico-alveolar	n	t	d	s	z	ṱ	ḓ
Apico-alveolar lateral	—	—	—	s^{l}	z^{l}	—	—
Apicopalatal retroflex	ɳ	ʈ	ɖ	ʂ	ʐ	—	—
Lamino-prepalatal[a]	ɲ	—	—	ʃ	ʒ	—	—
Tongue Dorsum Sounds							
Dorsopalatal	ŋ$^{+}$	k^{+}	g^{+}	ꝁ$^{+}$	ǥ$^{+}$	—	—
Dorsovelar	ŋ	k	g	ꝁ	ǥ	—	—
Dorso-uvular	ŋ$^{-}$	k^{-}	g^{-}	ꝁ$^{-}$	ǥ$^{-}$	k̭$^{-}$	g̭$^{-}$
Dorsopharyngeal	—	K	G	Ꝁ	Ǥ	—	—
Glottal Sounds							
Glottal	—	ʔ		h	ɦ		ʔ̭

[a]IPA uses this symbol for the dorsopalatal nasal, but Heffner (1952) uses it for the lamino-prepalatal nasal.

nological disorders are indicated. In conceptualizing the variations in position of articulation and in sound quality, it is helpful to group the descriptions into four categories: (1) sounds involving one or both lips; (2) sounds involving the tongue tip, or blade; (3) sounds involving the tongue dorsum; and (4) sounds involving the glottis.

Table 5–4 presents voiceless and voiced analogs for each articulatory position and manner except for nasals. It is possible to produce voiceless nasals by blocking the oral cavity at different locations and letting air flow out the nasal cavity. These sounds occur in the Burmese and Tibetan languages (Catford, 1977). Although voiceless nasals do not regularly occur in English, they may be produced when /m / or /n / follows /s / in words like 'smooth' and 'snow,' particularly in the speech of children.

Bilabial

Bilabial stops and a bilabial nasal occur as the usual allophones of phonemes in English. Bilabial fricatives occur only as somewhat infrequent allophones of the labiodental fricatives in words like 'comfort' and 'triumvirate.' Bilabial trills do not occur in any language, but they are sometimes used by children in play situations to represent motorboat-like sounds.

Apicolabial

No apicolabial sound occurs in any language. The stops and fricatives, however, can substitute for bilabial stops or labiodental fricatives for individuals with a radical loss of lower lip structure. The trill is commonly known as the raspberry or Bronx cheer, a sound demonstrating contempt or derision.

Labiodental

Labiodental fricatives occur as phonemes in English, but stops do not. The labiodental nasal is an allophone of the bilabial nasal in words like 'comfort.' Dentolabial stops and fricatives are potential substitutes for bilabial stops and labiodental fricatives for individuals with a prognathic lower jaw condition. No trill can be produced from this position.

Apico-interdental

The apico-interdental position (tongue tip protruding between the front teeth) is used in the production of English fricatives in words like 'thin' and 'them.' In addition, apico-interdental allophones of /t/, /d/, and /n/ are produced in words like 'eighth,' 'width,' and 'ninth.' If these sounds are produced as apico-interdentals in other contexts, the behavior is described as dentalizing and classified as a misarticulation. In one type of lisp, interdental fricatives are substituted for alveolar ones so that 'sin' becomes 'thin,' and 'tease' becomes 'teethe.' No trill is possible from this position.

Apicodental

Apicodental production involves tongue tip contact on the posterior surfaces of the upper teeth. As in the case of apico-interdentals, apicodental stops and nasals are allophones of /t/, /d/, and /n/ when produced in words like 'eighth,' 'width,' and 'ninth.' If they are substituted for other allophones, the dentalization pattern may be considered abnormal. Apicodental fricatives sound like /s/ and /z/, but the tongue tip interferes with the airstream. This results in dentalized /s/ and /z/ sounds, which are difficult to perceive without seeing the tongue position. No trill is possible from this position.

Apico-alveolar

The /t/, /d/, /n/, /s/, and /z/ phonemes are produced from the apico-alveolar position, with tongue tip contact for the stops and the nasal. /s/ and /z/ involve an approximation of the alveolar ridge by the tongue tip so that air is directed between the front teeth to produce frication noise. Many speakers orient the tongue tip toward the lower alveolar ridge rather than the upper one for /s/ and /z/ with no discernible difference in sound. Apico-alveolar voiced trills occur in Spanish words like *perro* 'dog' (Heffner, 1952). A very short trill, called a **flap,** frequently occurs in the pronunciation of American speakers in words like 'bitter' and 'bidder' (Bronstein, 1960; Tiffany & Carrell, 1977; Calvert, 1980). Such usage results in the loss of distinction between /t/ and /d/, especially in the intervocalic position of two-syllable words with stress on the first syllable. The alveolar flap contrasts phonemically with the alveolar trill in Spanish in words like *pero* 'but' (Heffner, 1952).

Apico-alveolar Lateral

For the apico-alveolar lateral position, the tongue tip contacts the alveolar ridge, but the margins of the tongue do not. This is basically the position for /l/ but with a closer approximation to the palate so that frication noise is produced as air flows over the sides of the tongue. These fricatives are used for /s/ and /z/ in lateral lisping. Because air can flow over the sides of the tongue, no stops, nasals, or trills are possible from this position.

Apicopalatal or Retroflex

As the term *retroflex* implies, the action of the tongue tip is to bend (*flex*) backward (*retro-*) to contact the hard palate for stops and nasals and to approximate the hard palate for fricatives. These sounds occur in some Indian languages (Heffner, 1952), and some Indian speakers of English may use them to substitute for alveolar consonants. No trill can be made from this position.

Lamino-prepalatal

The lamino-prepalatal position is similar to that used for /s/ and /z/, but the tongue blade rather than the tongue tip approaches the alveolar ridge for fricatives and contacts it for stops and nasals. In English the /ʃ/ and /ʒ/ fricatives are made from this position, but there are no lamino-prepalatal stop phonemes. The nasal occurs in French, Italian, and Spanish (Heffner, 1952). No trill can be made from this position.

Dorsopalatal

The anterior allophones of the English /k/ and /g/ stop phonemes are made from the dorsopalatal position in words like 'kill' and 'gill,' as is the anterior allophone of the nasal phoneme in words like 'sing.' The fricatives made from this position occur in German (Heffner, 1952). No trill can be made from this position.

Dorsovelar

The dorsovelar position is used for posterior allophones of the /k/ and /g/ stop phonemes of English in words like 'coal' and 'goal.' It is also the position for the posterior allophone of the nasal phoneme in words like 'song.' The fricatives occur in German (Heffner, 1952). No trill can be made from this position.

Dorso-uvular

Stops, fricatives, and nasals are produced from the dorso-uvular position in Eskimo (Heffner, 1952), but not in English. Voiced and voiceless uvular trills occur in French and German (Heffner, 1952). The trill requires vibrating the uvula as the airstream from the lungs passes between it and the tongue dorsum. The uvular trill is basically what happens during gargling.

Dorsopharyngeal

The dorsopharyngeal position requires some effort to draw the back of the tongue backward to contact or approximate the pharyngeal wall. Fricatives made from this position occur in Semitic and Hamitic languages (Heffner, 1952), but no stops. For some cleft-palate speakers, however, this position offers the possibility of using the airflow from the lungs to produce sounds before much of it escapes through the nasal cavity. For this reason, dorsopharyngeal stops and fricatives may substitute for dorsovelar sounds. No trill or nasal can be made from this position.

Glottal

An English fricative phoneme produced by approximating the vocal folds to create frication noise is made from the **glottal** position in words like 'hat.' A voiced analog may occur in intervocalic position in words like 'ahead,' but only as an allophone of the /h/ phoneme. A glottal stop regularly replaces /t/ intervocalically in the Brooklyn dialect and frequently in the speech of others as a substitute for /t/ in words like 'kitten.' The glottal trill does not occur as a phoneme in any language. It can occur as a substitute for the normal glottal tone, particularly at the end of phrases. Some speech pathologists have their voice disorder cases use the glottal trill as a therapy technique but refer to it as a *glottal fry.*

GLOSSARY

Affricate. A consonant produced by releasing a stop into a fricative, usually within the same syllable.

Apico-. Refers to the use of the tongue tip or apex in the production of sounds which involve contacts with the lips (apicolabial), teeth (apicodental), alveolar ridge (apico-alveolar), or hard palate (apicopalatal).

Approximant. A sound made by approximating two articulators not quite as closely as for fricatives; used to describe liquids and glides.

Aspirated. Describes a stop sound with a release of closure that precedes the onset of voicing of a following vowel long enough so that noise is produced during the interval.

Consonant. A sound produced by restricting or blocking the flow of air through the vocal tract.

Denasal. Describes the quality of sound produced when nasal resonance is influenced by a blockage in the nasal cavity.

Dental. Indicates a sound involving articulator contact with the teeth, as in *labiodental* and *interdental.*

Dento-. Refers to the use of the lower teeth in the production of sounds which involve contact with the upper lip (dentolabial).

Discontinuity. The abrupt change in formant levels on a spectrogram between nasal consonants and vowels.

Dorso-. Refers to the use of the tongue dorsum in the production of sounds which involve contacts with the hard palate (dorsopalatal), soft palate (dorsovelar), uvula (dorso-uvular), or pharyngeal wall (dorsopharyngeal).

Egressive. Describes the flow of air out of the vocal tract.

Ejective. An egressive stop produced by building up air pressure between laryngeal and lingual closures.

Explosive. Describes a mechanism for stop production by which relatively higher pressure within the vocal tract causes air to burst out of it after a closure is released.

Flap. A sound produced by very briefly interrupting voicing, as frequently occurs in words like 'bitter' and 'bidder.'

Fricative. A consonant produced by restricting the airflow through the vocal tract so that frication noise is produced.

Glottal. A sound produced by approximating the vocal folds, as for a glottal fricative, or closing them, as for a glottal stop.

Glottal fry. A trill-like sound produced by vibrating the vocal folds about 25 Hz; commonly known as vocal fry, creaky voice, or laryngealization when substituted for normal voice in speaking.

Glottalic. Describes sounds produced by changing the air pressure in the cavity extending from the glottis, or vocal folds, to an anterior closure.

Homorganic. Describes sounds made from the same place of articulation.

Implosive. Describes a mechanism for stop production by which relatively lower pressure within the vocal tract causes air to burst into it after a closure is released.

Ingressive. Describes the flow of air into the vocal tract.

Labial. Using the upper or lower lip in the production of sounds.

Labio-. Refers to the use of the lower lip in the production of sounds which involve contact with the teeth (labiodental).

Lamino-. Refers to the use of the tongue blade in the production of sounds which involve contact with the hard palate (lamino-prepalatal).

Manner of articulation. The nature of the interference with the airflow through the vocal tract in the production of speech sounds.

Nasal. A consonant produced by opening the velopharyngeal port so that airflow is through the nasal cavity instead of the oral cavity and nasal resonance is produced; the quality of resonance resulting from opening the velopharyngeal port.

Obstruent. A sound made with a complete closure or narrow constriction in the oral cavity so that airflow is stopped or frication noise is produced; used to describe stops, fricatives, affricates, and trills.

Oral. Describes the resonance characteristic of a relatively open oral cavity and a closed velopharyngeal port.

Place of articulation. The location in the vocal tract of the blockage or restriction of the airflow in the production of sounds.

Plosive. A term sometimes used instead of *stop,* particularly when there is a release of air pressure following a blockage of the vocal tract.

Pressure. Describes stops produced by increasing pressure within the vocal tract so that air bursts out of it after a closure is released.

Prevoicing. Vocal fold vibration that occurs during a stop closure.

Pulmonic. Describes sounds for which the expansion or contraction of the lungs provides the required airflow and change in air pressure.

Sibilant. A fricative sound characterized by higher frequency noise than other fricatives because of airflow directed against the edges of the teeth.

Sonorant. A sound made with a relatively open vocal tract so that cavity resonance occurs; used to describe nasal consonants, glides, and liquids.

Stop. A consonant produced by blocking the airflow through the vocal tract so as to increase air pressure, which may or may not be released.

Suction. Describes stops produced by decreasing air pressure within the vocal tract so that air bursts into it after a closure is released.

Trill. A consonant produced by about a 25 Hz vibration of an articulator, such as the tongue tip or the uvula.

Unaspirated. Describes a stop sound with release of closure that either slightly precedes or occurs simultaneously with voicing onset so that only brief or no aspiration noise is produced.

Voice bar. Low frequency bar in a spectrogram that looks like a formant but reflects low frequency energy of voicing.

REVIEW QUESTIONS

A. Match the acoustic cue with the physiologic event by inserting the appropriate letter.

1. Pressure buildup ______	a. Level formants
2. Frication ______	b. Spike
3. Aspiration ______	c. Voice bar
4. Pressure release ______	d. Formant discontinuity
5. Oral to nasal resonance shift ______	e. Gap
6. Closed cavity voicing ______	f. High F_1
7. No resonance change ______	g. Formant onset
8. Start of vocal fold vibration ______	h. Fill

****

Key: 1. e; 2. h; 3. h; 4. b; 5. d; 6. c; 7. a; 8. g

B. Indicate the status of each sound in English by inserting the appropriate letter.

1. Bilabial trill ______	a. Not in English
2. Apico-alveolar lateral fricative ______	b. Not possible
3. Dorsopharyngeal fricative ______	c. Misarticulated
4. Apico-alveolar stop ______	d. Normal
5. Dorsopharyngeal nasal ______	
6. Dorsovelar trill ______	
7. Dorsovelar stop ______	
8. Apicolabial fricative ______	

****

Key: 1. a; 2. c; 3. c; 4. d; 5. b; 6. b; 7. d; 8. c

C. Indicate the symbol for the English sounds described.

1. Voiced bilabial nasal ______
2. Voiceless alveolar stop ______
3. Voiced dorsovelar stop ______

4. Voiceless labiodental fricative ____________
5. Voiceless glottal fricative ________________
6. Voiceless interdental fricative ____________
7. Voiceless alveolar fricative ________________
8. Voiceless lamino-prepalatal fricative ________

****

Key: 1. /m/; 2. /t/; 3. /g/; 4. /f/; 5. /h/; 6. /θ/; 7. /z/; 8. /ʃ/

CHAPTER 6

Analysis of Stop Sounds

In Chapter 5, stops were differentiated from other consonant types on the basis of physiologic events and their acoustic cues as shown in spectrograms. The correspondence between acoustic cues and physiologic events was noted: gap and pressure buildup; spike and release of pressure; fill and frication or aspiration. The interval between the release of pressure and the onset of voicing, or VOT, was noted as an important measure for distinguishing voiced and voiceless stops. This chapter pays particular attention to differentiating stops on the basis of their articulatory characteristics. This requires consideration of the dynamics of stop production in three contexts: prevocalic, intervocalic, and postvocalic.

DYNAMICS OF PLACE OF ARTICULATION FOR STOPS

Table 6–1 presents minimal pairs of stops in prevocalic, intervocalic, and postvocalic positions in English words. These include voiceless and voiced bilabials, /p/ and /b/, apico-alveolars, /t/ and /d/, and dorsovelars, /k/ and /g/. By place of articulation and voicing, each of these sounds can be identified as unique.

Figure 6–1 includes palatograms and X-ray tracings of the articulatory structures involved in producing /p/, /t/, and /k/. For purposes of demonstrating differences in place of articulation, these illustrations apply as well to /b/, /d/, and /g/. Note that the lips are closed for the bilabial stop, but the tongue, which is not involved in its production, is free to move toward the position of the following vowel, which is /ɛ/. The alveolar contact for the apico-alveolar stop blocks the oral cavity completely, since the closure also involves contact by the margins of the tongue along the alveolar ridge of all

Table 6–1
Minimal pairs showing stop phonemes.

Phoneme	Prevocalic	Intervocalic		Postvocalic
/p/	pill	tapping	lapper	tap
/b/	bill	tabbing	—	tab
/t/	till	tatting	latter[a]	tat
/d/	dill	—	ladder [a]	tad
/k/	kill	tacking	lacquer	tack
/g/	gill	tagging	lagger	tag

[a] These words are pronounced alike. The difference between intervocalic /t/ and /d/ is minimal to nil in American English.

the teeth. Complete blockage of the oral cavity can be observed for the velar stop contact as well. The velar contact is forward because of the influence of the front /ɛ/ vowel.

The contact for each stop divides the vocal tract, which extends from the lips to the vocal folds, into anterior and posterior cavities. The velar stop closure creates the largest anterior cavity, as compared to the bilabial and alveolar stops, but the posterior cavity for it is the smallest. As the point of contact shifts forward in the mouth, the anterior cavity decreases in size and the posterior cavity increases. This is important since the resonance characteristics of the stop burst and contiguous vowels depend on this relationship.

Stop production is divided into three phases related to important physiologic events which precede closure and follow its release. The three phases are: (1) **precontact,** during which the articulators are moving toward contact; (2) **closure,** during which air pressure is built up; and (3) **postrelease,** during which the articulators are moving away from the contact position. The precontact phase can involve movement away from the position for a preceding sound, usually a vowel, or it can be preceded by silence. For example, the precontact phase for /t/ is preceded by a vowel in 'a tie' and 'attire' and by a consonant in 'sty' and 'necktie.' In the production of isolated words like 'tie,' no sound precedes precontact. The postrelease phase can involve movement toward a following vowel, as in 'eighty,' or else silence, as in 'eight'. Both precontact and postcontact phases can involve no sound.

In seeking cues to place of articulation, the obvious starting point is the physiologic events surrounding the contact of the articulators to produce closure. The release of this closure produces a spike and fill on a spectrogram. Because the articulators are in different positions for the bilabial, apico-alveolar, and dorsovelar stops, the articulatory configuration of the vocal tract is different for each. When the release occurs, the resonance of the oral cavity shapes pulse and frication noise differently for the three different positions.

Theoretically the frequency shaping of the noise represented by the spike and frication should reflect the size of the vocal tract anterior to the stop closure; that is, the smaller the cavity, the greater the concentration of energy at higher frequencies in the

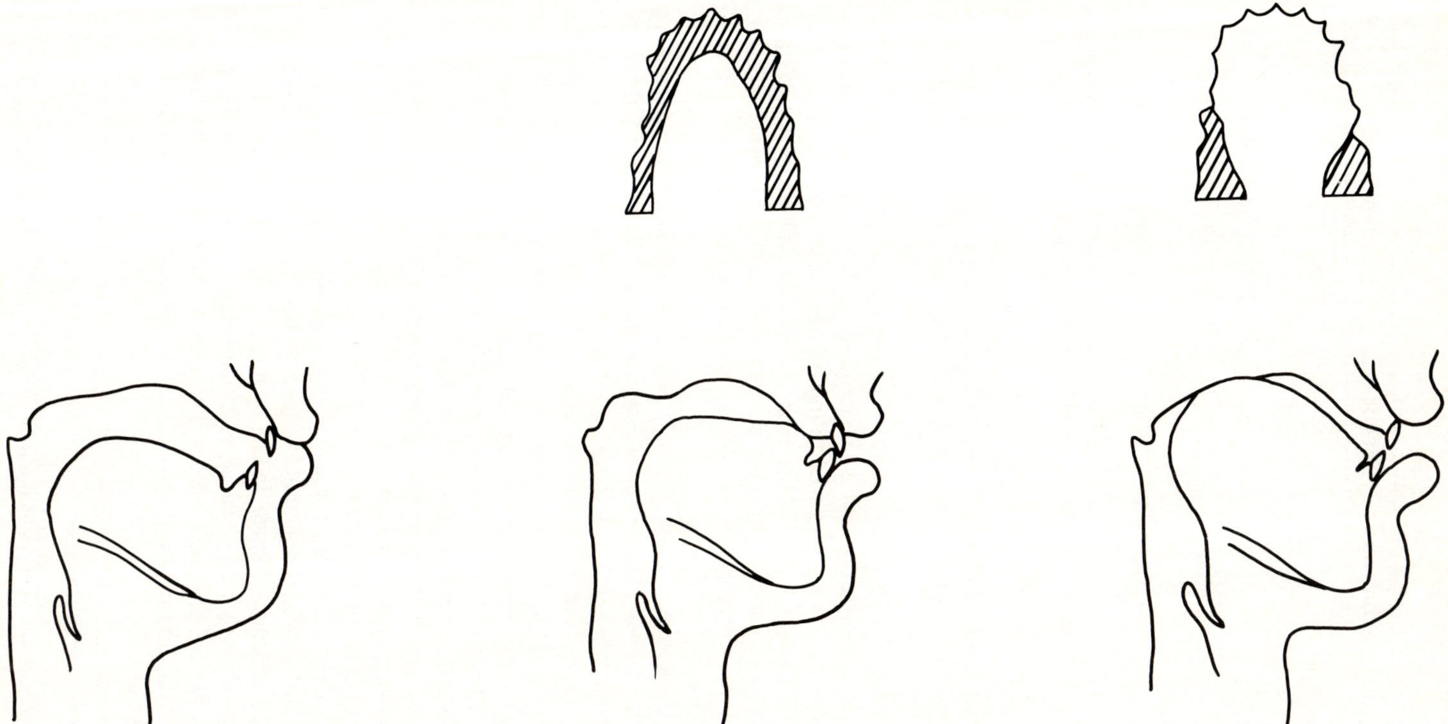

Figure 6–1
Palatograms of /t/ and /k/ and midsagittal X-ray tracings of /p/, /t/, and /k/ produced by an adult male. No palatogram is shown for /p/ because its production does not involve tongue contact. Contact areas are highlighted by dark bold lines. In each palatogram, the anterior part of the hard palate is at the top and the posterior part is at the bottom; the scalloped line shows the inner margins of the upper teeth. The X-ray tracings show the changing position of the tongue for /p/, /t/, and /k/.

noise. Concentration in sound energy should decrease in frequency from /p, b/ to /t, d/ to /k, g/. As you can see in figures 6–2 and 6–3 (spectrograms of a child and an adult speaker), this shift in frequency does not show clearly in the spectrograms of the stops. First, in the spectrograms of the voiced stops, /b, d, g/, the frication period is either very short or absent, so that there is little evidence of frequency variation. Second, the noise of the release is very weak even for the voiceless stops, /p, t, k/, so that it is difficult to see any variations in energy concentration.

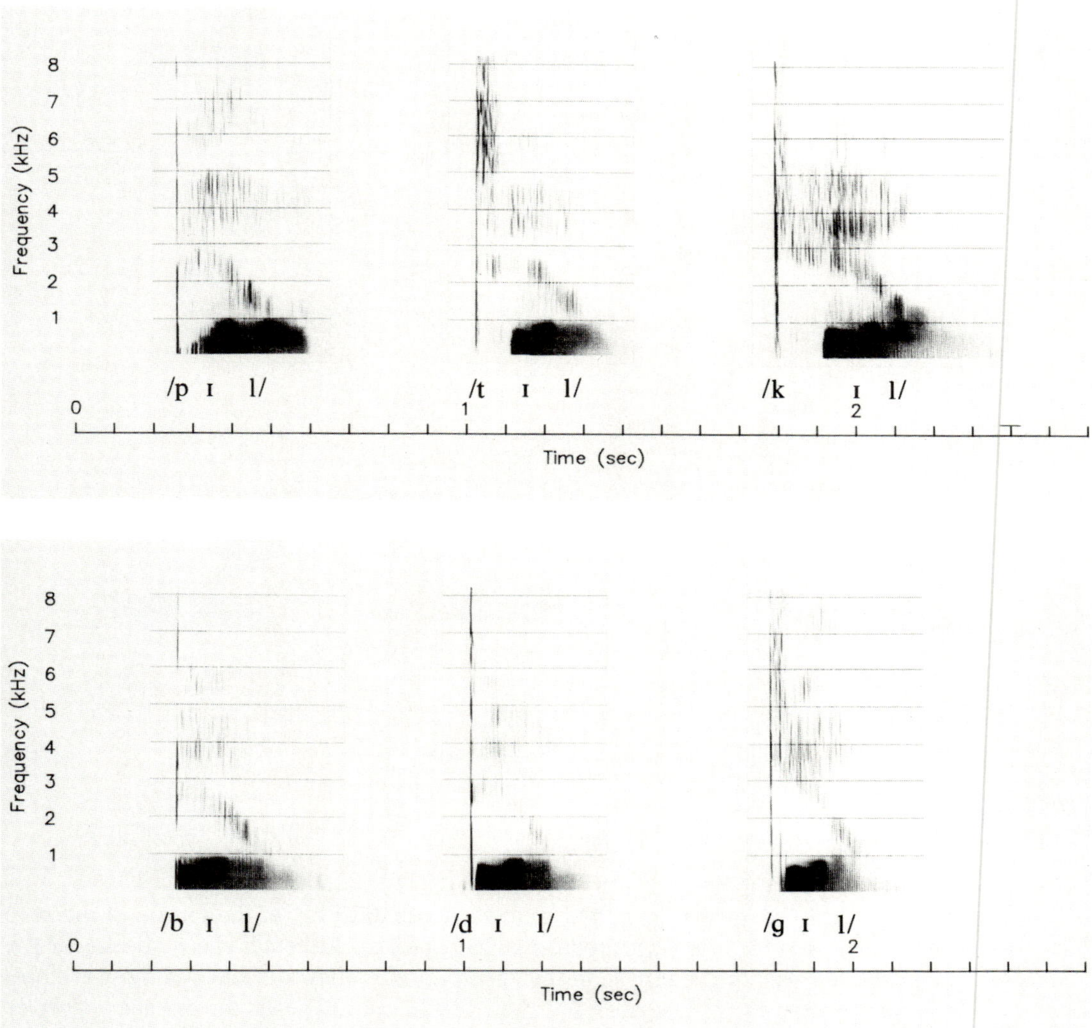

Figure 6–2
Spectrograms of a child's productions of 'pill,' 'till,' and 'kill' (top panel), and 'bill,' 'dill,' and 'gill' (bottom panel).

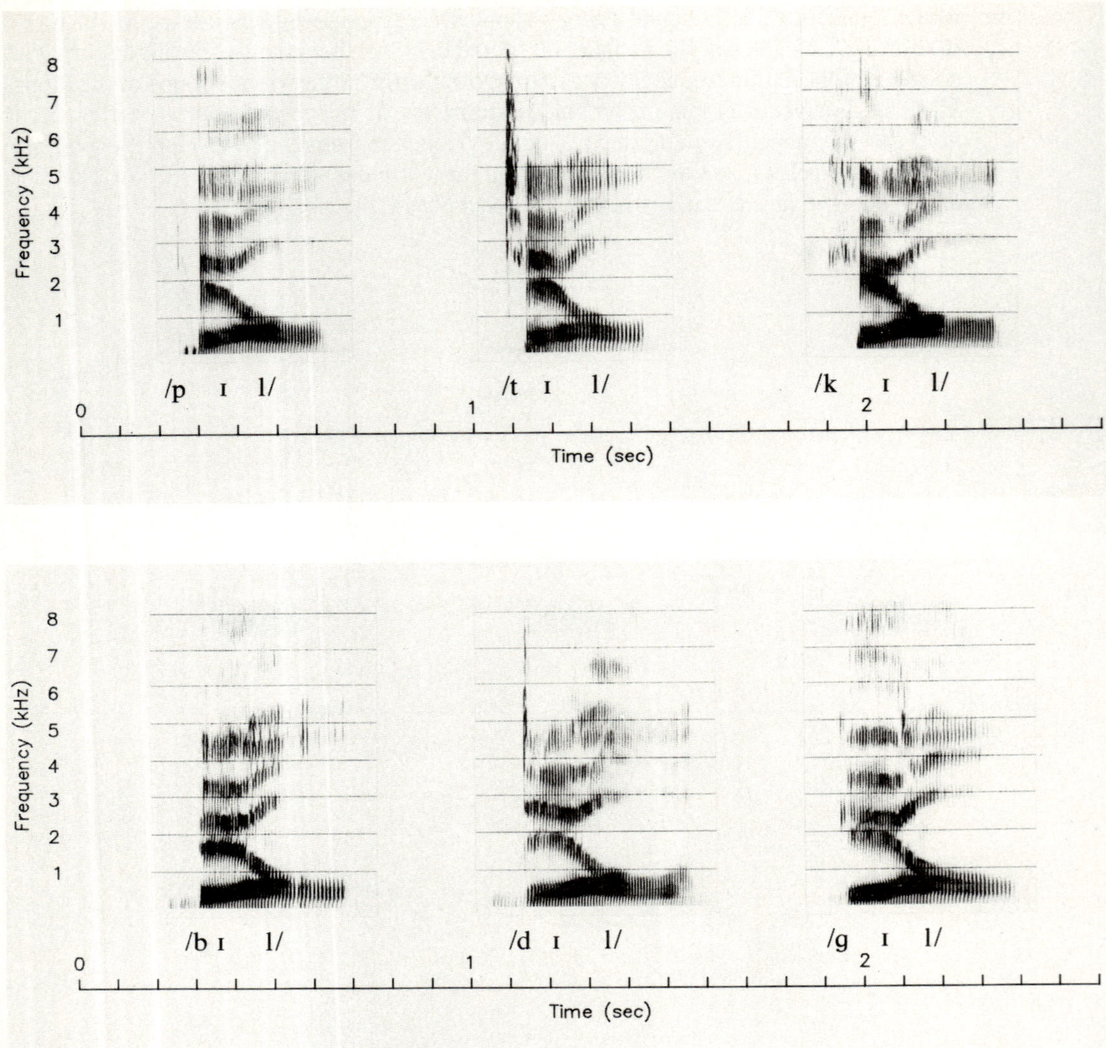

Figure 6–3
Spectrograms of an adult male's productions of 'pill,' 'till,' and 'kill,' (top panel), and 'bill,' 'dill,' and 'gill' (bottom panel).

In Figure 6–4, spectrographic and waveform analyses of the onsets of the stop consonants /p, t, k/ are illustrated for a child speaker. Although energy peaks for the stop releases are not discernible in the spectrograms, they are found in the waveform analyses (at arrows). These analyses show higher energy peaks for the apico-alveolar and dorsovelar stops and a lower energy peak for the bilabial stop. The prediction based on the size of the anterior cavity is not supported. But the frequency characteristic of the spike and frication can provide an auditory cue to place of stop articulation, as you can judge for yourself by whispering 'pill,' 'till,' and 'kill' and listening for the change in resonance characteristics in the bursts. Despite the difficulty in seeing the cues on spectrograms, studies of synthesized speech show that the place of articulation of stops can be differentiated on the basis of burst noise (Liberman, 1957).

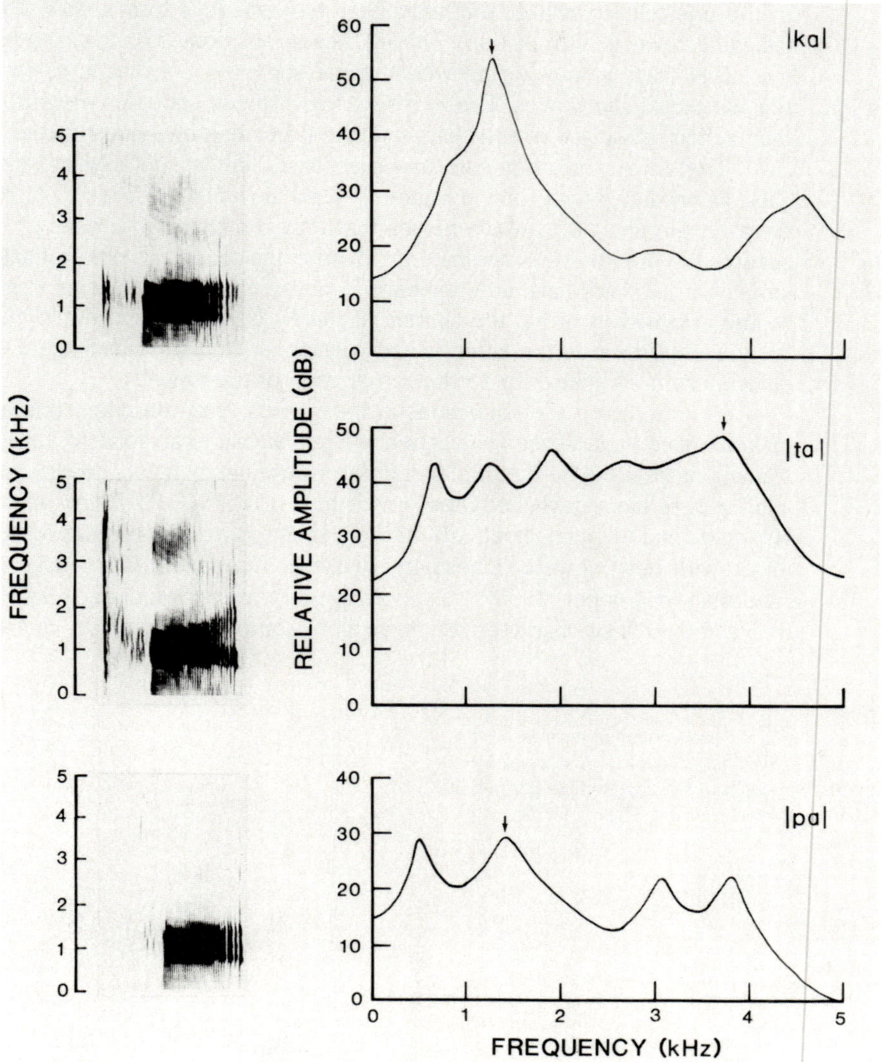

Figure 6–4
Spectrograms and waveforms of a child's productions of /pɑ/, /tɑ/, and /kɑ/. Arrows above the waveforms indicate the peak frequency of the burst. The waveforms were calculated using a 14-pole linear predictive coding algorithm and a 25.6-msec time window (half Hamming), with pre-emphasis of the higher frequencies.

Added to the difficulties the burst presents as a place cue is the fact that it is not always present. Many speakers do not release the stop when it occurs in final position in words like 'neck' produced in isolation or when another stop follows, as in 'necktie.' Fortunately there are other cues to place of articulation. One such cue is the acoustic representation of the precontact and postrelease phases. In the precontact phase, the articulator movement is from a preceding vowel toward a stop contact (VC transition). In the postrelease phase, the articulator movement is from a stop contact toward a following vowel (CV transition). During these transitions, the changing configurations of the vocal tract in moving between vowel and stop consonant positions modify the resonances of the vowel. These resonance changes shift the vowel formants so that they reflect the place of articulation of the preceding or following consonant.

The vowel transition cue can be observed in the spectrograms of 'pip,' 'pit,' and 'pick' as produced by a child in Figure 6–5 and an adult in Figure 6–6. Neither speaker released the final stop, which means that only the first two phases of stop production occurred. Thus, there is no spike or frication indicating the place of articulation of the stops. Yet listeners have little difficulty in differentiating them. One important cue may be the **transition** of F_2, the shifting of the F_2 frequency as the tongue changes from the vowel position to the different stop positions. In figures 6–5 and 6–6, you can see differences in F_2 just prior to the termination of the vowel.

By comparing the transitions in the vowels, you can differentiate place of articulation, since F_2 increases in frequency from bilabial to alveolar to velar positions. The transitions seem to be directed at a different frequency level. Research on synthesized adult speech has established these levels to be about 700 Hz for /p/ and /b/, about 1800 Hz for /t/ and /d/, and about 3300 Hz for /k/ and /g/ in the context of front vowels, and lower with back vowels (Liberman, Delattre, Cooper, & Gerstman, 1954; Delattre, Liberman, & Cooper, 1955); these values may vary in real speech, as shown in figures 6–5 and 6–6. The characteristic frequency location for each place of articulation is the

Figure 6–5
Spectrograms of a child's productions of unreleased final stop consonants in 'pip,' 'pit,' and 'pick.' Arrows along the *y* axis (ordinate) indicate the approximate position of F_2. Note that F_2 is lowest for /p/, highest for /k/.

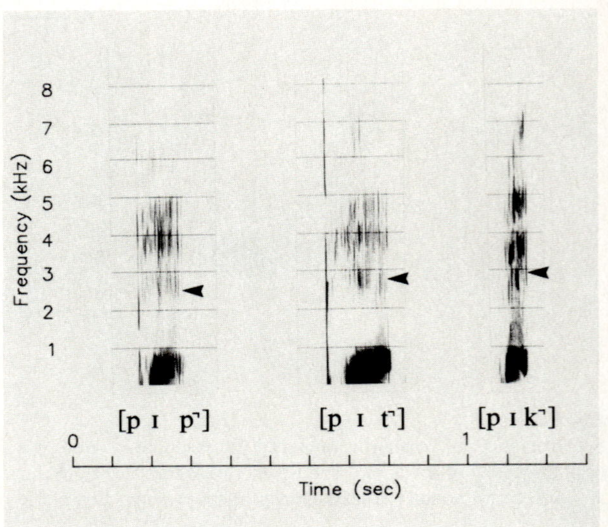

Figure 6–6
Spectrograms of an adult male's productions of unreleased final stop consonants in 'pip,' 'pit,' and 'pick.' Arrows along the *y* axis indicate the approximate position of F_2. Note that F_2 is lowest for /p/, highest for /k/.

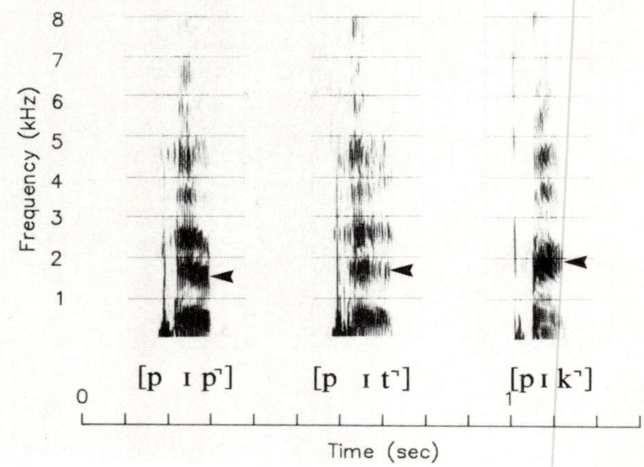

locus. Note that the locus generally increases in frequency as the articulatory position for the consonant moves farther back in the vocal tract, making the part of the tract behind the closure shorter. The locus varies this way in VCV, CV, and VC contexts.

More recent research has cast some doubt on the validity of the locus for differentiating the articulatory positions of consonants (Kewley-Port, 1982). Figure 6–7 is a schematic representation of the F_2 transitions for bilabial, alveolar, and velar stops in VCV utterances with a range of vowels. These diagrams are based on the results of the Kewley-Port (1982) study of CV transitions. The diagrams are somewhat idealized because CV transition values were used to generate VC transitions. The results show that the transitions do not point toward one locus for each place of articulation. Instead, the transitions differ depending on the F_2 level of the vowel. For example, note that the transition levels for the front vowels, /i/ and /æ/, decrease from the velar to the alveolar to the bilabial stops. This relationship holds for all the vowels except the rounded ones. As shown in Figure 6–7, transition levels for the /u/ vowel are still lowest for the bilabials, but they are reversed for the alveolar and velar sounds. Listeners can identify the place of articulation of stops just by hearing the vowel transitions, with no spike or aspiration noise (Liberman et al., 1954; Delattre et al., 1955; Sharf & Hemeyer, 1972). The same can be said for the place identification of fricatives and nasals. In the vowels of deaf adolescents, F_2 transitions are reduced in frequency and duration, which may be an important factor in the low intelligibility of their speech (Monsen, 1976a).

The cues and processes involved in stop consonant perception are a matter of controversy. Some studies of natural and synthetic speech have found F_2 transitions insufficient for place identification (Ohde & Sharf, 1977, 1981; Ohde, 1988b). Other researchers have proposed that place identification of stops is based on invariant acoustic properties that are independent of context (Blumstein & Stevens, 1979; Kewley-Port, 1983). These acoustic properties are similar to the spectral shapes illustrated in Figure 6–4.

Figure 6–7
A schematic representation of second formant transitions for bilabial /p, b/, alveolar /t, d/, and velar /k, g/ stops in a VCV context, where V is /i/ (upper panel), /æ/ (middle panel), or /u/ (lower panel). In each diagram, the horizontal lines represent F_2. The extensions of each line represent the vowel-to-consonant (VC) transitions and the consonant-to-vowel (CV) transitions.

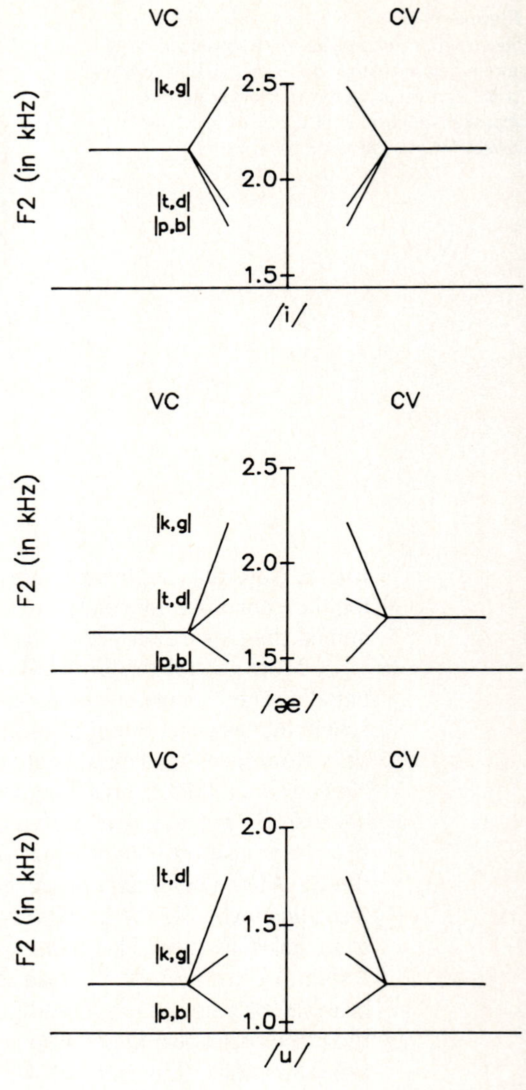

VOICING OF STOP CONSONANTS

Voiced and voiceless stop consonants can be differentiated. This distinction relates to the presence or absence of vocal fold vibration during stop production, particularly during closure. When the oral cavity is completely closed, vibrating the vocal folds is a problem for the articulatory system. In order for the folds to vibrate, there must be a continuing flow of air from the lungs. With the vocal tract closed, the flow cannot be continued unless the vocal tract is expanded. There are a few ways that this can be done. One you can observe for yourself. Place your finger on your thyroid cartilage and say 'boy,' making sure that you phonate right after you bring the lips together and before you release the closure. During the closure, you will feel the cartilage being lowered, which indicates the lowering of the larynx. The vocal tract between the level of the larynx and the bilabial closure is being elongated. This elongation mechanism, perhaps together with others, permits continuing phonation even into a closed oral cavity.

Phonation during closure is a cue to voicing in stops, and was observed in the earliest spectrographic analyses of speech (Potter, Kopp, & Green, 1947). It has been noted that making a glottal tone in a closed oral cavity in stop production is difficult for foreign speakers of English (Tiffany & Carrell, 1977). It is apparently not too easy for native speakers, either, because there is some question as to how frequently they start vocal fold vibration before the release for voiced stops. Some phoneticians believe that vocal fold vibration is present during at least part of the closure period (Heffner, 1952; Tiffany & Carrell, 1977). On the other hand, Bronstein (1960) indicates that prevocalic voiced stops are devoiced. On the basis of spectrographic analysis, it has been suggested that a voice bar occurs only occasionally (Dew & Jensen, 1977), occurs often (Shriberg & Kent, 1982), or is only faintly visible (Monsen, 1978) during the voiced stop gap. On the basis of the presence or absence of a voice bar, Lisker and Abramson (1967) found that /p, t, k/ were always voiceless, but /b, d, g/ were voiced or unvoiced. The absence or presence of vocal fold vibration during the closure phase may not be a reliable cue to differentiating prevocalic voiced and voiceless stops. It is easy to understand how the inconsistency of this cue might be a problem for children in the acquisition of a distinction between voiced and voiceless stops. It should be noted that prevoicing frequently occurs for voiced stops preceded by a vowel or a voiced consonant. Although prevoicing is not considered a primary cue in distinguishing voiced and voiceless stops, it is probably perceptually relevant (Klatt, 1975).

VOT, the time between the release of a stop closure and the onset of voicing, is a more reliable cue to stop voicing distinction than the prevoicing represented by the voice bar (Lisker & Abramson, 1967; Winitz, LaRiviere, & Herriman, 1975). For voiced stops, this interval is relatively short, usually between 0 and 20 msec. VOT of this duration is called **short-lag** VOT. If voicing starts before the release, VOT has a negative value. For voiceless stops, VOT is relatively long, usually between 50 and 80 msec. VOT of this duration is called **long-lag** VOT. As was pointed out in Chapter 5, this difference is about what would occur in minimal pairs like 'tie' and 'die.' Studies have shown that VOT differences of this magnitude are reliable cues for distinguishing voiced and voiceless stops. The noise that occurs between the stop release and the onset of voicing is frication and aspiration, and it is, of course, longer in voiceless stops than in voiced stops (Klatt, 1975; Zue, 1976). When preceded by /s/ in words like 'spy,' 'sty,' and 'sky,' the frication and aspiration intervals of voiceless stops are greatly reduced, and VOT is almost the same as for voiced stops.

Clinicians are especially interested in VOT values for children because of children's use of the phonological process of **prevocalic consonant voicing.** The use of this process reduces the distinction between voiced and voiceless consonants, but it is not clear whether the distinction is completely eliminated. There is evidence that

Table 6–2
Stages in the acquisition by children of the normal VOT distinction between voiced (+VD) and voiceless (−VD) stops (Macken & Barton, 1980).

Stage	VOT Distinction
I	No significant difference between VOT for +VD and −VD; both fall within short range appropriate for +VD
II	Significant difference between VOT for +VD and −VD; both fall within short range appropriate for +VD, but at opposite ends
III	VOT is appropriately short for +VD and appropriately long for −VD

children produce voiced and voiceless stops with VOT values that are short and not statistically different (Zlatin & Koenigsknecht, 1976; Macken & Barton, 1980). According to the three-stage model (Macken & Barton, 1980) of VOT development shown in Table 6–2, children first go through a stage in which they make no significant distinction between voiced and voiceless stops, then a stage in which there is a significant difference between stops that falls within the short range of VOT appropriate for voiced stops, and finally a stage in which the stops are distinguished by VOT in a manner that is analogous to that used by adults. Even though a distinction is made by the children, detecting the difference in the second stage is still difficult because the limited range of VOT makes all the stops sound voiced to adults.

Although VOT appears to be a primary cue to stop consonant voicing in prevocalic position, the situation is quite different in postvocalic position, as in 'heat' and 'heed.' If the stop is produced with a release, then the pressure buildup and postrelease phases include voicing cues. This is evident from Figures 6–8 and 6–9, which show spectrograms of /t/ and /d/ produced with releases. During the stop closure following the end of the vowel, there is a voice bar for /d/ but not for /t/. Also, the releases are quite different. The spike for /t/ is followed by fill, which reflects the frication expected at the release of a voiceless stop. The spike for /d/ is followed almost immediately by formants, which reflect the schwa-like vowel produced at the release of a voiced stop.

If the stops are not released, then the cues in the release are missing, as you can see in the spectrograms of 'heat' and 'heed' spoken without releases. With no release, there is no buildup phase and, of course, no voicing during it. The obvious difference between the two vowels is that the one preceding /d/ is considerably longer than the one preceding /t/. This difference was discussed in describing the allophones of the vowel phonemes. As was noted in Chapter 4, vowels are longer preceding voiced than preceding voiceless consonants (House & Fairbanks, 1953; Peterson & Lehiste, 1960; House, 1961). This difference is a substantial cue to distinguishing voiced and voiceless stops (Raphael, 1972; Krause, 1982b; Lehman, 1988).

Another difference between the vowels preceding voiced and voiceless stops is that the F_1 offset frequency of the vowel is typically lower for voiced than for voiceless stops. This cue interacts with vowel height, so that lower F_1 energy at vowel offset is more salient perceptually for low vowels than for high vowels (Hillenbrand, Ingrisano,

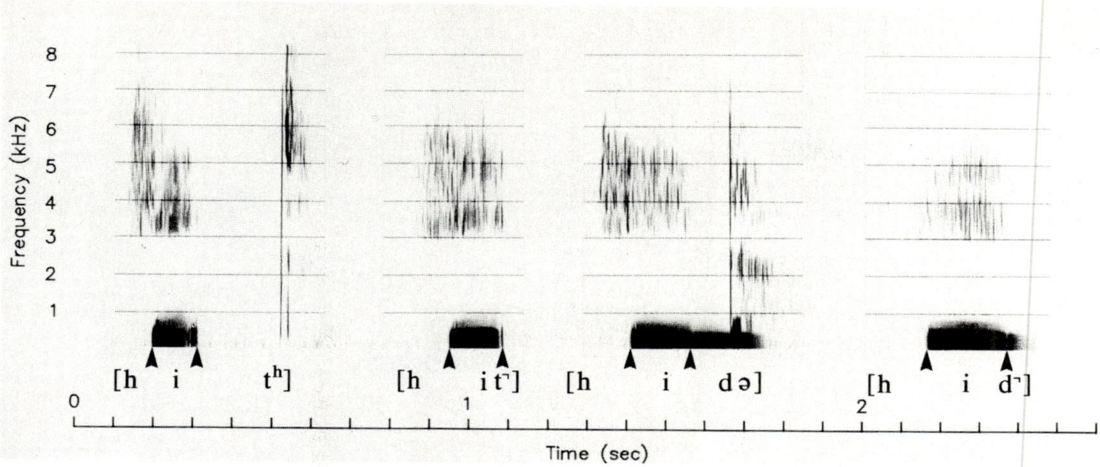

Figure 6–8
Spectrograms of a child's productions of released and unreleased stops in 'heat' and 'heed.' Arrows along the *x* axis indicate onsets and offsets of vowels.

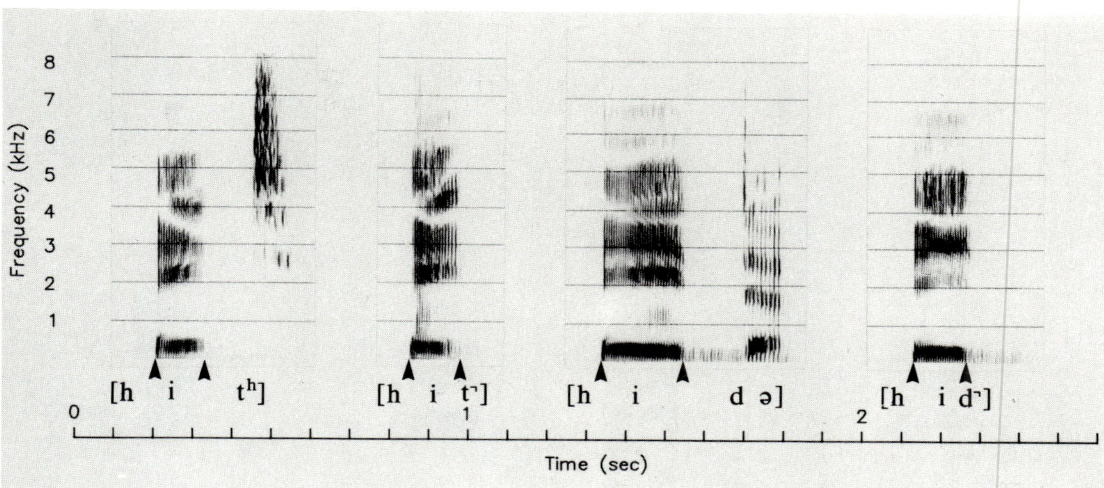

Figure 6–9
Spectrograms of an adult male's productions of released and unreleased stops in 'heat' and 'heed.' Arrows along the *x* axis indicate onsets and offsets of vowels.

Smith, & Flege, 1984; Fischer & Ohde, 1985, 1986). Comparing figures 6–8 and 6–9 for the /i/ vowel with figures 6–10 and 6–11 for the /æ/ vowel shows that the difference between F_1 offset frequency for voiced and voiceless stops is considerably greater for /hæd/ and /hæt/ than for /hid/ and /hit/.

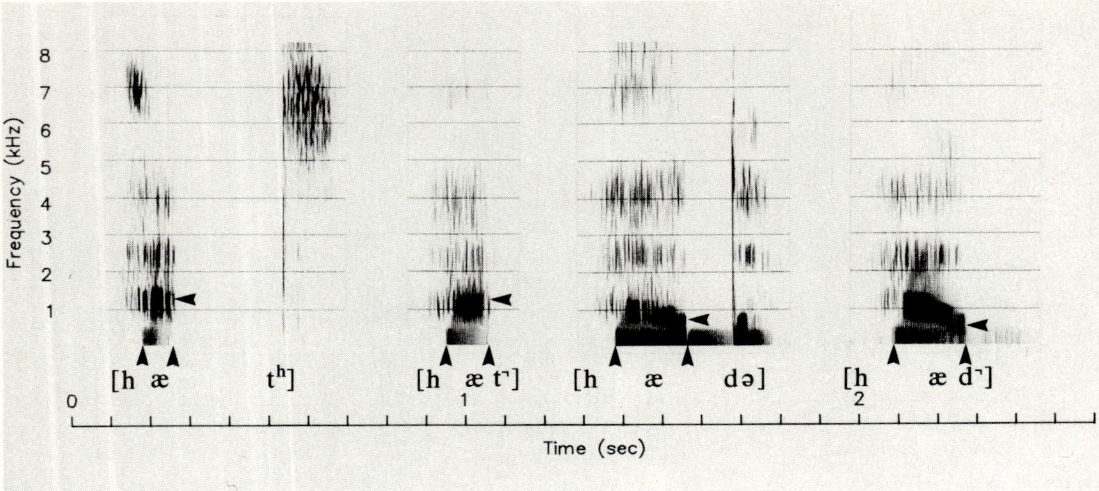

Figure 6–10
Spectrograms of a child's productions of released and unreleased stops in 'hat' and 'had.' Arrows along the *x* axis indicate onsets and offsets of vowels. Arrows along the *y* axis indicate the approximate position of F_1.

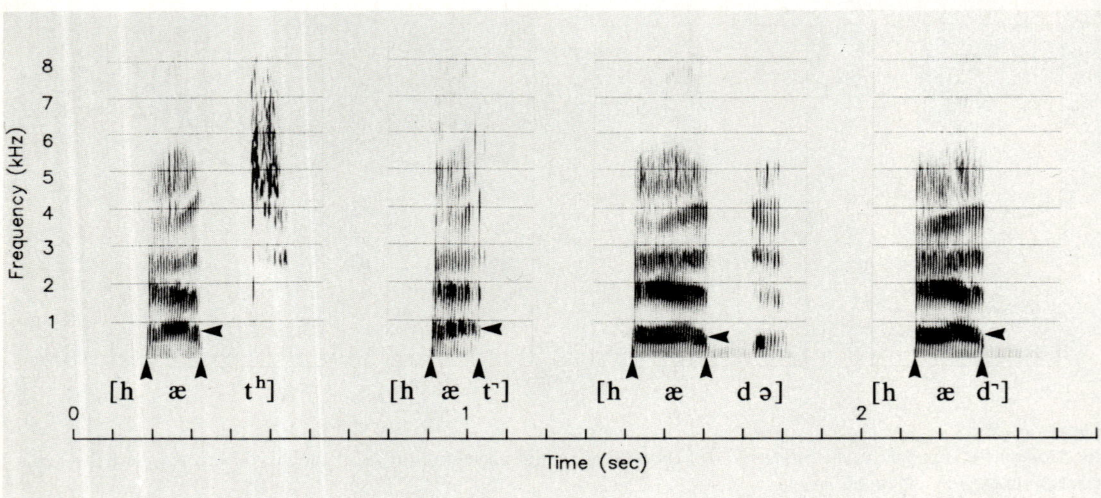

Figure 6–11
Spectrograms of an adult male's productions of released and unreleased stops in 'hat' and 'had.' Arrows along the *x* axis indicate onsets and offsets of vowels. Arrows along the *y* axis indicate the approximate position of F_1.

ALLOPHONES OF STOPS

Variants of All Stops

Table 6–3 gives examples of contextual influences that produce **variants** of all stops. All voiced stops are normally unaspirated in English, but voiceless stops are aspirated and unaspirated. As indicated in Table 6–3, /p, t, k/ are generally aspirated in words like 'peel,' 'appeal,' 'tire,' 'attire,' 'count,' and 'account.' When /s/ precedes any of these stops in the same syllable, however, the stop is unaspirated, as in 'spy' and 'aspire'; 'sty' and 'astound'; and 'sky' and 'askew.' Aspiration is indicated with a superscript /h/, as in [p^{h}ɑɪ] 'pie.' Absence of aspiration can be indicated by using no diacritic or by using a raised equal sign, as in [sp$^{=}$ɑɪ] 'spy.' Although the occurrence of unaspirated stops can be predicted following /s/ in English, it may be useful to note a lack of aspiration in children who voice prevocalic stops. Aspirated and unaspirated stops are allophones of their phonemes.

Released and unreleased allophones occur for each of the stops. In postvocalic position at the end of words produced in isolation, or at the end of a phrase or sentence, these allophones are in free variation. This means that context does not compel the speaker to use either variant, but some speakers release the stops, while others do not. It appears that most speakers do not release stops in these contexts. Doing so tends to sound overprecise. An unreleased stop can be indicated by a superscript angle bracket symbol, as in [sit˺] 'seat' or [sid˺] 'seed.' Release of a voiceless stop can be shown by a superscript /h/, as in [sit^{h}] 'seat,' and release of a voiced stop can be shown by using a schwa vowel symbol, as in [sidə] 'seed.' The schwa of the release can be more or less prominent. If it tends to be weak, you may use a superscript schwa.

Table 6–3
Contexts that produce common allophones of all stop sounds of American English. [C^{h}] represents aspirated stop release, [C$^{=}$] unaspirated stop release, [C˺] unreleased stop, and [Cə] voiced stop release.

	Context		
Phoneme	Syllable Onset	Preceded by /s/	Word-final[a]
/p/	[p^{h}] peal, appeal	[p$^{=}$] spy, aspire	[p˺]; [p^{h}] hop
/b/	[b] bout, about	–	[b˺]; [bə] hub
/t/	[t^{h}] tire, attire	[t$^{=}$] sty, astound	[t˺]; [t^{h}] hut
/d/	[d] do, ado	–	[d˺]; [də] had
/k/	[k^{h}] count, account	[k$^{=}$] sky, askew	[k˺]; [k^{h}] hack
/g/	[g] go, ago	–	[g˺]; [gə] hog

[a]Released and unreleased variants are in free variation, but the unreleased variant may be more common.

There are two contexts in which released stops are unlikely to occur. They are: (1) word-final position in the first morpheme of a compound word in which the following sound is a consonant, like /p/ in 'cupcake,' /b/ in 'rubdown,' /t/ in 'hotdog,' /d/ in 'bedbug,' /k/ in 'lockjaw,' and /g/ in 'ragtime'; and (2) syllable-final position in the first syllable in words of two or more syllables in which the following sound is a consonant, like /p/ in 'aptitude,' /b/ in 'abdicate,' /t/ in 'atmosphere,' /d/ in 'advertise,' /k/ in 'active,' and /g/ in 'ignore.' In all of these cases, the transition between stop and following consonant is simplified by not releasing the stop and shifting the articulators to the following consonant before continuing the flow of speech. You can appreciate the difference by saying these examples both ways. Speakers rarely release stops in these contexts.

Variants of Alveolar and Velar Stops

Table 6–4 presents allophones of alveolar and velar stops. When alveolar stops precede /θ/ and /ð/, the articulatory system anticipates the apico-interdental contact, and the tongue contact for /t/ and /d/ changes to an interdental or dental one. This change occurs in words like 'eighth' and 'width' and in phrases like 'hit the ball' and 'feed the pigeons.' This allophone is indicated by using the IPA dentalization diacritic, as in [et̪θ] 'eighth' and [wɪd̪θ] for 'width.' These dentalized allophones facilitate the transition between /t/ and /d/ and apico-interdental fricatives, as you can observe by trying to say 'eighth' with an apico-alveolar /t/.

In intervocalic position following a stressed syllable, the distinction between /t/ and /d/ has been greatly reduced in the American English pronunciation of minimal pairs like 'kitty'/'kiddie,' 'medal'/'metal,' 'matter'/'madder,' and 'waiting'/'wading.' As illustrated by the spectrograms of 'bitter,' 'bidder,' 'matter,' and 'madder' in figures 6–12 and 6–13, the closure for /t/ is generally no longer than it is for /d/ (Zue & Laferriere, 1979), there is no more voicing during the closure for /d/ than for /t/, and there is no more frication/

Table 6–4
Contexts that produce allophones of alveolar and velar stops of American English.

Phoneme	Context and Variant			
	Front Vowels Palatal	Back Vowels Velar	Preceding /θ/ and /ð/ Dental	Intervocalic[a] Voiced
/t/	–	–	[t̪] eighth; hit the ball	[ɾ]; [tʰ] bitter, catty
/d/	–	–	[d̪] width; feed the pigeons	[ɾ]; [d] bidder, caddy
/k/	[k⁺] key	[k] coo	–	–
/g/	[g⁺] geese	[g] goose	–	–

[a][ɾ] is much more common than [tʰ] or [d].

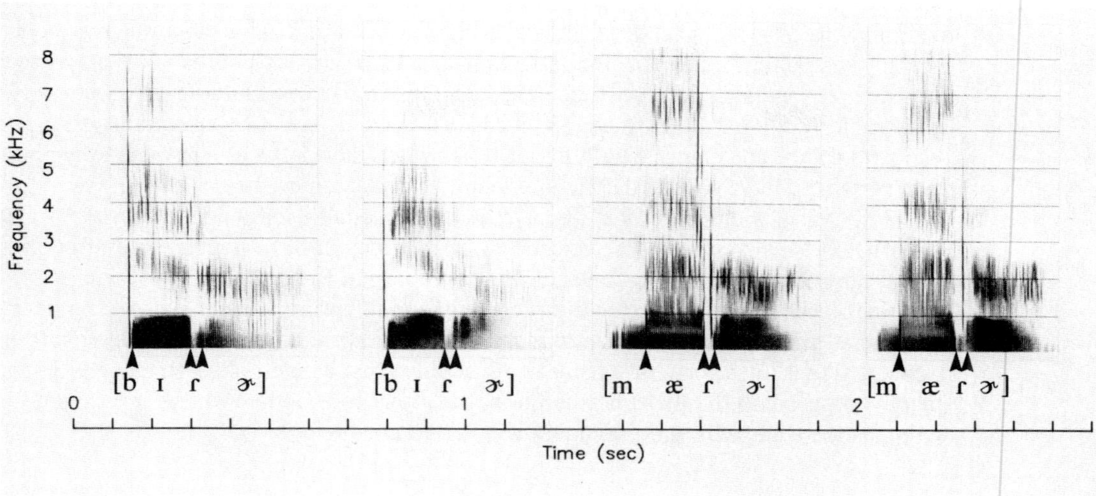

Figure 6–12
Spectrograms of a child's productions of 'bitter,' 'bidder,' 'matter,' and 'madder.' The first and second arrows along the x axis indicate vowel durations: 152 msec for 'bitter,' 148 msec for 'bidder,' 152 msec for 'matter,' and 144 msec for 'madder.' The second and third arrows indicate consonant closure durations of 24 msec for all four words.

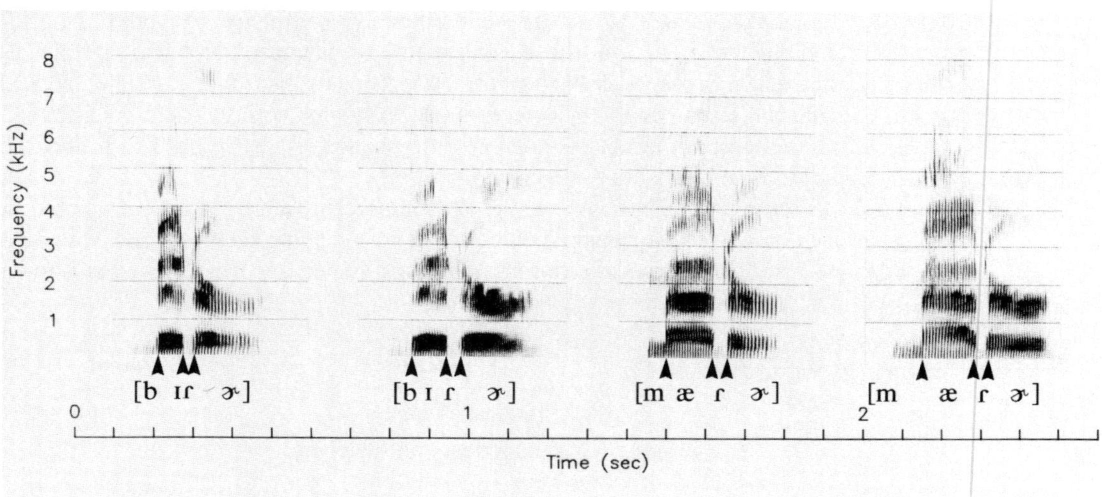

Figure 6–13
Spectrograms of an adult male's productions of 'bitter,' 'bidder,' 'matter,' and 'madder.' The first and second arrows along the x axis indicate vowel durations of 64 msec for 'bitter,' 88 msec for 'bidder,' 120 msec for 'matter,' and 136 msec for 'madder.' The second and third arrows indicate consonant closure durations of 24 msec for 'bitter,' 32 msec for 'bidder,' 40 msec for 'matter,' and 32 msec for 'madder.'

aspiration on the release of /t/ than on the release of /d/. The changes are not restricted to minimal pairs. They also occur in words like 'city,' 'lady,' 'batter,' and 'muddy.' About the only distinction that remains between /t/ and /d/ in this context is that vowels preceding /t/ are shorter than those preceding /d/ for many adults (Sharf, 1962). No comparable study has been made of children's speech, but it is interesting that the child's utterances in Figure 6–12 do not reflect the adult pattern. This same phenomenon of reduction in voicing distinction does not occur for /p, b/ or /k, g/.

Phoneticians differ in their description of the sound used for intervocalic /t/ and /d/. It has been described as a "voiced /t/" (Bronstein, 1960), though more often as a flap (Tiffany & Carrell, 1977; Calvert, 1980; Shriberg & Kent, 1982). The contact is so brief that vocal fold vibration for the preceding and following vowels may not be interrupted, and not enough air pressure is built up to produce a burst when the closure is released. The IPA symbol for a flap can be used for this variant (see Table 6–4). Thus, [læɾɚ] represents the pronunciation of both 'latter' and 'ladder' when they cannot be distinguished except by the preceding vowel duration.

PHONOLOGICALLY ABNORMAL VARIANTS

Prevocalic Voicing

As part of normal speech development, children produce voiceless stops that do not differ from voiced stops in VOT, so that adults perceive /b/ for /p/, /d/ for /t/, and /g/ for /k/. Some children persist in these errors and are diagnosed as having misarticulations. Traditionally, errors of this type were classified as substitutions. In phonological process terminology, however, these errors are examples of prevocalic voicing (see Table 6–5). This process is not confined to stop sounds; it also applies to prevocalic fricatives, as in /zup/ for 'soup.'

As with other phonological processes, it is important to have evidence whether a child is aware of the need for a distinction between voiced and voiceless stops. One type of evidence is the child's use of different VOTs for voiced and voiceless stops, even

Table 6–5
Stop changes due to phonological processes.

Process	Change
Prevocalic voicing	/du/ or [t⁼u] for 'to'
Final consonant deletion	[pɪː] or /pɪ/ for 'pig'
Final consonant devoicing	[pɪːk] or /pɪk/ for 'pig'
Fronting	/do/ for 'go'
Labial assimilation	/bebu/ for 'table'
Alveolar assimilation	/dɔdi/ for 'doggie'
Velar assimilation	/kek/ for 'take'

though all fall within the short range normally used by adults for voiced stops. In other words, a child might be at Macken and Barton's (1980) stage II of VOT development (shown in Table 6–2).

The distinction between stops with small VOT differences is difficult for speakers of English to hear since there is no phonemic difference between them. Maxwell and Weismer (1982) describe the case of a boy with many substitutions of voiced for voiceless obstruents, which include stops and fricatives. The boy's word-initial productions of voiceless obstruents were identified by eleven speech pathology students as 70% voiced. Yet spectrographic analysis revealed statistically significant differences between the mean VOT durations of the voiced and voiceless productions, which were 9 msec and 43 msec, respectively; 43 msec falls slightly beyond the range adults use for voiced stops.

It would be most desirable if each speech pathologist could determine that a particular child was really differentiating voiced and voiceless stops even if they sounded alike to the undiscriminating listener. Careful comparison of many words with intended voiced and voiceless stops is needed, particularly if no sound spectrograph is available. The discrimination exercises at the end of this chapter should help you learn to perceive the distinction between stops varying in VOT.

Practically it may be easier to approach the problem as one of differentiating between aspirated and unaspirated rather than between voiceless and voiced (Compton & Hutton, 1980). You can use your own pronunciation of words like 'spy,' 'sty,' and 'sky' in order to learn the distinction between aspirated and unaspirated stops. For example, by elongating the /s/ sound in 'spy' and then bringing the lips together to produce the rest of the word, you will produce an unaspirated voiceless stop. Your production can be improved even more by preparing to say /s/ in 'spy' but shifting to the /p/ position and saying the word without /s/. This should sound different from how you say 'pie' and 'buy.' The same approach can be used with 'sty,' 'tie,' and 'die,' and with 'skill,' 'kill,' and 'gill.'

The same approach can be used to evaluate the speech of a child who is suspected of voicing initial stops. You need to decide if his/her productions of /p/, /t/, and /k/ words really sound like intended /b/, /d/, and /g/ words. Have the child say minimal pairs like 'tie'/'die,' 'pie'/'buy,' and 'kill'/'gill' and listen very carefully for any distinction in the duration of VOT. If there is a consistent difference, no matter how small, then the child may be making a voicing distinction.

If the child also omits the /s/ of words like 'spy,' then compare his/her productions of 'spy,' 'pie,' and 'buy.' According to Bond and Wilson (1980), children who delete /s/ in words like 'spy' use an aspirated or unaspirated /p/. If 'pie' sounds more like 'spy' than 'buy,' then the child is either producing the stop in 'pie' correctly or making a minimal VOT distinction, stage II in the VOT development model (Macken & Barton, 1980). When a child omits the /s/ of words like 'spy,' it is worthwhile noting whether the /p/ is aspirated, [pʰɑɪ], or unaspirated, [p⁼ɑɪ].

In addition to VOT, fundamental frequency (f_0) serves to differentiate voiced and voiceless stops. As illustrated in figures 6–14 and 6–15, f_0 at vowel onset is relatively high when preceded by voiceless aspirated and unaspirated stops and relatively low when preceded by voiced stops (Ohde, 1984, 1985). This f_0 cue is perceptually impor-

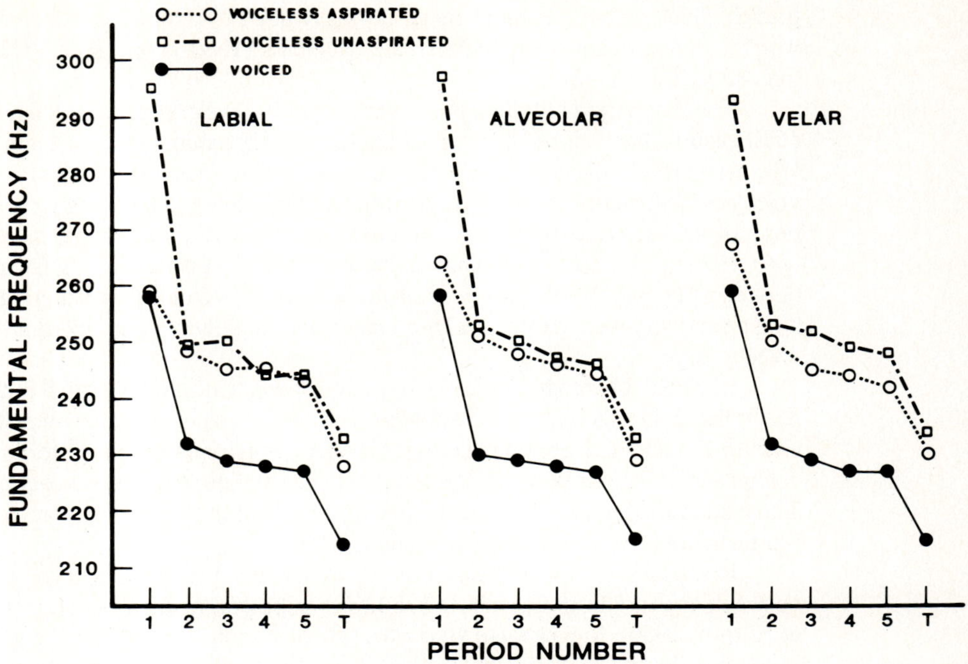

Figure 6–14
Mean fundamental frequency (f_0) of 8- to 9-year-old children from voicing onset to vowel target (T) for voiceless aspirated, voiceless unaspirated, and voiced stops, according to place of articulation. Each period number refers to one cycle of vocal fold vibration after voicing onset.
Source: "Fundamental Frequency Correlates of Stop Consonant Voicing and Vowel Quality in the Speech of Preadolescent Children" by R.N. Ohde, 1985, *Journal of the Acoustical Society of America, 78,* p. 1557. Copyright 1985 by the Acoustical Society of America.

tant for both adult and child listeners (Haggard, Summerfield, & Roberts, 1981; Bernstein, 1983). Although it is not clear if VOT or f_0 is more important in differentiating voiced from voiceless stops, speech and language pathologists should be aware of their cue potential and should learn to perceive these distinctions.

Final Consonant Deletion

In traditional analysis, **final consonant deletion** is classified as an omission of each phoneme affected, and therapy more than likely focuses on achieving correct production of each phoneme. With a phonological process approach the stress is initially placed on achieving syllable closure, no matter what consonant is used (Weiner, 1981). In working for closure on a word like 'pig,' /pɪd/ would be accepted as an initial improvement over /pɪ/ even though the place of articulation is incorrect.

Deletion of final stops, as, for example, in the use of /bi/ for 'bead,' involves the elimination of the contrast between closed and open syllables 'bee' and 'bead' as well as the elimination of the voicing contrast between 'bead' and 'beat.' This process is commonly found in the speech of misarticulating children (Ingram, 1976). Acoustic studies

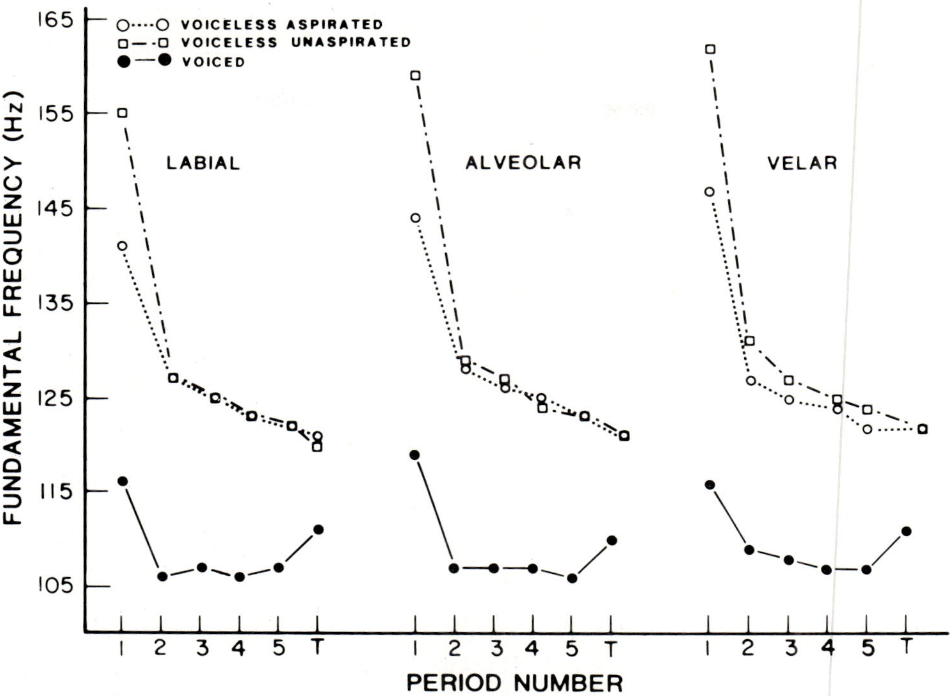

Figure 6–15
Mean fundamental frequency (f_0) of adult males from voicing onset to vowel target (T) for voiceless aspirated, voiceless unaspirated, and voiced stops, according to place of articulation. Each period number refers to one cycle of vocal fold vibration after voicing onset.
Source: "Fundamental Frequency as an Acoustic Correlate of Stop Consonant Voicing" by R.N. Ohde, 1984, *Journal of the Acoustical Society of America, 75,* p. 227. Copyright 1984 by the Acoustical Society of America.

have shown that some of these children use differential vowel duration to signal the voicing characteristics of final stops (Weismer, Dinnsen, & Elbert, 1981; Weismer, 1984). This evidence, plus the use of morphophonemic alternations like [pɪː] for 'pig' and /pɪgi/ for 'piggy,' suggests that the children have an underlying knowledge that 'pig' includes a final consonant (Weismer et al., 1981; Elbert & Gierut, 1986).

Acoustic evidence for an underlying knowledge of final stops is indirect. The presumption is that use of any feature of a consonant indicates underlying knowledge of it. Thus a child who omits final consonants but makes the vowel longer when the following consonant is voiced than when it is voiceless is presumably demonstrating awareness of final consonants. Evidence of this kind was presented by Weismer (1984) for five children who omitted final stops. Four of the children produced vowels that were significantly longer preceding intended voiced stops than those preceding intended voiceless stops. The mean differences between vowels were as substantial as those found in normal speech, and the mean ratio of prevoiceless stop vowel duration over prevoiced stop vowel duration was 0.65, which is very close to what is expected in the normal speech of children and adults (Peterson & Lehiste, 1960; Naeser, 1970b;

Lehman, 1988). The important point for the phonetic analysis of the speech of children who delete final stops is to note whether the vowels preceding omitted final consonants are comparable in duration to those for vowels preceding voiced and voiceless stops. Saying [pɪ:] for 'pig' and [pɪ] for 'pick' indicates awareness of an appropriate vowel duration differential for stop consonant voicing.

It is also possible for children who omit final consonants to move the articulators toward the correct closure positions for bilabial, alveolar, and velar stops, even though the contacts are not made. This has been referred to as "groping" toward final consonants (Weismer, 1984). One way of noting this kind of behavior is to use superscript stop symbols after the vowels, which generally denotes uncertainty on the part of the transcriber whether the sound was produced or only attempted. Weismer (1984) proposes the use of spectrographic analysis to measure the vowel formant transitions of children who omit final consonants. By assuming loci for bilabial, alveolar, and velar stops, an attempt could be made to differentiate the transitions for the target sounds on the basis of their trajectories. Do the transitions for each stop phoneme point in the direction of its appropriate locus? Unfortunately, the sophistication of the analysis required to answer this question is beyond the acoustic knowledge of children's normal speech and perhaps also the perceptual ability of speech and language pathologists. Variability in locus values across speakers and vowel contexts is an additional problem in using this measure.

Another indication that a child may be aware of the need for syllable closure is the use of glottal stops to terminate vowels in CV utterances so that the vowel ends abruptly without any auditory cues to the place of articulation. This type of termination can be transcribed as in [pɪˀ] for 'pig.' Since glottal stops can only be voiceless, their use to replace other stops may reflect an awareness of the stop manner but not of its voicing or place characteristics.

Final Consonant Devoicing

In **final consonant devoicing,** children neutralize the distinction between final stops, and 'pick' and 'pig' are both pronounced /pɪk/. This process is apparently not common among children with the most severe articulatory disorders (Hodson & Paden, 1983). Evidence that a child is aware of the voicing distinction would be his/her lengthening of the vowel preceding a target voiced stop, as in [pɪ:k] for 'pig.' There are examples of this type of awareness for some children (Ingram, 1976; Compton & Hutton, 1980). But there is no acoustic evidence to indicate the magnitude of the difference in vowel duration used by children, nor are there sufficient data for conclusions about the significance of the differences. As suggested for final consonant deletion, any vowel duration differences that occur in minimal pairs like 'pig' and 'pick' should be noted.

Fronting, Labial Assimilation, Alveolar Assimilation, and Velar Assimilation

Fronting, labial assimilation, alveolar assimilation, and velar assimilation are grouped together to highlight their similarities and differences (see Table 6–5). Each involves a change in place of consonant articulation, and each is relatively common among children with the most severe articulatory disorders (Hodson & Paden, 1983). In **fronting,** alveolar consonants replace velar ones. For example, /dʌn/ replaces /gʌn/ 'gun.' Nothing in the context explains the substitution. By comparison, labial and velar assimilations (**assimilation** is a phenomenon in which one sound changes to be more like another in the same or a contiguous word) are influenced by other sounds in the same word. **Labial assimilations** involve the substitution of a bilabial for another consonant in the context of a bilabial consonant. For example, in /bebu/ for 'table,' /b/ is substituted for /t/ under the influence of the succeeding /b/.

In back or **velar assimilation,** alveolars change to velars. For example, in /gɔg/ for 'dog,' /g/ is substituted for /d/ because of the /g/ at the end of the word. The same change occurs for the voiceless stop in /kek/ for 'take.' Although this is an unexpected substitution, since it involves the use of a later developing speech sound in preference to an earlier developing one, it occurs commonly in normally developing children. A more expected substitution occurs with the phonological process of alveolar assimilation, which involves the use of alveolars for velars. For example, /t/ replaces /k/ in 'cat' due to the influence of the final /t/, and /d/ replaces /g/ in 'doggie' due to the influence of the initial /d/.

STOP VARIANTS IN CLEFT-PALATE SPEECH

The stop productions in the speech of individuals with cleft palate are so unique that they are dealt with separately (see Table 6–6). Since people with cleft palates cannot produce normal velopharyngeal closure, stop production is very difficult. First, air pressure buildup behind the stop closure is precluded by the flow of air through the nasal cavity. Second, air released after the stop burst also tends to flow out of the nasal

Table 6–6
Stop variants in cleft-palate speech.

	Release Variant		Contact Variant	
Phoneme	Nasal Plosion	Nasal Friction	Glottal[a]	Pharyngeal
/p/	[p̃ʰũ]	[ʰp̃ʰũ]	[ʔp̃ʰũ]	–
/b/	[b̃ũ]	[ʰb̃ũ]	–	–
/t/	[t̃ʰũ]	[ʰt̃ʰũ]	[ʔt̃ʰũ]	–
/d/	[d̃ũ]	[ʰd̃ũ]	–	–
/k/	[k̃ʰũ]	[ʰk̃ʰũ]	[ʔk̃ʰũ]	[K̃ʰũ]
/g/	[g̃ũ]	[ʰg̃ũ]	–	[G̃ũ]

[a]Glottal stops may accompany or replace bilabial, alveolar, and velar stops; omit stop symbol to indicate replacement.

cavity. The escape of air during the stop closure can be shown by using a superscript /h/ preceding the stop symbol, as in [^{h}t^{h}u] 'two'; the occurrence of this escape of air depends on the severity of the cleft-palate problem. Air escaping through the nasal cavity after the burst and nasalization of the vowel can be transcribed with the nasalizing diacritic above the stop and vowel symbols, as in [t̃^{h}ũ] 'two.' Due to the loss of air pressure and the flow of air through the nasal cavity, stop sounds produced in cleft-palate speech are very weak. These problems relating to the manner of stop articulation are primary since they result from efforts to build up pressure.

An alternate way to cope with a deficient velopharyngeal mechanism is used by some individuals with cleft palates. Since the problem in producing normal bilabial, alveolar, and velar stops is that air escapes posterior to these closures, some individuals produce stops using closures posterior to the leaky velopharyngeal port. Two articulatory closures are used, the glottal and the dorsopharyngeal, which may be called glottalization and pharyngealization. In each case, air pressure can be built up by blocking air before it has a chance to escape through the nasal cavity. In using a glottal stop, cleft-palate speakers may or may not make the expected articulatory contact. In Table 6–6, the possibilities are shown, as in [ʔt^{h}u] 'two,' which can be simplified to [ʔu] if there is no alveolar contact.

Although the dorsopharyngeal contact may seem difficult to make, the effort may be a small price to pay for achieving some degree of control over air pressure. The sounds made from this position are probably more like normal /k/ and /g/ than are glottal stops.

ABNORMAL VARIANTS OF HEARING-IMPAIRED SPEECH

Early studies of the speech of the deaf were in agreement that omission and substitution errors are frequent in the production of stops (Hudgins & Numbers, 1942; C. R. Smith, 1973) but disagreed as to the direction of the substitution. On the basis of acoustic evidence, it was found that hearing-impaired children and adolescents produce both voiced and voiceless stops with VOT durations that are more appropriate for voiced stops (Monsen, 1976b). The problem is compounded because /p/ and /t/ are consistently produced without aspiration, so they sound like /b/ and /d/, but both /k/ and /g/ are sometimes produced with and sometimes without aspiration (Monsen, 1976b). Unlike normally hearing children, there is no indication that hearing-impaired children use the lower range of short-lag VOT for voiced stops and the upper range of long-lag VOT for voiceless stops.

In light of the fact that voicing distinction is a problem for more severely hearing-impaired children, it is interesting that some of these individuals also substitute implosive and ejective stops for normal ones. As was pointed out in Chapter 5, an implosive stop reverses normal production. Air bursts into rather than out of the vocal tract when the closure is released. The physiological mechanism for achieving this reversal is not clear for the hearing-impaired speaker, but it undoubtedly involves enlarging the vocal tract during closure. This could be accomplished by lowering the larynx. Since enlargement of the vocal tract decreases air pressure, air bursts into the vocal tract when the closure is released. Ejective stops use double closures, one at the usual place of articulation and another at the vocal folds. Pressure is built up within the vocal tract by raising the larynx so that the vocal tract is made smaller. When the anterior closure at the lips, alveolar ridge, or palate is released, the air bursts out of the oral cavity. These stop sounds are highly unusual in English, and it may be, as suggested by Monsen (1976b), that they are the consequence of exaggerated attempts to produce vocal fold vibration during stop closure. Although the use of ejectives and implosives is abnormal in English, the pattern of their usage may be systematic, that is, they may always be used to substitute for voiced stops.

In regard to place of articulation, the problem stops for hearing-impaired individuals are the velar and alveolar ones. Omissions of these stops are frequent (Hudgins & Numbers, 1942; C. R. Smith, 1973). Of particular interest is the observation of extensive variation in the place of articulation for /k/ and /g/, from an anterior contact at the hard palate to a posterior one at the uvula (Monsen, 1976b). This type of variation, which may be called uvularization, may not cause any problems for intelligibility, but uvular sounds are perceived as misarticulations.

GLOSSARY

Assimilation. The change of one sound to be more like another in the same context.

Closure. A phase in stop consonant production during which the articulators block the oral cavity so that air pressure is increased within it.

Final consonant deletion. A phonological process that results in the omission of word-final consonants; also called postvocalic consonant deletion.

Final consonant devoicing. A phonological process that results in the omission of voicing on word-final consonants; also called postvocalic consonant devoicing.

Fronting. A phonological process that results in the substitution of alveolar consonants for velar consonants.

Labial assimilation. A phonological process that results in a consonant becoming labial due to the contextual influence of a labial consonant.

Locus. Location of the second formant frequency in a vowel transition that is characteristic of a particular place of articulation.

Long-lag. A relatively long VOT, characteristic of voiceless stop consonants.

Postrelease. A phase in stop consonant production during which articulators are moving away from the contact position.

Precontact. A phase in stop consonant production during which articulators are moving toward contact for closure.

Prevocalic consonant voicing. A phonological process that results in the voicing of voiceless consonants in prevocalic position.

Short-lag. A relatively short VOT, characteristic of voiced stop consonants.

Transition. Articulator movement to a consonant from a vowel or to a vowel from a consonant.
Variant. A variation in the production of a speech sound.
Velar assimilation. A phonological process that results in a consonant becoming velar due to the contextual influence of a velar consonant; also called back assimilation.

REVIEW QUESTIONS

A. Insert the word that would result from the following processes.

1. Final consonant devoicing in 'sag' ________________
2. Fronting of first consonant in 'coal' ________________
3. Prevocalic voicing in 'time' ________________
4. Final consonant deletion in 'like' ________________
5. Velar assimilation in 'took' ________________
6. Labial assimilation in 'tumble' ________________
7. Fronting in 'get' ________________
8. Prevocalic voicing in 'coal' ________________

****

Key: 1. sack; 2. toll; 3. dime; 4. lie; 5. cook; 6. bumble; 7. debt; 8. goal

B. Indicate whether the locus for the first sound in a front vowel context is higher (H), lower (L), or the same (S) as for the second sound in each pair.

1. /p/, /k/ ______
2. /t/, /d/ ______
3. /k/, /t/ ______
4. /b/, /g/ ______
5. /p/, /g/ ______
6. /p/, [pʰ] ______
7. /p/, /t/ ______
8. /d/, /p/ ______

****

Key: 1. L; 2. S; 3. H; 4. L; 5. L; 6. S; 7. L; 8. H

C. Indicate the contexts in which the following allophones would occur by inserting the correct letter.

1. [k^{h+}] ________ a. skip
2. [t̪] ________ b. hotdog
3. [ɾ] ________ c. school
4. [$k^{=+}$] ________ d. step
5. [k^{h}] ________ e. sitting
6. [$t^{=}$] ________ f. cool
7. [t˺] ________ g. can
8. [$k^{=}$] ________ h. eighth

****

Key: 1. g; 2. h; 3. e; 4. a; 5. f; 6. d; 7. b; 8. c

D. Indicate typical errors for hearing-impaired (H) and cleft-palate (C) speakers, or those that are typical of both (B) or of neither (N) types by inserting the correct letter.

1. Prevocalic voicing ________
2. Pharyngeal stops ________
3. Nasalized bursts ________
4. Glottal stops ________
5. Fronting ________
6. Ejectives ________
7. Implosives ________
8. Labial assimilation ________

****

Key: 1. H; 2. B; 3. C; 4. C; 5. N; 6. H; 7. H; 8. N

LABORATORY ASSIGNMENT

Tape II, Side B
Sections 1–4: Stop Consonants
IIB1: Prevocalic Stops (Tape running time: 5:47; Elapsed time: 0:00–05:47)

a. Prevocalic Stop Models

Listen to the stop consonants produced in a /Cɪ l/ context by an adult and a child. If necessary, stop the tape at any time, rewind, and listen again.

1. Adult: /pɪ l/; /t ɪ l/; /k ɪ l/
2. Child repeats above.
3. Adult: /bɪ l/; /dɪ l/; /gɪ l/
4. Child repeats above.

b. Transcription of Prevocalic Stops in Minimal Contrast Context

Transcribe the prevocalic stop as it is pronounced by an adult and a child in a minimal contrast context /Cɪ l/.

1. ________ 2. ________ 3. ________ 4. ________ 5. ________

6. ________ 7. ________ 8. ________ 9. ________ 10. ________

11. ________ 12. ________

****

Consensus: 1. /p/ 2. /b/ 3. /d/ 4. /t/ 5. /g/ 6. /k/ 7. /b/ 8. /k/ 9. /d/ 10. /t/ 11. /p/ 12. /g/

Variants: None.

c. Transcription of Prevocalic Stops in a Sentence

Transcribe the prevocalic stop consonant as it is pronounced by an adult and a child in syllables in the sentence 'Say ________ again.'

1. ________ 2. ________ 3. ________ 4. ________ 5. ________

6. ________ 7. ________ 8. ________ 9. ________ 10. ________

11. ________ 12. ________

****

Consensus: 1. /k/ 2. /b/ 3. /d/ 4. /t/ 5. /p/ 6. /g/ 7. /b/ 8. /g/ 9. /t/ 10. /d/ 11. /p/ 12. /k/

Variants: None.

d. Transcription of Prevocalic Stops in Words in Isolation

Transcribe only the prevocalic stop consonants in the words pronounced by an adult and a child.

1. bowl ________ 2. cap ________ 3. time ________ 4. bat ________

5. deal ________ 6. gain ________ 7. calf ________ 8. pail ________

9. tame ________ 10. dole ________ 11. pot ________ 12. game ________

****

Consensus: 1. /b/ 2. /k/ 3. /t/ 4. /b/ 5. /d/ 6. /g/ 7. /k/ 8. /p/ 9. /t/ 10. /d/ 11. /p/ 12. /g/

Variants: None.

e. Transcription of Prevocalic Stops in Words in Sentences

Transcribe only the prevocalic stop consonants as they are pronounced by an adult and a child in words in the following sentences: 'I can say ______'; 'Say the name ______'; '______ is the name.'

1. boy ________	2. ban ________	3. top ________	4. king ________
5. pear ________	6. goat ________	7. cap ________	8. deem ________
9. pet ________	10. dime ________	11. gave ________	12. tome ________

****

Consensus: 1. /b/ 2. /b/ 3. /t/ 4. /k/ 5. /p/ 6. /g/ 7. /k/ 8. /d/ 9. /p/ 10. /d/ 11. /g/ 12. /t/

Variants: None.

IIB2: VOT Distinction (Tape running time: 9:52; Elapsed time: 05:47–15:39)

The purpose of this section is to train students to discriminate and identify the difference between stops with relatively short /b, d, g/ and relatively long [p$^{=}$, t$^{=}$, k$^{=}$] VOT durations.

a. Models of Relatively Short and Long VOT

Listen to the stop consonants as they are pronounced by a child. If necessary, stop the tape at any time, rewind, and listen again.

1. [p$^{=}$ɪl]; /bɪl/
2. [t$^{=}$ɪl]; /dɪl/
3. [k$^{=}$ɪl]; /gɪl/

b. Discrimination of Relatively Short and Long VOT

Listen to the following pairs of syllables produced by a child and indicate if they are the same (S) or different (D).

1. ________	2. ________	3. ________	4. ________	5. ________
6. ________	7. ________	8. ________	9. ________	10. ________
11. ________	12. ________	13. ________	14. ________	15. ________
16. ________	17. ________	18. ________	19. ________	20. ________
21. ________	22. ________	23. ________	24. ________	25. ________
26. ________	27. ________	28. ________	29. ________	30. ________
31. ________	32. ________	33. ________	34. ________	35. ________
36. ________				

****

Key: 1. D 2. S 3. D 4. S 5. D 6. S 7. S 8. D 9. S 10. D 11. S 12. D 13. D
14. D 15. S 16. S 17. D 18. S 19. D 20. S 21. D 22. S 23. S 24. D 25. S
26. D 27. D 28. S 29. D 30. S 31. D 32. S 33. D 34. S 35. D 36. S

c. Transcription of Prevocalic Stops in Minimal Contrast Context

Transcribe only the prevocalic stops pronounced by a child in a minimal contrast context /Cɪl/.

1. ________ 2. ________ 3. ________ 4. ________ 5. ________

6. ________ 7. ________ 8. ________ 9. ________ 10. ________

11. ________ 12. ________ 13. ________ 14. ________ 15. ________

16. ________ 17. ________ 18. ________

****

Consensus: 1. [p˭] 2. /b/ 3. [k˭] 4. /d/ 5. [p˭] 6. [t˭] 7. /g/ 8. [t˭]
9. [k˭] 10. [t˭] 11. /b/ 12. [p˭] 13. /d/ 14. [p˭] 15. [t˭]
16. [p˭] 17. /d/ 18. [k˭]

Variants: 7. [k˭] 9. /g/ 10. /d/ 12. [t˭] 14. /b/ 17. [t˭] 18. /g/

d. Transcription of Prevocalic Stops in a Sentence

Transcribe the prevocalic stops pronounced by a child in the sentence 'Say /Cɪl/ again.'

1. ________ 2. ________ 3. ________ 4. ________ 5. ________

6. ________ 7. ________ 8. ________ 9. ________

****

Consensus: 1. [k˭] 2. [t˭] 3. /b/ 4. /d/ 5. [p˭] 6. [t˭] 7. [k˭] 8. [p˭]
9. /g/

Variants: 2. [p˭]

e. Transcription of Prevocalic Stops in Words

Transcribe the prevocalic stops pronounced by a child in words in isolation.

1. bowl ________ 2. tock ________ 3. cap ________ 4. time ________

5. Kate ________ 6. bat ________ 7. deal ________ 8. gain ________

9. pill ________ 10. calf ________ 11. pail ________ 12. pin ________

13. tame ________ 14. dole ________ 15. teal ________ 16. pot ________

17. game ________ 18. Kate ________

****

Consensus: 1. /b/ 2. $[t^{=}]$ 3. $[k^{=}]$ 4. $[t^{=}]$ 5. $[k^{=}]$ 6. /b/ 7. /d/ 8. $[k^{=}]$ 9. $[p^{=}]$ 10. $[k^{=}]$ 11. $[p^{=}]$ 12. $[p^{=}]$ 13. $[t^{h}]$ 14. /d/ 15. $[t^{=}]$ 16. $[p^{h}]$ 17. /g/ 18. $[k^{=}]$

Variants: 8. $[k^{h}]$ 17. $[k^{=}]$

f. Transcription of Prevocalic Stops in Words in Sentences

Transcribe the prevocalic stops pronounced by a child in words in one of the following sentences: 'I can say ________'; 'Say the word ________'; '________ is the word.'

1. boy ________ 2. peek ________ 3. cape ________ 4. ban ________

5. top ________ 6. king ________ 7. pin ________ 8. pear ________

9. goat ________ 10. core ________ 11. cap ________ 12. deem ________

13. pet ________ 14. tamp ________ 15. dime ________ 16. gave ________

17. tore ________ 18. tome ________

****

Consensus: 1. /b/ 2. $[p^{=}]$ 3. $[k^{=}]$ 4. /b/ 5. $[t^{h}]$ 6. $[k^{=}]$ 7. $[p^{=}]$ 8. $[p^{=}]$ 9. /g/ 10. /g/ 11. $[k^{=}]$ 12. /d/ 13. $[p^{=}]$ 14. $[t^{=}]$ 15. /d/ 16. /g/ 17. $[t^{=}]$ 18. $[t^{=}]$

Variants: 6. /g/ 7. $[p^{h}]$ 10. $[k^{=}]$ 11. $[t^{=}]$

IIB3: Postvocalic Stops (Tape running time: 8:11; Elapsed time: 15:39–23:50)

The purpose of this section is to train students to discriminate and identify place of articulation of released and unreleased postvocalic stop consonants.

a. Stop Consonant Models

Listen to the released and unreleased stop consonants as they are pronounced in a minimal contrast context by an adult and a child.

1. Adult: /tæp/; [tæp̚]; /tæt/; [tæt̚]; /tæk/; [tæk̚]
2. Child repeats above.
3. Adult: /tæb/; [tæb̚]; /tæd/; [tæd̚]; /tæg/; [tæg̚]
4. Child repeats above.

b. Discrimination of Place of Articulation of Unreleased Stops

Listen to the following pairs of syllables produced by a child and indicate if they are the same (S) or different (D).

1. ________ 2. ________ 3. ________ 4. ________ 5. ________
6. ________ 7. ________ 8. ________ 9. ________ 10. ________
11. ________ 12. ________ 13. ________ 14. ________ 15. ________
16. ________ 17. ________ 18. ________ 19. ________ 20. ________
21. ________ 22. ________ 23. ________ 24. ________ 25. ________
26. ________ 27. ________ 28. ________ 29. ________ 30. ________

****

Key: 1. D 2. D 3. D 4. D 5. S 6. S 7. S 8. D 9. D 10. S 11. D 12. D 13. D 14. D 15. S 16. S 17. D 18. D 19. D 20. D 21. S 22. D 23. D 24. D 25. D 26. D 27. D 28. D 29. D 30. S

c. Transcription of Postvocalic Stops in Minimal Contrast Context

Transcribe each postvocalic stop as it is pronounced by an adult and a child in a minimal contrast context. You do not need to indicate whether or not the stop is released.

1. ________ 2. ________ 3. ________ 4. ________ 5. ________
6. ________ 7. ________ 8. ________ 9. ________ 10. ________
11. ________ 12. ________

****

Consensus: 1. /p/ 2. /g/ 3. /t/ 4. /g/ 5. /t/ 6. /b/ 7. /k/ 8. /d/ 9. /k/ 10. /b/ 11. /p/ 12. /d/

Variants: None.

d. Transcription of Postvocalic Stops in a Sentence

Transcribe each postvocalic stop as it is pronounced by an adult and a child in a minimal contrast context in a sentence. You do not need to indicate whether or not the stop is released.

1. ________ 2. ________ 3. ________ 4. ________ 5. ________

6. ________ 7. ________ 8. ________ 9. ________ 10. ________

11. ________ 12. ________

****

Consensus: 1. /p/ 2. /t/ 3. /g/ 4. /b/ 5. /g/ 6. /t/ 7. /d/ 8. /k/ 9. /b/ 10. /k/ 11. /d/ 12. /p/

Variants: None.

e. Transcription of Postvocalic Stops in Words in Isolation

Transcribe each postvocalic stop as it is pronounced in a word by an adult and a child. You do not need to indicate whether or not the stop is released.

1. robe ________ 2. hug ________ 3. back ________ 4. chip ________

5. cob ________ 6. bag ________ 7. duck ________ 8. mud ________

9. dog ________ 10. boot ________ 11. web ________ 12. cup ________

****

Consensus: 1. /b/ 2. /g/ 3. /k/ 4. /p/ 5. /b/ 6. /g/ 7. /k/ 8. /d/ 9. /g/ 10. /t/ 11. /b/ 12. /p/

Variants: 12. /0/

f. Transcription of Postvocalic Stops in Words in Sentences

Transcribe each postvocalic stop as it is pronounced by an adult and a child in words in the following sentences: 'I can say ________ '; 'Say the word ________ '; ' ________ is the word.' You do not need to indicate whether or not the stop is released.

1. head ________ 2. brag ________ 3. log ________ 4. rub ________

5. hat ________ 6. glad ________ 7. clock ________ 8. sop ________

9. mop ________ 10. lock ________ 11. cab ________ 12. date ________

****

Consensus: 1. /d/ 2. /g/ 3. /g/ 4. /b/ 5. /t/ 6. /d/ 7. /k/ 8. /p/ 9. /p/ 10. /k/ 11. /b/ 12. /t/

Variants: None.

IIB4: Vowel Duration Distinction (Tape running time: 5:18; Elapsed time: 23:50–29:08)

The purpose of this section is to train students to discriminate and identify the difference between postvocalic voiced and voiceless stops based on preceding vowel duration differences. Target utterances are synthesized speech.

a. Models of Relatively Short and Long Vowel Durations

Listen to the voiced and voiceless stops with vowels of relatively long [bɪ:k] and relatively short /bɪk/ vowel durations pronounced by a child.

1. /bɪk/; [bɪ:k]

b. Discrimination of Relatively Short and Long Vowel Durations

Listen to the following syllable pairs produced by a child and indicate if they are the same (S) or different (D).

1. ________	2. ________	3. ________	4. ________	5. ________
6. ________	7. ________	8. ________	9. ________	10. ________
11. ________	12. ________	13. ________	14. ________	15. ________
16. ________	17. ________	18. ________	19. ________	20. ________
21. ________	22. ________	23. ________	24. ________	25. ________
26. ________	27. ________	28. ________	29. ________	30. ________

****

Key: 1. S 2. D 3. S 4. S 5. S 6. D 7. S 8. D 9. S 10. D 11. S 12. S 13. D 14. S 15. S 16. S 17. S 18. D 19. D 20. S 21. S 22. S 23. S 24. D 25. S 26. S 27. D 28. S 29. D 30. S

c. Transcription of Postvocalic Stops in Minimal Contrast Context

Transcribe each postvocalic stop as either /k/ (short vowel) or /g/ (long vowel) as it is pronounced by a child in a minimal contrast context.

1. ________	2. ________	3. ________	4. ________	5. ________
6. ________	7. ________	8. ________	9. ________	10. ________

****

Consensus: 1. /k/ 2. /k/ 3. /g/ 4. /k/ 5. /g/ 6. /g/ 7. /k/ 8. /g/ 9. /k/ 10. /g/

Variants: None.

d. Transcription of Postvocalic Stops in Syllables in Context

Transcribe each postvocalic stop as either /k/ (short vowel) or /g/ (long vowel) as it is pronounced by a child in a minimal contrast context in the phrase, 'Say ________.'

1. ________ 2. ________ 3. ________ 4. ________ 5. ________

6. ________ 7. ________ 8. ________ 9. ________ 10. ________

****

Consensus: 1. /g/ 2. /k/ 3. /g/ 4. /k/ 5. /g/ 6. /g/ 7. /k/ 8. /g/ 9. /k/ 10. /k/

Variants: None.

e. Transcription of Postvocalic Stops in Syllables in Sentences

Transcribe each postvocalic stop as either /k/ (short vowel) or /g/ (long vowel) as it is pronounced by a child in a minimal contrast context in the following sentences: 'I can say '; 'Say the word ________.'

1. ________ 2. ________ 3. ________ 4. ________ 5. ________

6. ________ 7. ________ 8. ________ 9. ________ 10. ________

****

Consensus: 1. /k/ 2. /g/ 3. /g/ 4. /k/ 5. /k/ 6. /g/ 7. /k/ 8. /k/ 9. /g/ 10. /g/

Variants: None.

Tape III, Side A
IIIA1: Words with Vowels, Glides, and Stops (Tape running time: 3:25; Elapsed time: 00:00–03:25)

The purpose of this section is to provide students with practice in transcribing complete words that include the sounds covered so far—vowels, glides, and stops. Transcribe each word below as it is produced by a child, reversing the tape as needed to listen to an utterance again. You do not need to indicate whether or not the stops have aspiration or are released or unreleased. After you have finished with all the words, check your transcriptions.

1. leaf ________________ 2. belly ________________

3. parrot ________________ 4. cattle ________________

5. bird ________________ 6. let ________________

7. boat ________________ 8. belly ________________

9. tail ________________ 10. dairy ________________

11. lot ____________ 12. dairy ____________

13. bird ____________ 14. wade ____________

15. coat ____________ 16. get ____________

17. lot ____________ 18. dog ____________

19. ray ____________ 20. doctor ____________

21. dairy ____________ 22. leg ____________

23. coat ____________ 24. yellow ____________

25. raid ____________

****

Consensus: 1. /lif/ 2. /bɛwi/ 3. /pɛr˔ət/ 4. [kætl̩] 5. /bɝd/ 6. /jɛt/ 7. /bot/ 8. /bɛwi/ 9. /teo/ 10. /dɛri/ 11. /lɑt/ 12. [dɛr˔i] 13. /bʊd/ 14. /wed/ 15. /kot/ 16. /gɛt/ 17. /wɑt/ 18. /dɔg/ 19. /we/ 20. /dɑktɚ/ 21. /dɛwi/ 22. /lɛg/ 23. /kot/ 24. /jɛlo/ 25. [r˔ed]

Variants: 4. [kærl̩] 8. [bɛr˔i] 13. [wʊd̥] 16. /gɪt/ 17. /wɑp/ 18. /dɑg/ 21. [dɛr˔i] 22. /leg/

IIIA2: Phonological Processes Affecting Stops (Tape running time: 5:27; Elapsed time: 03:25–08:52)

The purpose of this section is to train students to identify the occurrence of common phonological processes that affect stops: fronting, labial assimilation, and velar assimilation.

a. Velar Fronting Process

Indicate whether the stops in the following words produced by a child are fronted (Y) or not (N): 'cup' /kʌp/; 'bigger' /bɪgɚ/; 'back' /bæk/; 'vacuum' /vækjum/; 'king' /kɪŋ/; 'gum' /gʌm/; 'wagon' /wægən/.

1. gum ________ 2. vacuum ________ 3. cup ________

4. back ________ 5. wagon ________ 6. bigger ________

7. vacuum ________ 8. king ________ 9. back ________

10. gum ________ 11. cup ________ 12. king ________

13. back ________ 14. king ________ 15. cup ________

16. gum ________ 17. vacuum ________ 18. bigger ________

****

Consensus: 1. N 2. Y 3. N 4. Y 5. Y 6. N 7. N 8. N 9. N 10. Y 11. Y 12. N 13. N 14. Y 15. N 16. N 17. N 18. N

b. Labial Assimilation Process

Indicate whether the stops in the following words produced by a child are characterized by labial assimilation (Y) or not (N): 'pig' /pɪg/; 'two' /tu/; 'dive' /daɪv/; 'pot' /pɑt/; 'step' /stɛp/; 'muddy' /mʌdi/.

1. muddy ________ 2. two ________ 3. step ________
4. pot ________ 5. dive ________ 6. pig ________
7. pot ________ 8. muddy ________ 9. two ________
10. pig ________ 11. two ________ 12. muddy ________
13. dive ________ 14. step ________ 15. dive ________
16. pig ________ 17. step ________ 18. pot ________

****

Consensus: 1. Y 2. N 3. N 4. Y 5. N 6. N 7. N 8. N 9. Y 10. Y 11. N 12. N 13. Y 14. Y 15. N 16. N 17. N 18. N

c. Velar Assimilation Process

Indicate whether the stops in the following words produced by a child are characterized by velar assimilation (Y) or not (N): 'truck' /trʌk/; 'duck' /dʌk/; 'bag' /bæg/; 'goat' /got/; 'kitten' /kɪtən/; 'grape' /grep/.

1. grape ________ 2. truck ________ 3. bag ________ 4. kitten ________
5. duck ________ 6. bag ________ 7. goat ________ 8. kitten ________
9. truck ________ 10. goat ________ 11. truck ________ 12. duck ________
13. grape ________ 14. goat ________ 15. duck ________ 16. bag ________
17. kitten ________ 18. grape ________

****

Consensus: 1. N 2. N 3. Y 4. N 5. N 6. N 7. N 8. Y 9. Y 10. N 11. N 12. Y 13. N 14. Y 15. N 16. N 17. N 18. Y

CHAPTER 7

Analysis of Fricatives and Affricates

Chapter 6 described physiologic events and acoustic cues that differentiate fricatives from stops and nasals. Like stops, **fricatives** involve interference with airflow through the oral cavity, so they are classified as obstruents. The fricative constriction restricts airflow so that frication noise is produced. This noise appears as fill on sound spectrograms. When vocal fold vibration occurs for voiced fricatives, there are two sound-producing mechanisms operating simultaneously, the glottal production of a tone and the articulatory production of frication noise. As a result, voiced fricatives may display one or more formants representing oral cavity resonance, as well as fill. The relative prominence of fill and formants in spectrograms depends on the relative strength of the two sound sources. Since individual utterances have varying degrees of emphasis on the two sound sources, spectrographic patterns also vary.

DYNAMICS OF PLACE OF ARTICULATION

Fricatives

In Table 7–1, the fricative phonemes of English are shown in minimal pairs. It was necessary to use several different vowel contexts to show contrasts between all the fricatives in prevocalic, intervocalic, and postvocalic positions, even more than were needed for stop contrasts. One reason for this is that there are more fricatives (nine) than there are stops (six). In addition, a few of the fricatives are limited in their occurrence. The phoneme /ʒ/ does not occur prevocalically and only rarely postvocalically; /h/ does not occur postvocalically, and /ð/ occurs in all positions, but not in many words.

Table 7–1
Minimal pair word analysis of the fricative phonemes.

Phoneme	Prevocalic		Intervocalic			Postvocalic		
/f/	fie	—	leafing	—	—	—	roof	leaf
/v/	vie	—	leaving	—	—	—	—	leave
/θ/	thigh	—	—	ether	—	teeth	Ruth	—
/ð/	thy	—	—	either	—	teethe	—	—
/s/	sigh	sue	leasing	—	messer	—	ruse	lease
/z/	—	zoo	—	easer	—	tease	rues	lees
/ʃ/	shy	shoe	leashing	—	mesher	—	ruche	leash
/ʒ/[a]	—	—	—	—	measure	—	rouge	—
/h/[b]	high	who	—	—	—	—	—	—

[a]Does not occur in prevocalic position.
[b]Does not occur in postvocalic position; a partially voiced /h/ occurs in intervocalic position in words like 'ahead.'

Figure 7–1 includes palatograms and X-ray tracings of the articulatory structures involved in the production of /θ/, /s/, /ʃ/, /f/, and /h/. For demonstrating differences in place of articulation, the /θ/, /s/, /f/, and /ʃ/ illustrations apply as well to /ð/, /z/, /v/, and /ʒ/. The lower lip and upper teeth touch for /f/ and /v/. The airflow between the lip and the teeth produces frication noise. Because the tongue is not involved in saying /f/ and /v/, it is free to move toward its position for the following vowel. This process is similar to the articulatory pattern described in Chapter 6 for bilabial stops. Because their articulatory configurations are similar, the acoustic cues in the consonant noise and the vowel transitions are alike for the labiodental fricatives and the bilabial stops.

For the production of /θ/ and /ð/, the tongue tip is inserted between the teeth, which are approximated. The extent of tongue protrusion is not critical as long as the tip approximates the cutting edges of the upper teeth. Frication noise is produced by airflow between the tongue and the upper teeth. For /f/ and /θ/, the soft tissues of the lip and tongue, respectively, contact the cutting edges of the teeth. This type of articulation produces weak fricatives. Probably because they share this acoustic characteristic, /f/ often replaces /θ/, and /v/ often replaces /ð/ in children's speech.

In the production of /s/ the margins of the tongue touch the hard palate, but the middle part and tongue tip do not. If you compare the palatogram for /s/ in Figure 7–1 with the palatogram for /t/ in Figure 6–1, you will see that the contacts are very similar—except that there is tongue tip contact at the alveolar ridge for /t/ but not for /s/. For both /s/ and /z/ a channel is formed between the upper surface of the tongue and the hard palate. Air flows out through this channel and between the cutting edges of the front teeth. Phoneticians differ as to whether the characteristic frication noise of /s, z/ is due to the constriction formed by the teeth (Bronstein, 1960) or to the one formed between the tongue tip and the alveolar ridge (Tiffany & Carrell, 1977). It seems clear, however, that dental problems like underbite, overbite, irregular teeth, and open bite are associated with defective /s, z/ production (Bronstein, 1960; Tiffany & Carrell, 1977). One can infer from this that the cutting edges of the upper and lower teeth need to be approximated for normal /s, z/ articulation. In forming the channel for airflow, it is important that the tongue tip be kept out of the way, for if it touches the teeth or the upper alveolar ridge, the resulting frication noise will be lower in frequency and intensity than is expected for these sounds.

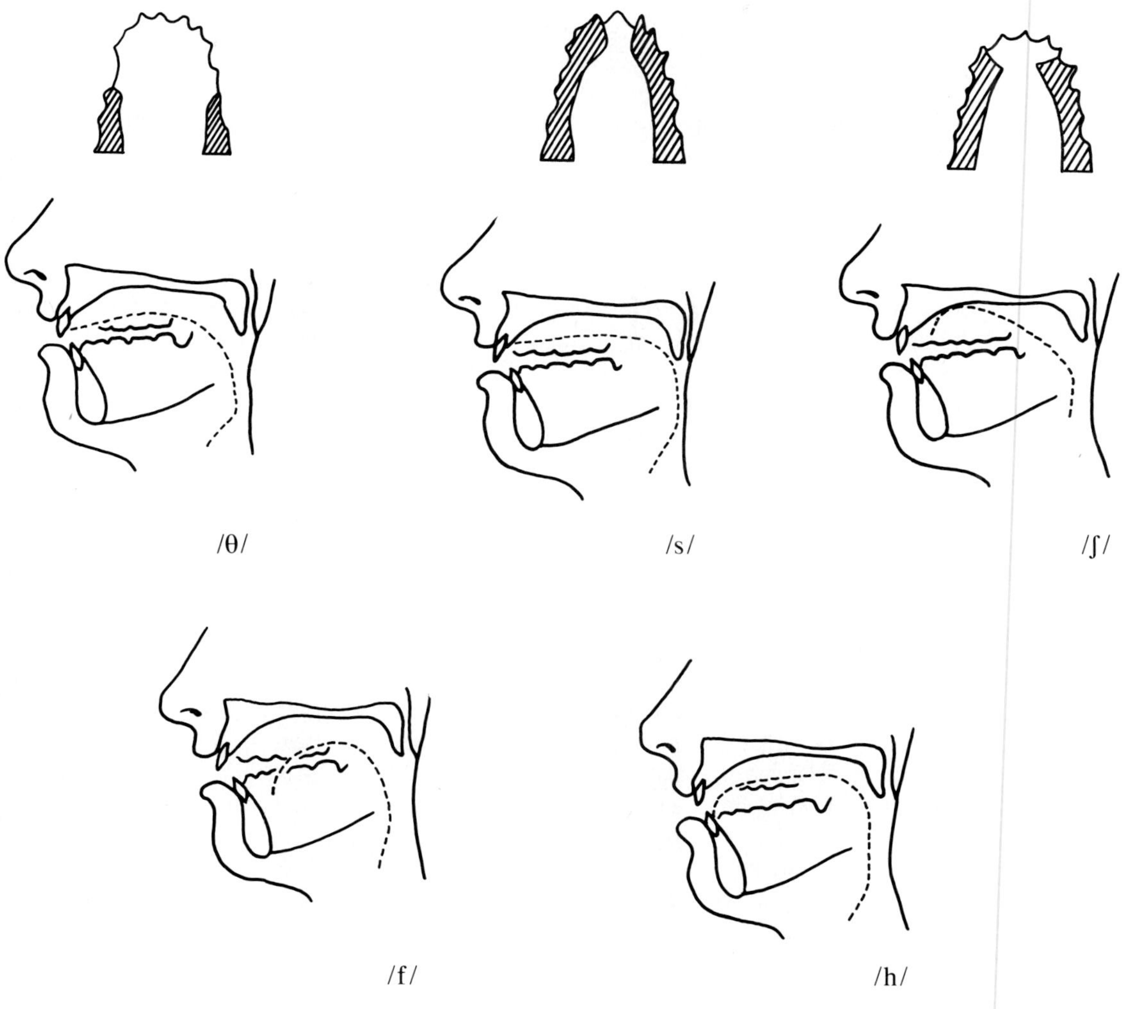

Figure 7–1
Midsagittal X-ray tracings and palatograms of /θ/, /s/, and /ʃ/, and midsagittal tracings of /f/ and /h/. No palatograms are shown for /f/ and /h/ because no tongue contact occurs in their production. The contact areas are highlighted by bold lines in the palatograms. The scalloped line shows the inner margins of the upper teeth. The dashed lines in the X-ray tracings show the changing position of the tongue for these sounds.

Different speakers use two tongue tip positions to maintain a free flow of air for /s/ and /z/. Some position the tongue tip just posterior to the upper alveolar ridge and teeth. Others place the tongue tip just posterior to the lower alveolar ridge. You can determine your own tongue tip position by repeating 'sigh' a number of times to get the feel of where your tongue is during the /s/. There are no accurate figures, but it is likely that 50% of American English speakers use each type; according to Bronstein (1960), many speakers use the lower tongue position. One position does not seem to be preferable in producing acceptable /s/ and /z/ sounds. If the lower tongue position results in a wider opening of the constriction, one would expect its noise to be lower in frequency (Bronstein, 1960). Limited palatographic evidence, however, indicates that the channel formed by the tongue and palate is alike for both sounds (Jones, 1956). Some phoneticians imply that the difference is perceptible (Bronstein, 1960); others maintain that it is not (Jones, 1956). The authors' experience is that it is very difficult, if not impossible, to determine which position is being used just by listening. In training someone with defective /s/ and /z/ to make the sounds correctly, it is worthwhile trying both positions to determine which works best for the individual.

Another aspect of /s, z/ production that needs clarification is whether or not the tongue needs to be **grooved** for normal production. Some individuals can stick out their tongue and make a groove in it, but this ability is genetically determined, and many individuals cannot groove the tongue. No relationship has been established between this ability and normal /s, z/ production. As long as a narrow channel, slit, or groove is formed between the tongue and the hard palate, it is not necessary for the tongue itself to form a groove.

As one can observe from the X-ray tracings and palatograms of /ʒ/ in Figure 7–1, the lamino-prepalatal fricatives involve contact by the tongue margins with the hard palate, no contact by the tip or middle part of the tongue, and close approximation of the cutting edges of the upper and lower teeth. In these aspects, /ʃ, ʒ/ are similar to /s, z/. But unlike /s, z/, the anterior opening for the channel between the upper surface of the tongue and the hard palate for /ʃ, ʒ/ is formed by the tongue blade just posterior to the alveolar ridge. The constriction for /ʃ, ʒ/ is wider than for /s, z/, and the airflow directed between the upper and lower teeth is more diffuse. If you say the following minimal pairs several times, you can feel the shift in tongue position for the apico-alveolar and lamino-prepalatal sounds: 'sigh'/'shy,' 'bays'/'beige.' If you are like many other speakers, you may also feel the lips rounding for /ʃ/ and /ʒ/ in words like 'she' and 'beige,' but not for /s/ and /z/ in words like 'see' and 'zip' (Bronstein, 1960; Singh & Singh, 1976; Tiffany & Carrell, 1977; Shriberg & Kent, 1982).

One of the most unusual sounds of English is /h/, because it involves producing noise at the vocal folds while the tongue is in position for any following vowel. It is the only fricative that does not have a voiced cognate. In making this glottal fricative, the vocal folds are approximated, and frication noise is produced as air flows between them. This is also the position for whispering. The resonator for /h/, then, is the entire vocal tract anterior to the vocal folds. Unlike other fricatives, /h/ involves no constriction in the oral cavity. Because the tongue assumes the position for whatever vowel follows, the /h/ phoneme actually is a series of whispered vowels. The /h/ sounds in 'heat,' 'hat,' and 'hoot' could be transcribed as whispered /i/, /æ/, and /u/ vowels. /h/ cannot have a truly voiced cognate, although a partially voiced allophone can occur intervocalically.

Affricates

Simply defined, an **affricate** is a combination of a stop and a fricative. More specifically, an affricate is a stop that is released into a fricative in the same syllable. Thus 'my chair' is transcribed as [mɑɪ+tʃɛr], and 'might share' is transcribed as [mɑɪt+ʃɛr]. Only 'my chair' contains the /tʃ/ affricate; 'might share' contains the /t/ stop plus the /ʃ/ fricative. In the ideal affricate the two sounds are homorganic so as to facilitate the transition between stop and fricative. According to some phoneticians, **homorganic** means that two sounds involve the same articulator and the same place of articulation. Thus, /p, b, m/, /t, d, n/, and /k, g, ŋ/ are three sets of homorganic sounds, an observation you can test for yourself by comparing the tongue contacts for the following threesomes: 'pie,' 'buy,' and 'my'; 'tie,' 'die,' and 'nigh'; 'rack,' 'rag,' and 'rang.' Compare also the palatograms and X-rays for these sounds in the chapters on stops and nasals. According to other phoneticians, homorganic means that two sounds involve the same articulator and similar places of articulation. Thus, /t, d, n, s, z/ would be considered homorganic. Affricates are easily produced even with nonhomorganic sounds, because approximation by the tongue of the fricative position is not precluded during stop production, as for /ps/ in 'caps,' or because only a release of the tongue contact is required to shift from the stop to the fricative, as for /tʃ/ in 'itch.'

Table 7–2 presents examples of words that include the affricates of English. The most frequent affricates in normal speech involve combinations of /p, t, k/ with the *s* morpheme in words like 'cups,' 'cats,' and 'backs,' and combinations of /b, d, g/ with the *s* morpheme in words like 'cubs,' 'beds,' and 'bags.' When the *s* morpheme follows a voiced consonant like /b/ in 'cubs,' it is pronounced as /z/ instead of /s/. As indicated in Table 7–2, an individual with an interdental lisp substitutes /θ/ for /s/ and /ð/ for /z/ in pronouncing the /ts/ and /dz/ affricates. These affricates occur rarely in word-initial position in English, for example, in 'tsetse.' They are uncommon in medial position.

Table 7–2
Examples of English words with affricates. Only /tʃ/ and /dʒ/ are considered phonemes.

	Fricative					
Stop	/s/		/θ/		/ʃ/	
/p/	/ps/	cups	/pθ/	depth; cups[a]		–
/t/	/ts/	cats	/tθ/	eighth; cats[a]	/tʃ/	chin; rich
/k/	/ks/	backs	/kθ/	backs[a]		–
	Fricative					
	/z/		/ð/		/ʒ/	
/b/	/bz/	cubs	/bð/	cubs[a]		–
/d/	/dz/	beds	/dð/	width; beds[a]	/dʒ/	gin; ridge
/g/	/gz/	bags	/gð/	bags[a]		–

[a]s morpheme as pronounced by speakers with an interdental lisp.

'Pizza,' 'nazi,' 'waltzing,' 'curtsy,' 'patsy,' 'tsetse,' 'hotsy-totsy,' and 'itsy-bitsy' are exceptions.

Two frequent stop plus fricative combinations used in forming affricates are /t/ with /ʃ/ and /d/ with /ʒ/ in words like 'chin' and 'gin.' Unlike other affricates, /tʃ/ and /dʒ/ occur in all environments. On the basis of this phonological distinction, /tʃ/ and /dʒ/ are classified as the only affricate phonemes in English. According to Bronstein (1960), /ts/ and /dz/ are clusters containing two distinctive sounds; /tʃ/ and /dʒ/ are single phonemic entities. But /ts/ and /dz/ are no different phonetically from the other affricates in that they are stops released into fricatives, and children who use the phonological process of fronting treat affricates the same whether or not they are considered phonemes. For example, /ts/ is substituted for /tʃ/ in 'watch' by such children.

For each of the affricates covered in Table 7–2, the transition between stop and fricative is facilitated because the tongue can anticipate the fricative position. In the case of /ps/, /bz/, /pθ/, and /bð/, the tongue is completely free to move into position for the following fricative during the stop. For /ts/, /tθ/, /tʃ/, /dz/, /dð/, and /dʒ/, only a slight adjustment of the tongue tip or tongue blade is required after the stop release. For /ks/, /kθ/, /gz/, and /gð/, the tongue tip is free to approximate the fricative position during stop production.

ACOUSTIC CUES TO FRICATIVES AND AFFRICATES

Fricative sounds vary considerably in their acoustic characteristics, depending on the configuration of the vocal tract and the constriction used in their production. The intensity and the frequency concentration of the noise produced vary as a function of the restrictions on airflow and pressure, and of the size of the resonance cavity. The following factors influence the characteristics of fricative noise: (1) A soft tissue constriction or obstruction anterior to the constriction opening produces lower intensity noise than a hard tissue constriction or obstruction; (2) a larger resonating cavity anterior to the opening of the constriction produces lower frequency noise than a smaller one; and (3) a larger opening of the constriction produces a lower frequency and less intense noise than a smaller opening.

On the basis of the articulators involved in their production, fricatives can be classified as sibilants /s, z, ʃ, ʒ/ and nonsibilants /f, v, θ, ð, h/. For sibilant production, airflow is directed by the tongue so that it passes between the teeth. Opinion varies among phoneticians as to whether the airstream for sibilants is directed against the upper teeth (Tiffany & Carrell, 1977), the lower teeth (Bronstein, 1960), or the closely approximated upper and lower teeth (Catford, 1977; Calvert, 1980). In any case, the mechanism for sibilant production results in a very distinctive frication noise. Nonsibilants are produced either by approximating the lower lip to the upper teeth or by putting the tongue tip between the teeth. Nonsibilants have lower intensity levels and less energy below 8000 Hz than sibilants have. You can see these differences if you compare the following nonsibilant and sibilant pairs in figures 7–2, 7–3, 7–4, and 7–5: 'high'/'sigh,' 'high'/'shy,' 'fie'/'sigh,' 'fie'/'shy,' 'thigh'/'sigh,' 'thigh'/'shy' (figures 7–2 and 7–4), 'veal'/ 'zeal,' 'bathe'/'beige' (figures 7–3 and 7–5). (In these figures, vowels were truncated and nonfricative final consonants were deleted from spectrograms in order to save space.) In general the fill is not as dark for nonsibilants as it is for sibilants. In some cases, nonsibilant intensity is so low that fill is absent or very faint. The distribution of energy is substantially higher in frequency in the child's fricatives than in the adult's,

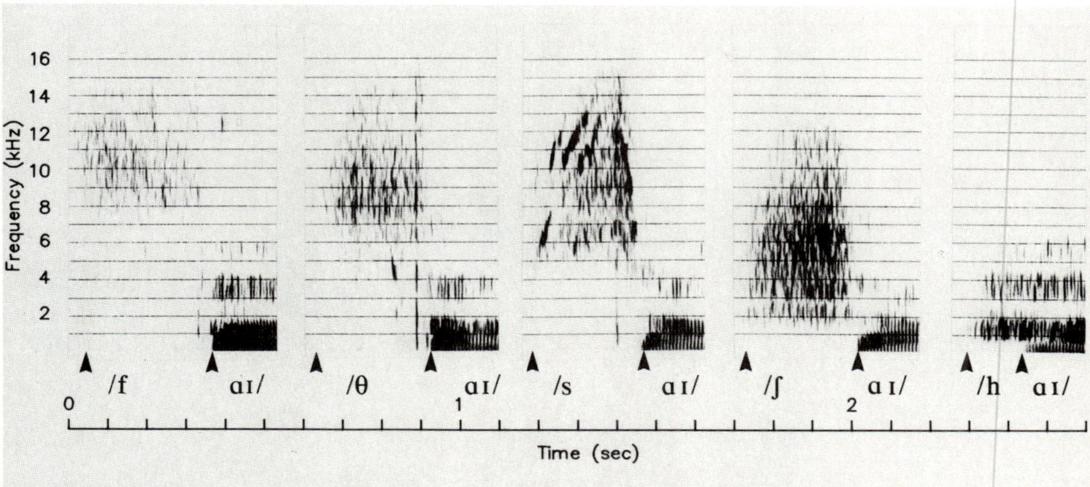

Figure 7–2
Spectrograms of a child's productions of 'fie,' 'thigh,' 'sigh,' 'shy,' and 'high.' Arrows along the *x* axis (abscissa) indicate onset and offset of frication noise. The vowels were truncated to save space. The frequency range for analysis was 16 kHz, and the filter bandwidth 600 Hz. This filter setting was used for all 16 kHz analyses of a child's speech.

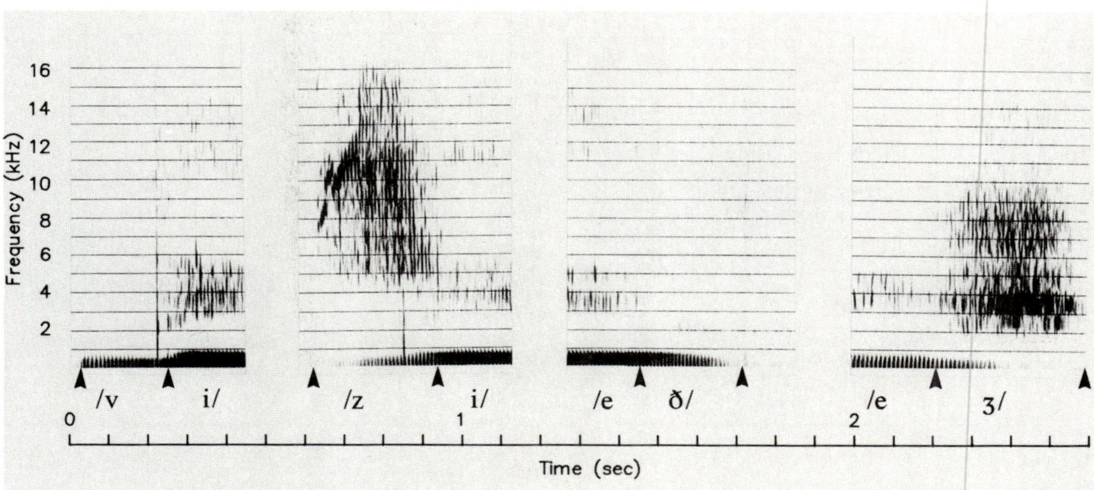

Figure 7–3
Spectrograms of a child's productions of 'veal,' 'zeal,' 'bathe,' and 'beige.' Arrows along the *x* axis indicate onset and offset of frication noise. Vowels were truncated and final consonants deleted to save space.

which is consistent with research on fricative production in children and infants (Pentz, Gilbert, & Zawadzki, 1979; Bauer & Kent, 1987).

Fricatives can also be differentiated on the basis of their place of articulation. Since the size of the cavity in front of the constriction increases as position shifts from

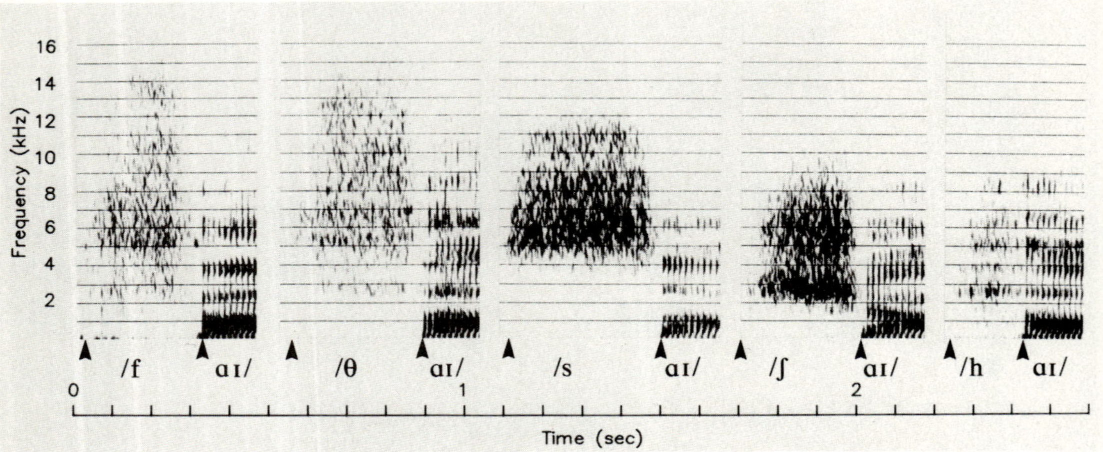

Figure 7–4
Spectrograms of an adult male's productions of 'fie,' 'thigh,' 'sigh,' 'shy,' and 'high.' Arrows along the *x* axis indicate onset and offset of frication noise. Vowels were truncated in order to save space. The standard 300 Hz wide band filter setting was used for both 8 kHz and 16 kHz frequency range analyses of adult speech.

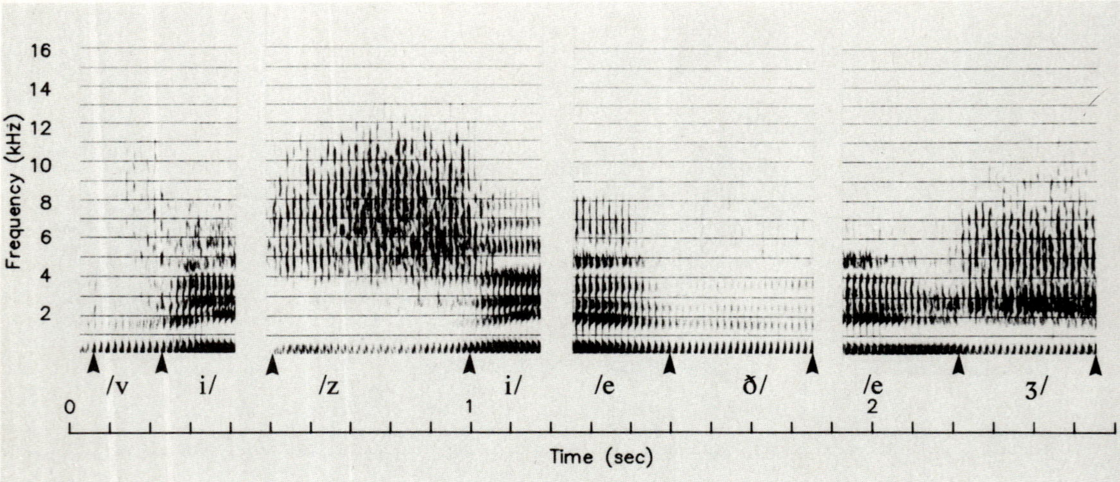

Figure 7–5
Spectrograms of an adult male's productions of 'veal,' 'zeal,' 'bathe,' and 'beige.' Arrows along the *x* axis indicate onset and offset of frication noise. Vowels were truncated and final consonants deleted to save space.

labiodental to lamino-prepalatal, the frequency of fricative noise should decrease. For nonsibilants, the resonance frequency should decrease as the place of articulation shifts from front to back. If you compare the front and back fricatives in the minimal pairs 'fie' and 'thigh,' 'thigh' and 'high,' you can see that it is difficult to detect this change in figures 7–2 and 7–4. The problem is due to the fact that the difference between place of articulation is so small and the intensity of all these sounds is so weak. For sibilants the frequency of fricative noise should decrease as the place of articulation shifts from front to back, because the anterior cavity increases in size and the airstream is more diffuse for /ʃ, ʒ/ than for /s, z/. You can observe this change in figures 7–2, 7–3, 7–4, and 7–5 by comparing the front and back minimal pair 'sigh' and 'shy.' Note that the fill for /ʃ/ extends to lower frequency levels than it does for /s/.

Fricatives do not present the problem that occurs in certain contexts with stops, the absence of the burst noise as a place cue. Frication noise is always present, but it may be very weak, particularly in nonsibilants. For example, it is very difficult to differentiate /f/ and /θ/ from just the noise. As suggested for stops, vowel transitions are cues to place of articulation, and they may be more reliable cues than frication noise for nonsibilants. In spectrograms, VC transitions are acoustic representations of articulator movement from a preceding vowel to a fricative constriction, and CV transitions are acoustic representations of articulator movement from a fricative constriction toward a following vowel. During these transitions the changing configurations of the vocal tract between vowel and fricative positions modify vowel resonances. These resonance changes shift the vowel formants so that they reflect the place of articulation of the preceding or following consonant.

Since F_2 is supposed to increase in frequency from labial to alveolar to palatal positions, one can try to differentiate place of articulation by comparing vowel transitions. Some of the transitions in figures 7–6 and 7–7 seem to be directed at different frequency levels, or loci. Research on synthetic speech has established stop loci at about 700 Hz for /p/ and /b/, about 1800 Hz for /t/ and /d/, and about 3000 Hz for /k/ and /g/ (Liberman, Delattre, Cooper, & Gerstman, 1954; Delattre, Liberman, & Cooper, 1955). More recent research on real speech by Kewley-Port (1982) has cast doubt on the invariability of loci for stops, and it seems likely that research on real speech fricatives would produce similar results. You can see that some transitions are quite similar in the real speech transitions shown in figures 7–6 and 7–7 even though they should reflect different places of articulation. Listeners can identify the place of articulation of fricatives just from the vowel transitions, with no frication noise (Liberman et al., 1954; Delattre et al., 1955). F_2 transitions for fricatives are reduced in frequency and duration in the vowels of deaf adolescents, which may be an important factor in the low intelligibility of their speech (Monsen, 1976a).

Figures 7–8 and 7–9 include spectrograms of 'church' and 'judge,' which contain the /tʃ/ and /dʒ/ affricates, respectively, each in both pre- and postvocalic position. Since /tʃ/ is a combination of a voiceless stop and fricative, its pattern is characterized by a gap, a spike, and fill. The gap can be observed clearly in the postvocalic /tʃ/ in 'church.' Since /dʒ/ is a combination of a voiced stop and a voiced fricative, its pattern is characterized by a gap with a voice bar, a spike, and fill with varying degrees of formant representation.

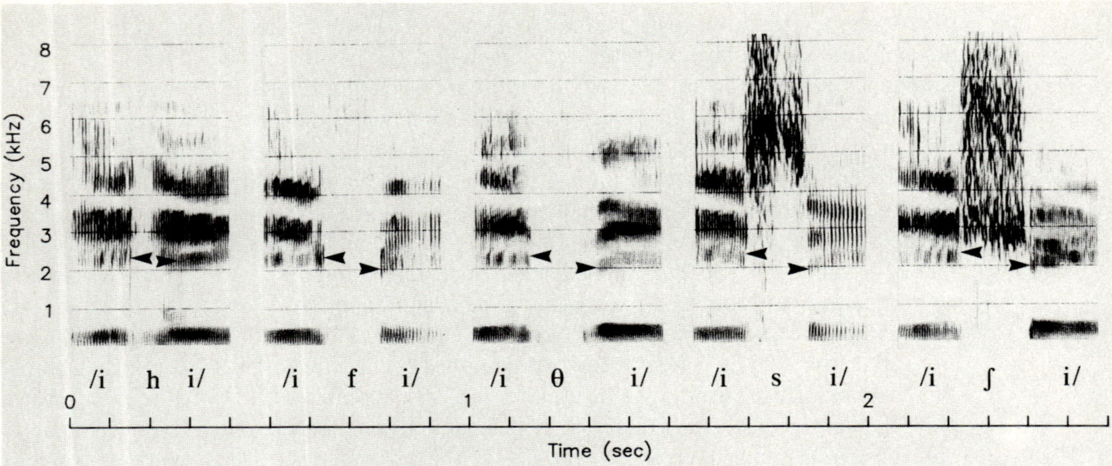

Figure 7–6
Spectrograms of an adult male's productions of intervocalic voiceless fricatives with /i/. Arrows along the *y* axis indicate the approximate position of F_2 at the onset and offset of fricative closure.

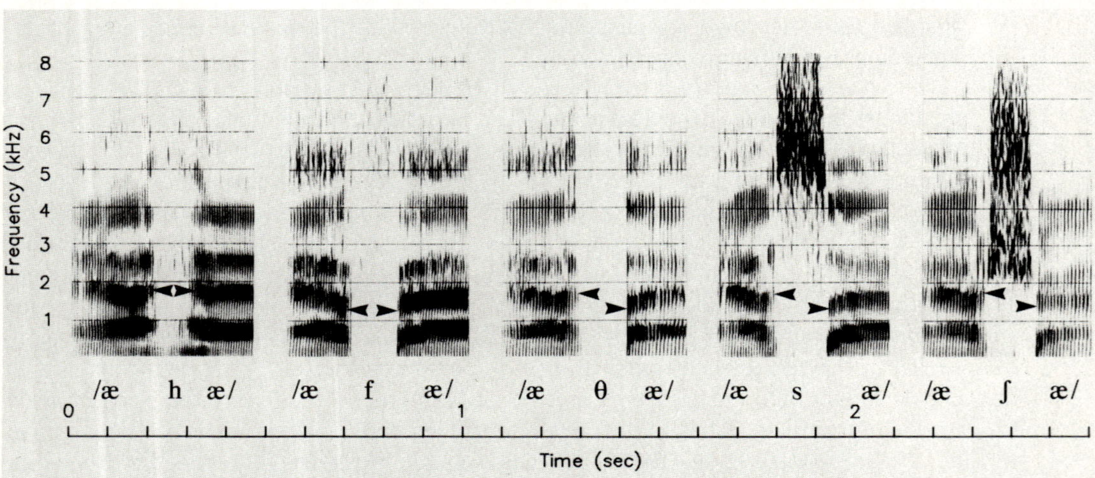

Figure 7–7
Spectrograms of an adult male's productions of intervocalic voiceless fricatives with /æ/. Arrows along the *y* axis indicate the approximate position of F_2 at the onset and offset of fricative closure.

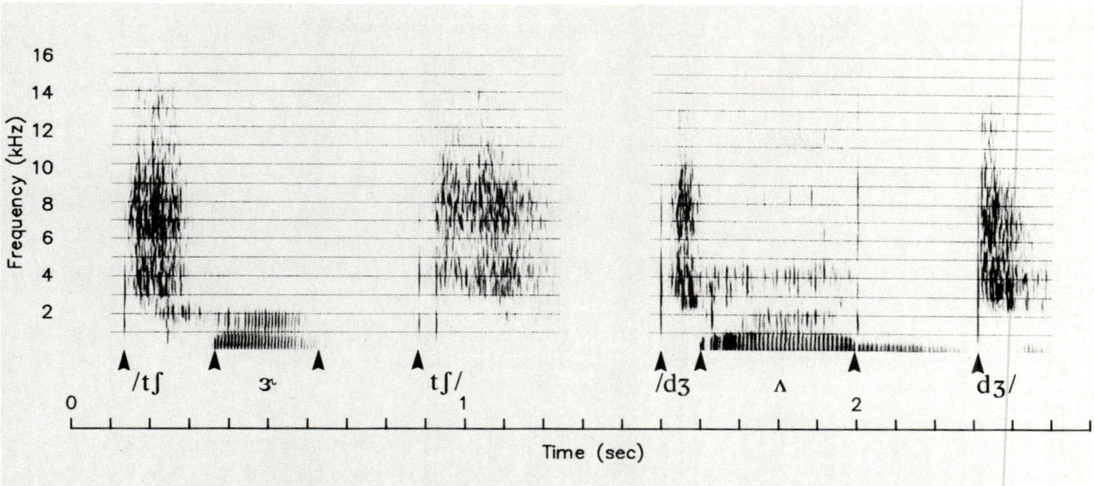

Figure 7–8
Spectrograms of a child's productions of /tʃɝtʃ/ and /dʒʌdʒ/. The first pair of arrows along the *x* axis indicates the spike release of the prevocalic affricate and the onset of the vowel. The second pair of arrows indicates the offset of the vowel and the spike release of the postvocalic affricate.

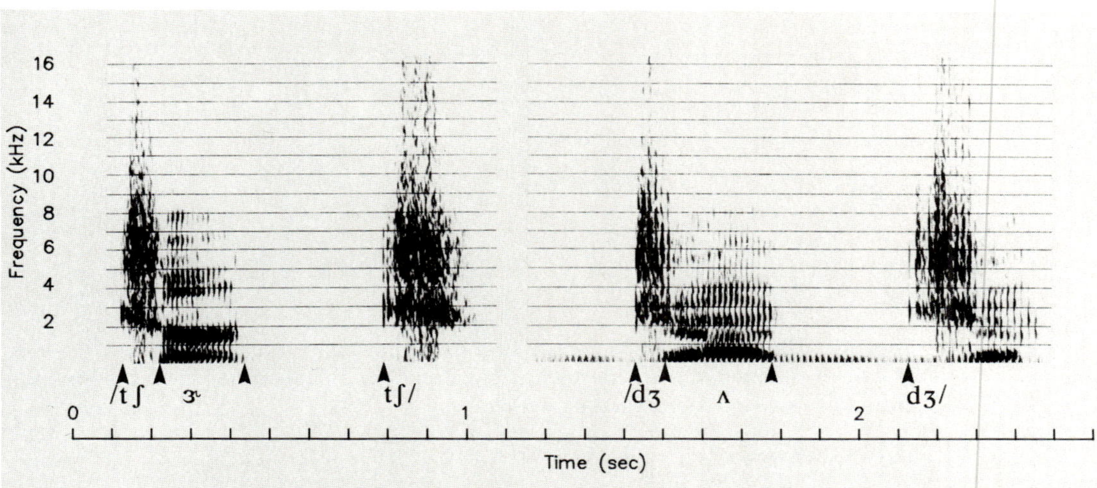

Figure 7–9
Spectrograms of an adult male's productions of /tʃɝtʃ/ and /dʒʌdʒ/. The first pair of arrows along the *x* axis (abscissa) indicates the spike release of the prevocalic affricate and the onset of the vowel. The second pair of arrows indicates the offset of the vowel and the spike release of the postvocalic affricate.

GLOSSARY

Affricate. A consonant produced by releasing a stop into a fricative, usually within the same syllable.

Fricative. A consonant produced by restricting the airflow through the vocal tract so that frication noise is produced.

Groove. The channel formed between the tongue and the hard palate that directs the flow of air out of the oral cavity.

Homorganic. Made with the same articulator and place of articulation, as /t, d, n/, or with the same articulator and similar places of articulation, as /t, d, n, s, z/.

REVIEW QUESTIONS

A. Indicate whether the cavity anterior to the constriction or closure for the first sound is larger (L), smaller (S), or no different (ND) than that for the second sound.

1. /f/, /s/ ______
2. /f/, /v/ ______
3. /s/, /ʃ/ ______
4. /v/, /t/ ______
5. /s/, /k/ ______
6. /s/, /p/ ______
7. /s/, /h/ ______
8. /θ/, /s/ ______
9. /t/, /k/ ______
10. /z/, /f/ ______

****

Key: 1. S; 2. ND; 3. S; 4. S; 5. S; 6. L; 7. S; 8. S; 9. S; 10. L

B. Indicate whether the locus for the first consonant is relatively higher (H), lower (L), or the same (S) as for the second consonant in each pair based on the findings from research on synthesized speech.

1. /fi/, /si/ ______
2. /si/, /zi/ ______
3. /si/, /ʃi/ ______
4. /vi/, /zi/ ______
5. /fi/, /zi/ ______
6. /fi/, /pi/ ______
7. /fi/, /ki/ ______
8. /ti/, /fi/ ______
9. /ki/, /si/ ______
10. /pi/, /ki/ ______

****

Key: 1. L; 2. S; 3. L; 4. L; 5. L; 6. S; 7. L; 8. H; 9. H; 10. L

C. Indicate whether the following pairs of sounds are homorganic (+) or not homorganic (−), using the strictest definition of homorganic.

1. /t/, /n/ ________
2. /t/, /s/ ________
3. /t/, /h/ ________
4. /p/, /f/ ________
5. /p/, /m/ ________
6. /k/, /ʃ/ ________
7. /d/, /t/ ________
8. /d/, /ʒ/ ________
9. /θ/, /f/ ________
10. /θ/, /t/ ________

****

Key: 1. +; 2. −; 3. −; 4. −; 5. +; 6. −; 7. +; 8. −; 9. −; 10. −

D. Indicate the spectrographic cues to the following sounds in word-initial position by inserting the letters for those that apply: (a) spike; (b) gap; (c) gap with voice bar; (d) fill; (e) fill with formants. More than one characteristic may occur.

1. /s/ ____________
2. /v/ ____________
3. /dʒ/ ____________
4. /ts/ ____________
5. /tʃ/ ____________
6. /ʃ/ ____________
7. /θ/ ____________
8. /h/ ____________

****

Key: 1. d; 2. e; 3. a, c, e; 4. a, b, d; 5. a, b, d; 6. d; 7. d; 8. d

LABORATORY ASSIGNMENT

Tape III, Side A
IIIA3: Fricatives and Affricates (Tape running time: 14:24; Elapsed time: 08:52–23:16)

a. Fricative and Affricate Models

Listen to the fricative and affricate consonants produced in a /Cɪ l/ context by an adult and a child. If necessary, stop the tape at any time, rewind, and listen again.

1. Adult: /fɪ l/; /θɪ l/; /sɪ l/; /ʃɪ l/; /hɪ l/; /tʃɪ l/
2. Child repeats above.
3. Adult: /vɪ l/; /ðɪ l/; /zɪ l/; /ʒɪ l/; /dʒɪ l/
4. Child repeats above.

b. Transcription of Fricatives and Affricates in Minimal Contrast Context

Transcribe the fricatives and affricates as they are pronounced by an adult and a child in a minimal contrast context /Cɪ l/.

1. ______ 2. ______ 3. ______ 4. ______ 5. ______

6. ______ 7. ______ 8. ______ 9. ______ 10. ______

11. ______ 12. ______ 13. ______ 14. ______ 15. ______

16. ________ 17. ________ 18. ________ 19. ________ 20. ________

21. ________ 22. ________

****

Consensus: 1. /f/ 2. /v/ 3. /z/ 4. /s/ 5. /ʒ/ 6. /tʃ/ 7. /θ/ 8. /h/ 9. /ʃ/ 10. /ð/ 11. /dʒ/ 12. /ð/ 13. /tʃ/ 14. /z/ 15. /s/ 16. /f/ 17. /dʒ/ 18. /ð/ 19. /θ/ 20. /ʒ/ 21. /h/ 22. /ʃ/

Variants: 14. [z̪] 15. [s̪] 16. /θ/

c. Transcription of Fricatives and Affricates in a Sentence

Transcribe the fricative and affricate consonants as they are pronounced by an adult and a child in syllables in the sentence 'Say ________ again.'

1. ________ 2. ________ 3. ________ 4. ________ 5. ________

6. ________ 7. ________ 8. ________ 9. ________ 10. ________

11. ________ 12. ________ 13. ________ 14. ________ 15. ________

16. ________ 17. ________ 18. ________ 19. ________ 20. ________

21. ________ 22. ________

****

Consensus: 1. /f/ 2. /θ/ 3. /s/ 4. /tʃ/ 5. /h/ 6. /ʒ/ 7. /z/ 8. /θ/ 9. /ð/ 10. /ʃ/ 11. /dʒ/ 12. /h/ 13. /dʒ/ 14. /z/ 15. /ð/ 16. /v/ 17. /f/ 18. /θ/ 19. /s/ 20. /ʃ/ 21. /ʒ/ 22. /tʃ/

Variants: 7. [z̪] 8. /f/

d. Transcription of Fricatives and Affricates in Words in Isolation

Transcribe the initial fricative and affricate consonants as they are pronounced by an adult and a child in words.

1. shoe ________ 2. soap ________ 3. home ________ 4. fat ________

5. vote ________ 6. zoo ________ 7. that ________ 8. hop ________

9. thumb ________ 10. chick ________ 11. face ________ 12. sail ________

13. thin ________ 14. hole ________ 15. them ________ 16. vest ________

17. zipper ________ 18. chill ________ 19. shy ________ 20. joke ________

****

Consensus: 1. /ʃ/ 2. /s/ 3. /h/ 4. /f/ 5. /v/ 6. /z/ 7. /ð/ 8. /h/ 9. /θ/ 10. /tʃ/ 11. /f/ 12. /s/ 13. /θ/ 14. /h/ 15. /ð/ 16. /v/ 17. /z/ 18. /tʃ/ 19. /ʃ/ 20. /dʒ/

Variants: 2. [s̺]

e. Transcription of Prevocalic Fricatives and Affricates in Words in Context

Transcribe the prevocalic fricative and affricate consonants as they are pronounced by an adult and a child in words in the following sentences: 'I can say ________ '; 'Say the word ________ '; '________ is the word.'

1. thigh ________	2. fan ________	3. sop ________	4. ship ________
5. very ________	6. hotel ________	7. chap ________	8. gym ________
9. zone ________	10. thine ________	11. this ________	12. zap ________
13. jam ________	14. chin ________	15. hit ________	16. vine ________
17. shoot ________	18. supper ________	19. funny ________	20. thing ________

****

Consensus: 1. /θ/ 2. /f/ 3. /s/ 4. /ʃ/ 5. /v/ 6. /h/ 7. /tʃ/ 8. /dʒ/ 9. /z/ 10. /ð/ 11. /ð/ 12. /z/ 13. /dʒ/ 14. /tʃ/ 15. /h/ 16. /v/ 17. /ʃ/ 18. /s/ 19. /f/ 20. /θ/

Variants: 3. [s̺] 9. [z̺]

f. Transcription of Intervocalic Fricatives and Affricates in Words in Context

Transcribe the intervocalic fricative and affricate consonants as they are pronounced by an adult and a child in words in the following sentences: 'I can say ________ '; 'Say the word ________ '; '________ is the word.'

1. lesson ________	2. razor ________	3. cover ________
4. budging ________	5. dishing ________	6. behead ________
7. coughing ________	8. richer ________	9. bother ________
10. ether ________	11. pleasure ________	12. leisure ________
13. toothy ________	14. mother ________	15. itching ________
16. roofer ________	17. ahead ________	18. issue ________
19. edger ________	20. raving ________	21. dozen ________
22. tossing ________		

****

Consensus: 1. /s/ 2. /z/ 3. /v/ 4. /dʒ/ 5. /ʃ/ 6. /h/ 7. /f/ 8. /tʃ/
9. /ð/ 10. /θ/ 11. /ʒ/ 12. /ʒ/ 13. /θ/ 14. /ð/ 15. /tʃ/
16. /f/ 17. /h/ 18. /ʃ/ 19. /dʒ/ 20. /v/ 21. /z/ 22. /s/

Variants: 1. [s̺] 11. [ʒ̥] 19. [dʒ̥] 21. [z̥]

g. Transcription of Postvocalic Fricatives and Affricates in Words in Context

Transcribe the postvocalic fricative and affricate consonants as they are pronounced by an adult and a child in words in the following sentences: 'I can say ________ '; 'Say the word ________ '; '________ is the word.'

1. peace ________	2. days ________	3. love ________	4. edge ________
5. push ________	6. laugh ________	7. catch ________	8. bathe ________
9. cloth ________	10. garage ________	11. garage ________	12. both ________
13. teethe ________	14. rich ________	15. poof ________	16. rush ________
17. ledge ________	18. leave ________	19. has ________	20. touch ________

****

Consensus: 1. /s/ 2. /z̥/ 3. /v/ 4. /dʒ/ 5. /ʃ/ 6. /f/ 7. /tʃ/ 8. /ð/ 9. /θ/
10. /dʒ/ 11. /ʒ/ 12. /θ/ 13. /ð/ 14. /tʃ/ 15. /f/ 16. /ʃ/17. /dʒ/
18. /v/ 19. /z/ 20. /tʃ/

Variants: 1. [s̺] 11. [ʒ̥] 19. [ʤ̥] 21. [z̥]

CHAPTER 8

Normal and Misarticulated Fricatives and Affricates

Chapter 7 covered the physiological characteristics that differentiate fricatives and affricates and the acoustic cues that reflect them. Unlike other consonants, fricatives require near contact or contact just sufficient to form a constriction for generating their characteristic frication noise. Forming a constriction rather than a closure may cause problems for some individuals. Although fricatives can be differentiated as sibilants or nonsibilants, finer distinctions may cause problems because the noise of the nonsibilants is so weak. In this chapter, the allophones of fricatives and affricates are described, including their misarticulations, in particular lisping and phonological processes.

ALLOPHONES OF FRICATIVES AND AFFRICATES

Examples of common allophones of fricatives and affricates are shown in Table 8–1. These variations involve devoicing of voiced fricatives, lip rounding of all fricatives, and changing tongue configurations for /h/.

Devoicing

There is a tendency to devoice voiced fricatives in postvocalic position. The devoicing may be complete, as in the common pronunciation of 'have' as /h æ f/ in the phrase 'I have to,' in which a voiceless stop follows (see Figure 8–1), or it may be partial, with only the last part of the fricative being devoiced. The partially devoiced word may be transcribed [h æ v f], but [h æ v̥] is generally used to represent the pronunciation of a fricative whose last part is voiceless. Although devoicing occurs in postvocalic position,

Table 8–1
Contexts of common allophones of fricatives and affricates (V = vowel; C = consonant).

Phoneme	Pre-, Inter-, Post-Vocalic[a]	Preceding/Following[a] Rounded Vowels /u, ʊ, o, ɔ/
/f/	fail; affair; leaf	[f͗] foot; roof
/v/	veil; devise; leave	[v͗] vote; move
/θ/	thigh; ether; teeth	[θ͗] thought; youth
/ð/	they; mother; bathe	[ð͗] though; smooth
/s/	see; lesson; class	[s͗] sue; loose
/z/	zebra; easy; is	[z͗] zoo; lose
/ʃ/	she; fashion; wish	[ʃ͗] shoe; push
/ʒ/[b]	–; vision; beige	[ʒ͗] usual; rouge
/h/[c]	e.g., [i̥] he; [ɛ̥] ahead; –	[h͗] who; –
/tʃ/	chair; pitcher; catch	[t͗ʃ] chew; coach
/dʒ/	joy; major; age	[d͗ʒ] June; huge

[a]Voiced fricatives are sometimes devoiced [C̥] in postvocalic position.
[b]/ʒ/ does not occur in prevocalic position.
[c]/h/ is the whispered vowel [V̥] equivalent of each vowel it precedes. It does not occur in postvocalic position.

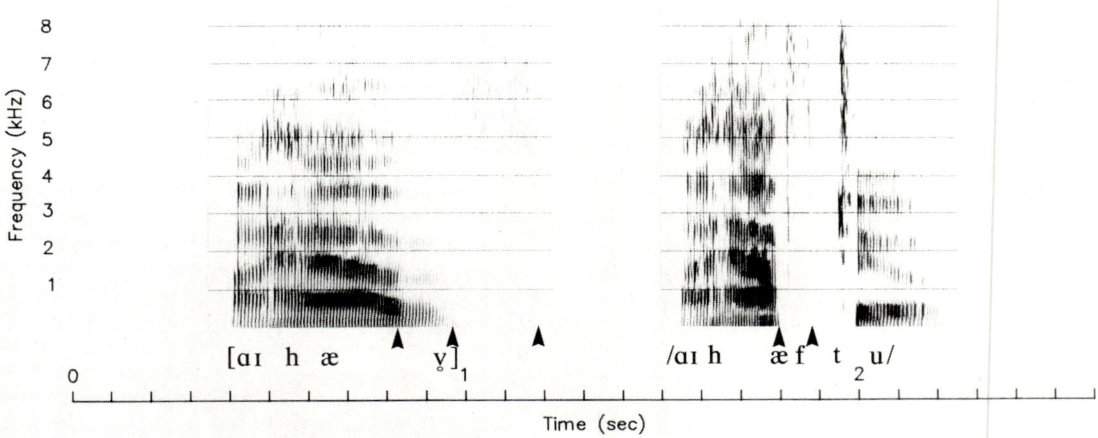

Figure 8–1
Spectrograms of an adult male's productions of 'I have' (left panel) and 'I have to' (right panel) illustrating partial and complete devoicing of /v/, respectively. The first and second arrows along the *x* axis (abscissa) of 'I have' indicate the duration of the voiced component of /v/; the second and third arrows indicate the duration of the voiceless component of /v/. For 'I have to,' the arrows along the *x* axis indicate that /v/ has only a voiceless component for this production.

it is not completely predictable. Some speakers may devoice more than others, and some fricatives and affricates may be devoiced more than others. For diagnostic purposes it is important to differentiate allophonic devoicing from the consistent devoicing that eliminates the distinction between such minimal pairs as 'safe' and 'save.'

Rounding

In the context of the rounded vowels /u, ʊ, o, ɔ/, fricatives and affricates may be rounded as indicated in Table 8–1. When the rounded vowel follows, lip rounding is anticipated during the production of the fricative or the affricate, as in [s͗u] 'sue' and [t͗ʃu] 'chew.' Rounding also occurs when the fricative and affricate follow the vowel, as in [uz͗] 'ooze' and [rot͗ʃ] 'roach,' where lip rounding is carried over from the vowel into the consonant. You can see and hear the difference by pronouncing pairs of words in which these consonants occur with rounded and unrounded vowels, for example, 'shoe'/'she' and 'choose'/'cheese.'

/h/ Variants

The glottal fricative /h/ involves anticipation by the tongue of the position for the following vowel. Thus, the voiceless /i/ at the beginning of 'heat' and the voiceless /u/ at the beginning of 'hoot' are allophones of the /h/ phoneme, as are all glottal fricatives preceding the other vowels of English. There is an /h/ allophone for each vowel of English, but they need not be transcribed because they can be predicted from context.

Bilabial /f, v/

As indicated in Table 8–2, one of the less common allophonic variants is the change from labiodental to bilabial articulation that occurs when /f/ and /v/ follow /p, b, m/. In these variants the bilabial position is carried over from the preceding sounds so that the fricatives are produced with bilabial constriction. A limited number of English words include the necessary sound sequence: 'amphibian,' 'amphitheater,' 'comfort,' 'comfortable,' 'camphor,' 'obvious,' 'obviate,' and 'cupful' are relatively common examples. The opposite change is much more likely to occur in such words, as the bilabial stop or nasal changes to a labiodental under the influence of the following /f/ or /v/.

Labiodentalized /s/ and /z/

Intrusions by the lower lip in the production of /s/ and /z/ result in labiodentalized versions of these consonants in the context of /f/ and /v/. For these variants, the usual tongue position is maintained for /s/ and /z/, but the upper and lower teeth are parted slightly and the lower lip approximates the upper teeth. The sibilant quality is still maintained, but the intrusion of the lip tends to decrease its intensity. As indicated in Table 8–2, this change occurs for words which add the morpheme *s* to /f/ and /v/, as

Table 8–2
Contexts that produce relatively infrequent fricative allophones.

Phonemes	Contexts, Allophones, and Examples
	Following bilabials /p, b, m/
/f/	[ɸ] comfort
/v/	[β] obvious
	Following labiodentals /f, v/
/s/	[$\overset{f}{s}$] coughs; cuffs
/z/	[$\overset{v}{z}$] caves; saves
	Following interdentals /θ, ð/
/s/	[s̪] paths; cloths
/z/	[z̪] breathes; soothes
	Preceding interdental /θ/
/s/	[s̪] sixth; aesthetic
	Preceding /j/
/h/	[$\overset{+}{ꝁ}$] hue; huge
	Intervocalic
/h/	[ɦ] ahead; behind

in 'coughs' and 'caves.' Other words in which the change occurs are 'cuffs,' 'muffs,' 'miffs,' 'laughs,' 'puffs,' 'saves,' 'loves,' 'raves,' 'roves,' and 'leaves.' These labiodentalized /s, z/ sounds are phonemic in the Bantu languages (Heffner, 1952).

Dentalized /s, z/

Tongue intrusion causes dentalization of /s/ and /z/ when they are preceded or followed by /θ/ and /ð/ (Table 8–2). These changes occur in words which add the *s* morpheme, like 'paths,' 'cloths,' and 'booths,' in which /s/ follows /θ/, and like 'breathes,' and 'soothes,' in which /z/ follows /ð/. The same phenomenon occurs in a few words in which /s/ precedes /θ/—'sixth,' 'aesthetic,' and 'anesthesia' are the most common ones. This type of intrusion tends to decrease the sibilant quality of /s/ and /z/ by decreasing their intensity.

Palatalized and Voiced /h/

Palatalized /h/ occurs in a few words like 'hue,' 'huge,' and 'humor.' The tongue constriction for the /h/ in the /hju/ sequence that begins each of these words may be increased, and frication noise is produced in the oral cavity. The result is a dorsopalatal fricative similar to the sound in the German word 'ich.' The voiced variant of /h/ occurs only in intervocalic position in a few words like 'ahead,' 'behind,' 'ahoy,' and 'behoove.' Although this variant is sometimes referred to as voiced /h/, it is not truly voiced. In the production of /h/, the vocal folds are approximated so that a glottal tone is produced with some escape of air. The resultant sound has the quality of a breathy voice.

LISPING: MISARTICULATIONS OF /s/ AND /z/

Lisping is the clinical disorder that specifically involves sibilants. Traditionally defined, it is the misarticulation of /s/ and /z/ by the **substitution** of /θ/ and /ð/. This type of error is commonly called a **frontal lisp.** The meaning of lisping has, however, been broadened to include not only these errors of tongue protrusion but any tongue tip deviation that results in a loss of sibilant quality. Thus, a **lateral lisp** and a **dental lisp** are also identified by speech and language pathologists. In addition, certain /s/ and /z/ misarticulations are classified as phonological process problems. The major types of sibilant misarticulations as they traditionally relate to lisping are described in this section. The errors that are identified as phonological processes are covered in the next section.

The basic requirements for /s/ and /z/ production are (1) a constriction formed between the tongue tip and alveolar ridge or between the tongue blade and the alveolar ridge with the tongue tip posterior to the lower teeth, and (2) airflow directed between the upper and lower teeth. Fulfillment of these specifications results in relatively high-intensity sibilant noise with relatively high spectral peaks of about 5000 and 8000 Hz for males, 6000 and 9000 Hz for females, and 6500 and 10,000 Hz for children (Daniloff, Wilcox, & Stephens, 1980). Correct production of the sibilants requires a certain articulatory precision. Otherwise, subtle but perceptible changes occur which make it difficult to identify sounds as sibilants or to accept them as normal. As indicated in Table 8–3, these alterations can be described as omitted, stopped, nasalized, protruded, dentalized, labiodentalized, lateralized, and retroflex. Protruded, dentalized, and lateralized /s/ and /z/ are considered lisping problems by most speech and language pathologists; retroflex and labiodentalized /s/ and /z/ are less frequently identified as lisps.

Omitted /s/ and /z/

Omission of /s/ and /z/ is a misarticulation characterized by the absence of frication noise or any other sound in place of /s/ and /z/ (see Table 8–3). This error can occur in any position, for example, prevocalically in /op/ for 'soap' or postvocalically in /hɑʊ/ for 'house' and /kɔ/ for 'cause.' Like all omission errors, the deletion of /s/ and /z/ is serious because no cues remain from which to identify the intended sound. Although this error is not included as a lisping problem, it is considered an error characteristic of a few phonological process problems. One of these, cluster reduction, was discussed in Chapter 2. This process includes the omission of /s/ in clusters like /st/ in 'stop' (see Figure 2–3).

Table 8–3
Misarticulations of the /s/ and /z/ phonemes (0 = omitted).

Symbol	Misarticulation	Description
[0] [0]	Omitted	No sound produced
/t/ /d/	Stopped	Tongue tip contacts alveolar ridge
[s̃] [z̃]	Nasalized	Air escapes through nasal cavity
/θ/ /ð/	Protruded[a]	Tongue tip protrudes between teeth
[s̪] [z̪]	Dentalized[a]	Tongue tip approximates back of teeth
$[\overset{f}{s}]$ $[\overset{v}{z}]$	Labiodentalized[b]	Lower lip approximates upper teeth
$[s^{l}]$ $[z^{l}]$	Lateralized[a]	Tongue tip contacts alveolar ridge with margins lowered
[s̢] [z̢]	Retroflex[b]	Tongue tip arches back to approximate palate

[a]These are the three major types of lisps.
[b]These are considered to be types of lisps by some speech and language pathologists.

Stopped /s/ and /z/

Stopping, the opposite error from omission, is the substitution of /t/ and /d/ for /s/ and /z/, as in /tip/ 'sleep' and /dibrə/ 'zebra.' If used consistently, these substitutions provide a cue to the place of articulation of the intended sound but still make for confusion between minimal pairs like 'sick'/'tick' and 'zip'/'dip,' as shown in Figure 8–2. These substitutions are not considered lisping errors; they are classified as part of the phonological process of stopping along with other substitutions for fricatives.

Nasalized /s/ and /z/

Nasalization of fricatives is most characteristic of cleft-palate speakers who are able to make the appropriate articulatory adjustments for /s/ and /z/ but cannot prevent air from escaping through the nasal cavity. The severity of the sibilant nasalization depends on how much air gets to the tongue constriction to produce oral frication and how much goes through the nasal cavity to produce nasal frication. Loss of oral airflow results in sibilants that are lower in intensity and frequency than normal ones. The presence of nasal frication adds to the perception of a loss of sibilant quality.

Lisping

The three major types of lisps are generally described in terms of the nature of the tongue interference with the normal constriction for /s/ and /z/. These are identified in Table 8–3 as protruded, dentalized, and lateralized sounds; in some classification systems, these are called frontal, dental, and lateral lisps. For the **protruded lisp,** the tongue tip is actually between the teeth so that /θ/ is substituted for /s/ and /ð/ is substituted for /z/. Evidence from studies of tongue contact and pressure indicates

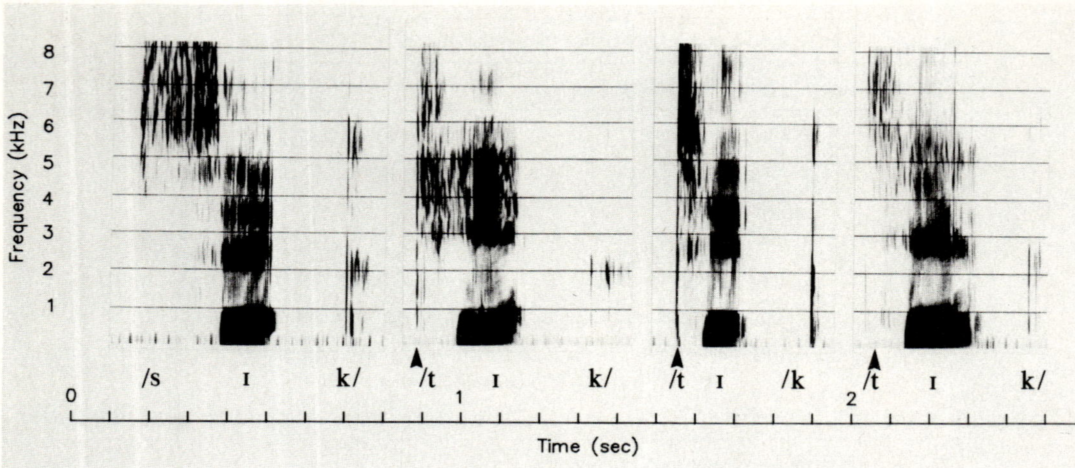

Figure 8–2

Spectrograms of a child's normal and stopped productions of 'sick' followed by a child's normal and stopped productions of 'tick.' Arrows along the *x* axis indicate the release of the stop. Since stopping does not affect /t/, the two patterns of 'tick' are similar.

close similarity between the frontal lisp and /θ/ (McGlone & Profitt, 1974). Moreover, /s/ and /θ/ produced by children with frontal lisps have significantly greater variability in duration than do /s/ productions by normally articulating children (Weismer & Elbert, 1982). The protruded lisp results in loss of phonemic distinction between minimal pairs like 'some' and 'thumb' and 'close' (verb) and 'clothe.' Figures 8–3 and 8–4 include spectrograms of these words spoken by a child with a protrusion lisp and another child without this problem. (In Figure 8–3 and other figures in this chapter, non-fricative consonants and parts of vowels were deleted to save space.) As you can observe, the lisp results in loss of the intensity of the high-frequency noise that is characteristic of sibilants (Daniloff et al., 1980).

For the dentalized lisp, the tongue tip is placed very close to the upper teeth so that the airstream is obstructed as it passes between the upper and lower teeth. This sound is similar to, if not the same as, the **dentalized** allophones of /s, z/ described in Table 8–2. These allophones occur in English only when /θ/ and /ð/ precede or follow /s/ and /z/. The use of dentalized variants is considered lisping when they occur in the production of sibilants not adjacent to /θ/ and /ð/. The quality of the dental lisp may vary depending on the degree to which the tongue tip approximates the teeth. Variations are described as whistling sounds, strident sounds, weakly articulated /ts/ or /dz/ affricates, or weak /s/ and /z/ sounds similar to /θ/ and /ð/. Figures 8–5 and 8–6 include spectrograms of a child's normal and dental productions of the minimal pairs 'some' and 'thumb' and 'close' (verb) and 'clothe.' The deviant /s/ and /z/ still retain their characteristic high-frequency energy, but they are weaker in intensity than the normal sibilants, almost as weak as the /θ/ and /ð/ sounds (Daniloff et al., 1980).

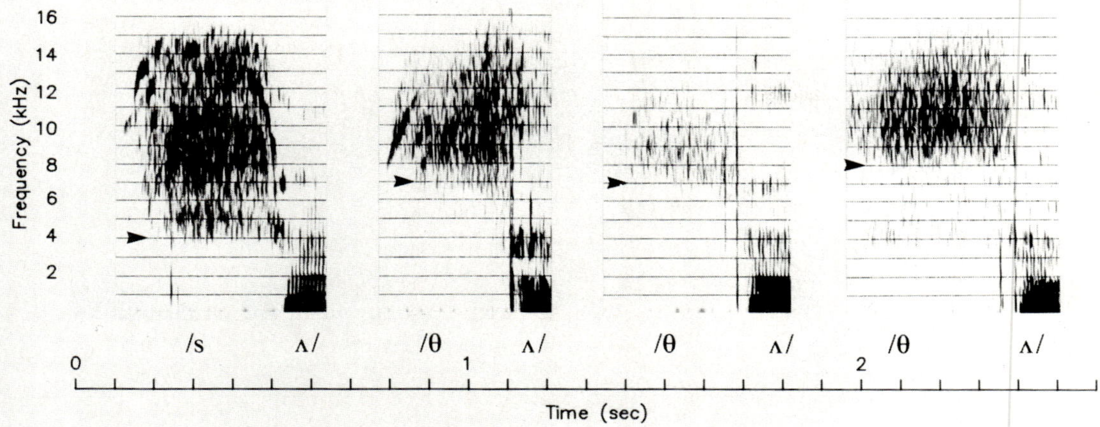

Figure 8–3
Spectrograms of a child's normal and protruded productions of 'some' followed by a child's normal and protruded productions of 'thumb.' The final consonant and part of the vowel were removed from each pattern to save space. Arrows along the *y* axis mark the lower border of relatively intense spectral energy for each fricative. Since lisping does not affect /θ/, the two patterns of 'thumb' are similar.

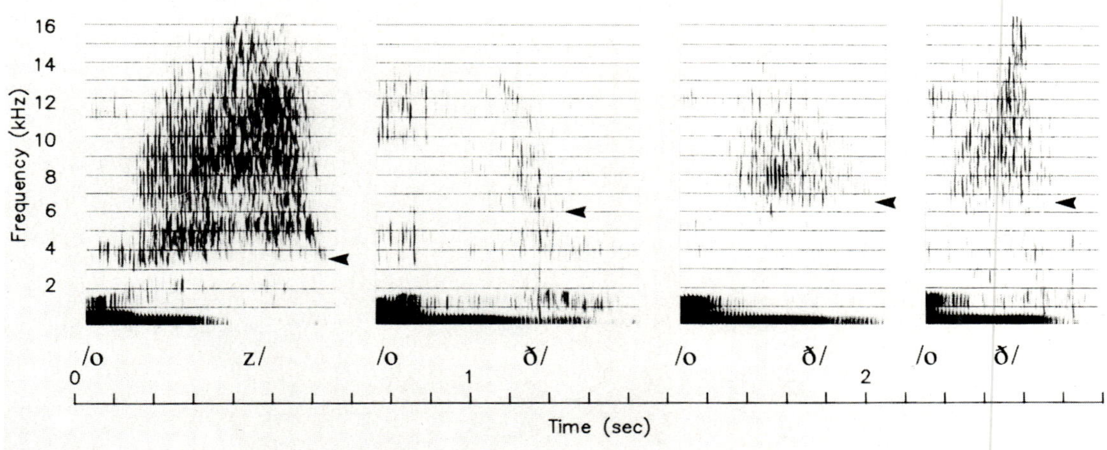

Figure 8–4
Spectrograms of a child's normal and protruded productions of 'close' followed by a child's normal and protruded productions of 'clothe.' The initial consonants and part of the vowel were removed from each pattern to save space. Arrows along the *y* axis mark the lower border of relatively intense spectral energy for each fricative. Since lisping does not affect /ð/, the two patterns of 'clothe' are similar.

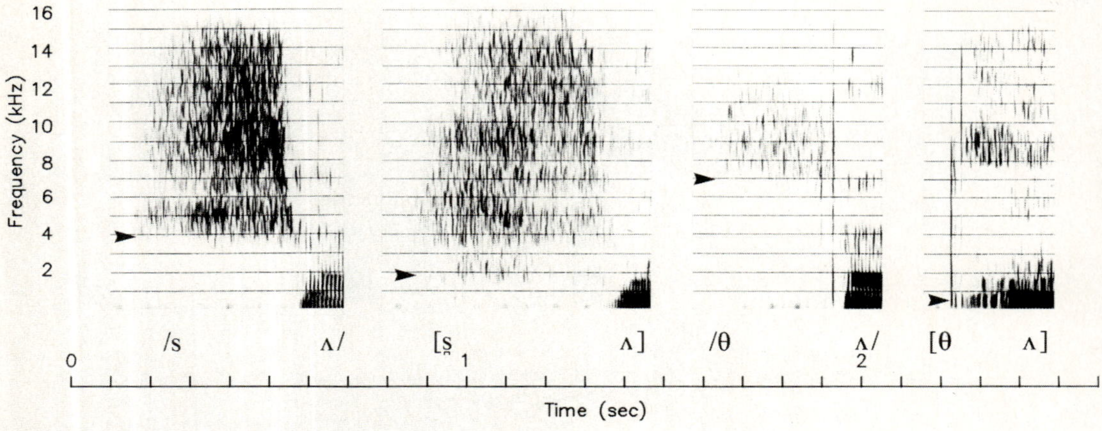

Figure 8–5
Spectrograms of a child's normal and dentalized productions of 'some' followed by a child's normal and dentalized productions of 'thumb.' The final consonant and part of the vowel were removed from each pattern to save space. Arrows along the *y* axis mark the lower border of relatively intense spectral energy for each fricative. Normally lisping does not affect /θ/, but the arrow in the lisper's 'thumb' pattern indicates a spike which reflects an affricate production /t θ/.

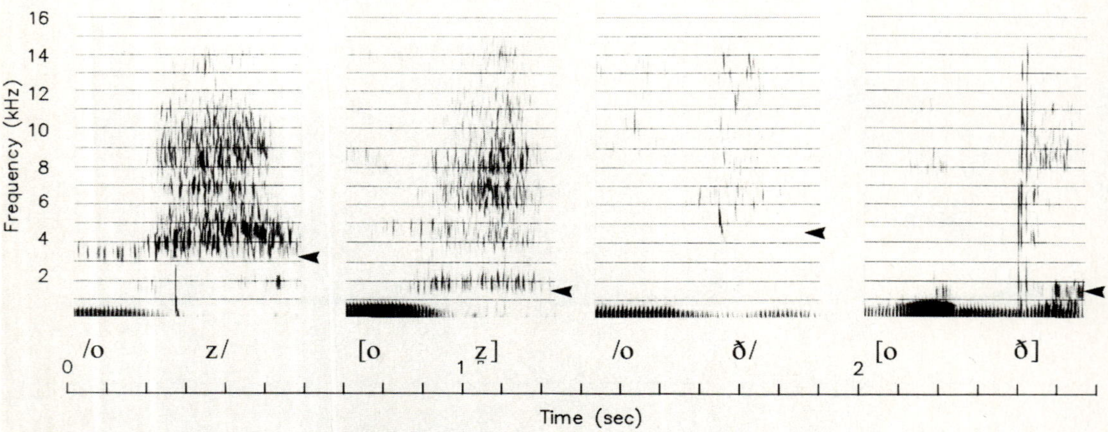

Figure 8–6
Spectrograms of a child's normal and dentalized productions of 'close' followed by a child's normal and dentalized productions of 'clothe.' The initial consonants and part of the vowel were removed from each pattern to save space. Arrows along the *y* axis mark the lower border of relatively intense spectral energy for each fricative. Since lisping does not affect /ð/, the two patterns of 'clothe' are similar.

Unlike the protruded lisp, the dental lisp does not result in the loss of phonemic distinction between sibilants and the /θ/ and /ð/ sounds. For this reason the dental lisp may not be considered as serious a problem as the frontal lisp. Some individuals with a dentalized lisp have a complex pattern of dentalization that includes the other apico-alveolar sounds /t, d, n, l/. Dentalized alveolar stops were described in Chapter 6, and dentalized /l/ was described in Chapter 4. The dentalization problem as it relates to /n/ is described in Chapter 9. Dentalization of all or any of the apico-alveolar sounds tends to make the dental lisp more noticeable. Since no phonemic substitution is involved, the dental lisp is traditionally described as a distortion, the use of a sound which is close to the correct one but has an unacceptable sound quality.

An understanding of the nature of the lateral lisp can be reached by considering the mechanism for the production of the lateral sound. By putting your tongue in the position for the first sound in 'lap,' you put it in the position to produce a lateral lisp. If you keep your tongue in this position and simply blow air out, air passes over the sides of the tongue. Some frication noise will be produced; it can be increased by raising the sides of the tongue slightly. The noise should have a slushy quality. Now, if you pronounce 'lap' with this slushy /l/, you produce a lateral lisp. Producing the voiced equivalent requires only that you add voicing to the frication noise. These sounds can be transcribed by using /s/ and /z/ followed by superscript /l/ (see Table 8–3). Figures 8–7 and 8–8 are spectrograms of a child's normal and lateralized productions of the minimal pairs 'sew'/'show' and 'bays'/'beige.' These words were chosen because some observers believe that lateral lisping makes 'sew' sound like 'show' and 'bays' sound like 'beige.' Notice that lateralizing tends to produce sibilants with much less intensity and somewhat lower frequency concentration than normal (Daniloff et al., 1980).

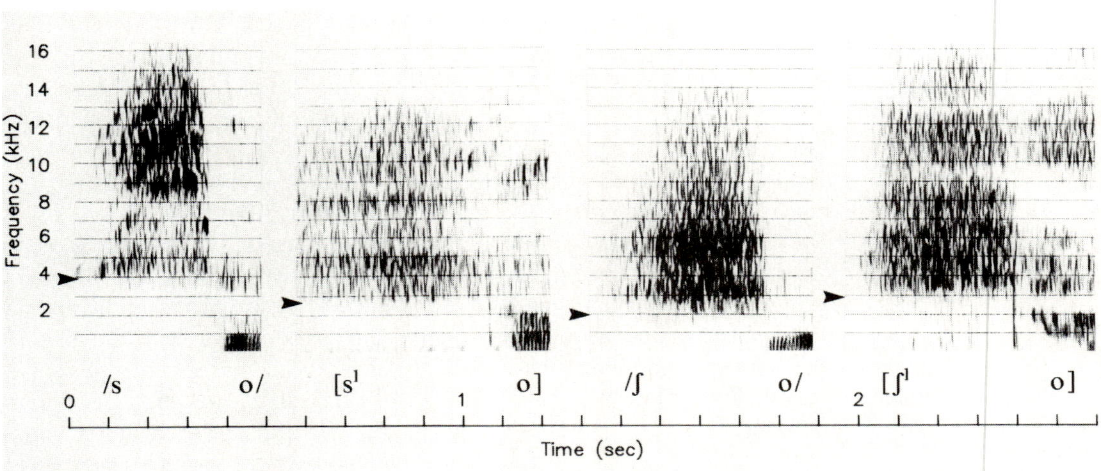

Figure 8–7
Spectrograms of a child's normal and lateralized productions of 'so' followed by a child's normal and lateralized productions of 'show.' Arrows along the *y* axis mark the lower border of relatively intense spectral energy for each fricative. Part of the vowel was deleted from each pattern to save space.

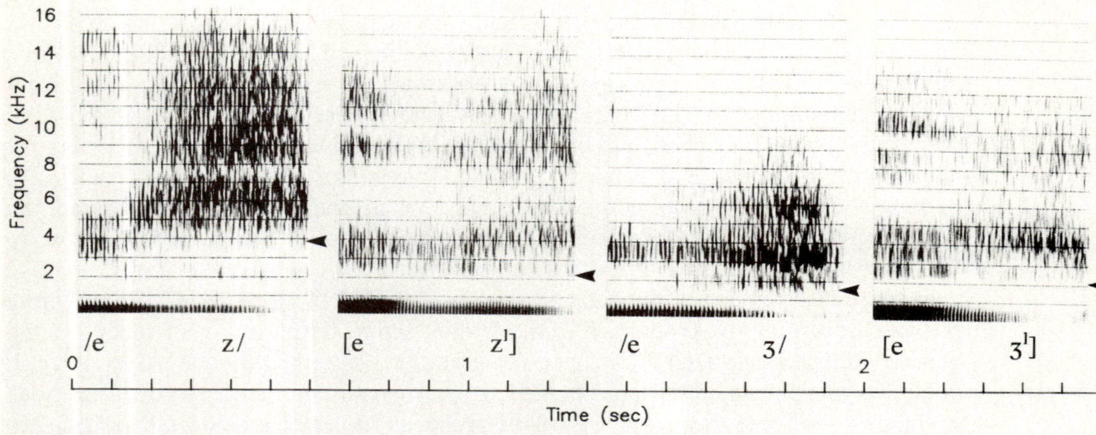

Figure 8–8
Spectrograms of a child's normal and lateralized productions of 'bays' followed by a child's normal and lateralized productions of 'beige.' The initial consonant and part of the vowel were removed from each pattern to save space. Arrows along the *y* axis mark the lower border of relatively intense spectral energy for each fricative.

The articulatory mechanism used in the production of a lateral lisp results in a diffuse or spread pattern of airflow between the teeth. You can check this for yourself by producing 'say' alternately with normal and lateral /s/ sounds. The air flows out between the upper and lower central incisor teeth for normal /s/ but more to either side of these teeth for lateral /s/. The same holds true for normal and lateral /z/ sounds. Lateral /s, z/ can be produced as bilateral or unilateral sounds, that is, with the air flowing over both sides or just one side of the tongue. Unilateral production involves raising either the right or the left margin of the tongue so as to block the airflow. Apparently, the occurrence of unilateral instead of bilateral lisps has no important implications for the rehabilitation of the problem.

As indicated in Table 8–3, some speech and language pathologists identify two additional types of lisp, the **retroflex lisp** and the **labiodentalized lisp.** Retroflex /s/ and /z/ are not commonly found among native English speakers (Shriberg & Kent, 1982). Although they are considered distortions in English, the retroflex sibilants occur as phonemes in some Indian languages (Heffner, 1952). They are produced by arching the tongue tip up and back so that it approximates the palate posterior to the alveolar ridge. For the retroflex sibilants, unlike the lateral lisp, the margins of the tongue contact the palate. The airflow, while not lateralized, is very diffuse because the opening is rather wide—more like /ʃ, ʒ/ than /s, z/. Figures 8–9 and 8–10 include spectrograms of an adult male's normal and retroflex productions of the minimal pairs 'sew'/'show' and 'bays'/'beige.' These pairs were selected so that /s/ could be compared with /ʃ/ and /z/ with /ʒ/, since some observers believe that this type of lisp makes the front sibilants sound like the back ones. Notice that this lisp produces a low-frequency concentration more characteristic of /ʃ/ and /ʒ/ than of /s/ and /z/.

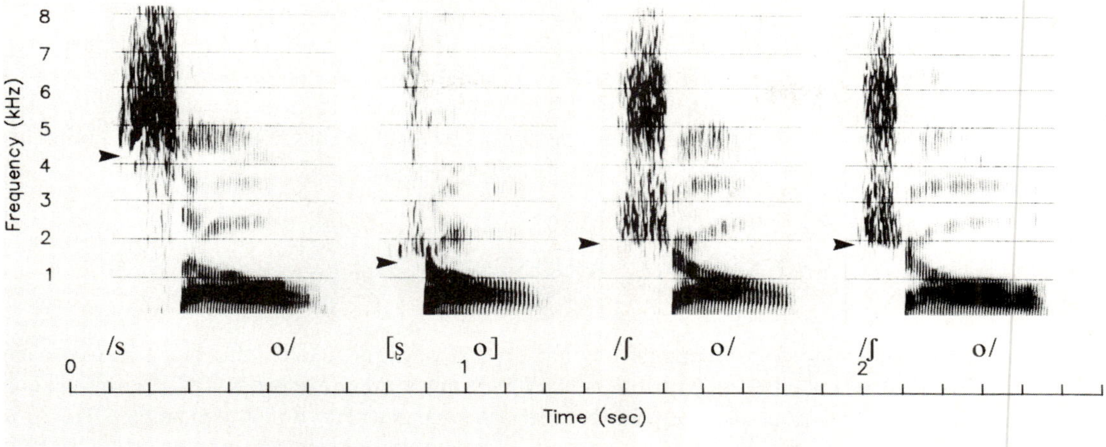

Figure 8–9
Spectrograms of an adult male's normal and retroflex productions of 'so' followed by an adult male's normal and retroflex productions of 'show.' Arrows along the *y* axis mark the lower border of relatively intense spectral energy for each fricative. Since a normal /ʃ/ was produced by the retroflexing speaker, the two patterns of 'show' are similar.

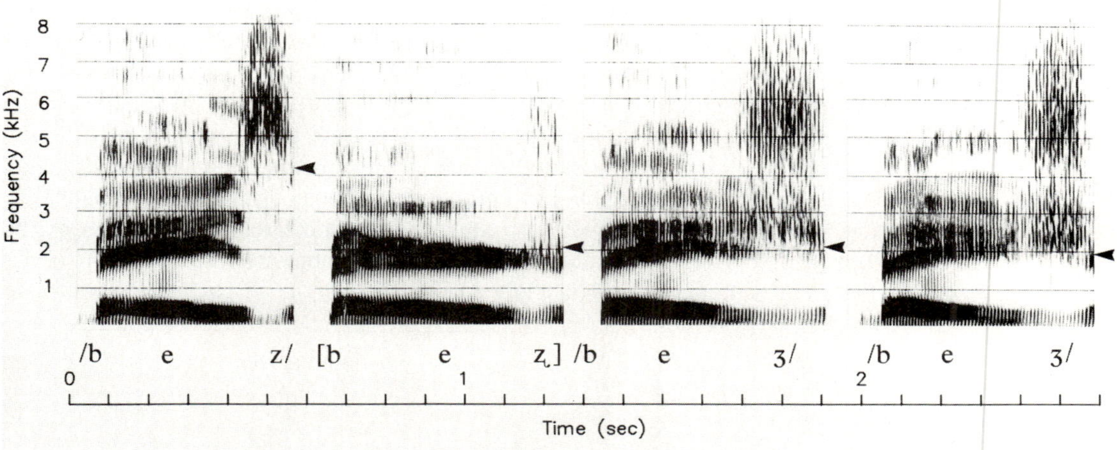

Figure 8–10
Spectrograms of an adult male's normal and retroflex productions of 'bays' followed by an adult male's normal and retroflex productions of 'beige.' Arrows along the *y* axis mark the lower border of relatively intense spectral energy for each fricative. Since a normal /ʒ/ was produced by the retroflexing speaker, the two patterns of 'beige' are similar.

The labiodentalized lisp, like the allophone of /s/ when preceded by /f/ and of /z/ when preceded by /v/, involves lower lip contact with the upper teeth. If the **labiodentalized** variants occur only in the context of /f/ and /v/, they are considered allophones of /s/ and /z/. If they occur in other contexts, their usage is described as a labiodentalized lisp. Although this lisp is commonly referred to as a labialized lisp, the more exact descriptive term *labiodentalized* is used in this book since IPA and many phoneticians use *labialized* to refer to rounded consonants.

PHONOLOGICALLY ABNORMAL VARIANTS

In the following descriptions of phonological processes that influence fricatives and affricates, examples of words in which the changes occur are presented. More than one process can influence the pronunciation of a particular word. For example, /bɪʃ/ for 'fish' demonstrates processes of both stopping and prevocalic voicing since /b/ is a voiced stop and /f/ is a voiceless fricative. One must be sure to look for each type of process that might be involved in a misarticulation.

Cluster Reduction

Although cluster reduction was covered in Chapter 2 in the discussion of syllable simplification processes, it is appropriate to review it here because of the large number of cluster reductions that involve /s/. The following are a few samples of the influence of cluster reduction on /s/: /dip/ for 'sleep'; /pɑt/ for 'spot'; /mɔ/ for 'small'; /dɛk/ for 'desk.' In each case, note that /s/ is the sound that is omitted from the cluster, which is what the markedness theory (Ingram, 1976) would predict. According to this theory, /s/ is more marked than the nondeleted sounds in the clusters, as may be determined from the criteria for designating the unmarked member of a cognate pair in a phonemic opposition. The unmarked member (1) requires less articulatory effort; (2) requires less complex acoustic representation; (3) is less ambiguous in perception; (4) is acquired first by children; and (5) is more likely to occur in all language inventories (Toombs, Singh, & Hayden, 1981).

Final Consonant Deletion

In traditional analysis, deletion of final consonants is classified as an omission of each phoneme affected. Therapy based on this classification usually focuses on achieving correct production of each phoneme. With a phonological process approach, the stress is placed on achieving syllable closure (Weiner, 1981). Deletion of final fricatives as, for example, in /lu/ for 'lose' involves elimination of the contrast between the closed and open syllables 'Lou' and 'lose,' as well as the elimination of the voicing contrast between 'lose' and 'loose.' This process is commonly found in the speech of misarticulating children (Ingram, 1976). There have been no acoustic studies to show that children use differential vowel duration to signal the voicing characteristic of final fricatives as they do for stops

(Weismer, Dinnsen, & Elbert, 1981; Weismer, 1984). Such evidence plus the use of morphophonemic alternations, as in [lu:] for 'lose' and /luzɚ/ for 'loser,' would indicate that a child has underlying knowledge of the existence of a final consonant in 'lose.'

In discussing the acoustic evidence presented to support an underlying knowledge of final stops, a study was described in which five children omitted final consonants but made the vowel longer when the omitted following consonant was a voiced one (Weismer, 1984). The mean difference between vowels preceding voiced and voiceless fricatives is as substantial as that for stops (Peterson & Lehiste, 1960; Naeser, 1970b; Lehman, 1988). There is no spectrographic evidence, however, to support the perception that the same pattern occurs for deleted fricatives. In analyzing the speech of children who delete final consonants, it is important to note as long or short those vowels preceding omitted final fricatives and affricates. Thus, [lu:] for 'lose' and /lu/ for 'loose' might indicate some awareness of an appropriate vowel duration differential for fricative voicing.

In referring to the omission of final stops in Chapter 6, it was noted that children may be "groping" toward the articulatory positions for those sounds (Weismer, 1984). This behavior involves moving the articulators from vowels toward appropriate constrictions for final consonants. If such approximations are heard, they can be noted by using vowel plus superscript fricative symbols. Weismer (1984) describes how spectrographic analysis of vowel formant transitions might be used to detect such "groping" in cases of final consonant deletion. But much research on children's normal speech must be done before such efforts are feasible.

Although children use glottal stops instead of other stops to terminate vowels in CVC words, there is no indication that they do the same for fricatives. But children may use a glottal stop to replace the voiceless affricate /tʃ/ in words like 'church' (Compton & Hutton, 1980).

Prevocalic Voicing

Prevocalic voicing occurs for fricatives as well as stops. (Its application to stops was covered in Chapter 6.) For fricatives as well as stops, the misarticulation may involve just voicing, as in /zup/ for 'soup.' Misarticulations that involve prevocalic voicing errors for fricatives frequently involve other errors as well. For example, /bɪʃ/ for 'fish' and /dʌm/ for 'thumb' also involve stopping of prevocalic consonants; /dʌpo/ for 'shovel' also involves stopping and fronting of a prevocalic consonant. Although it would be helpful if there were evidence that children use subtle acoustic cues to differentiate intended voiceless fricatives as they may do for stops, this is not the case. Prevocalic voicing of fricatives results in the loss of distinction of minimal pairs like 'sue'/'zoo.'

Final Consonant Devoicing

In devoicing final fricatives, children neutralize the distinction between, for example, 'loose' and 'lose,' which may both be pronounced /lus/. This process is apparently not common among children with the most severe articulatory disorders (Hodson & Paden,

1983). Evidence that a child is aware of the voicing distinction would be lengthening of the vowel preceding a target voiced fricative, as in [lu:s] for 'lose.' Some children show this type of awareness (Ingram, 1976; Compton & Hutton, 1980). But no acoustic evidence exists to indicate the magnitude of the difference in vowel duration used by these children, nor are there sufficient data for conclusions about the significance of any differences. As suggested for final consonant deletion, the clinician should note any vowel duration differences that occur for minimal pairs like 'loose' and 'lose,' in particular, any prolonged vowel preceding a voiceless consonant which has been substituted for a target voiced final consonant.

Stopping, Affrication, and Deaffrication

Stopping, affrication, and deaffrication, as indicated in Table 8–4, are related in that they involve changes in manner of production of fricatives and affricates by means of the substitution, addition, or deletion of a stop consonant. Reference was made earlier to the use of stops for sibilants, as in /tip/ for 'sleep' and /dibrə/ for 'zebra.' The substitution of a stop consonant can occur for any fricative, as in /təm/ for 'thumb,' /nɑɪp/ for 'knife,' and /dʌpo/ for 'shovel.' **Stopping** is a commonly used process among older children with unintelligible speech (Hodson & Paden, 1981); it results in

Table 8–4
Phonological processes influencing the production of fricatives and affricates.

Process	Change
Omissions	
Cluster reduction	/tɑp/ 'stop'; /lip/ 'sleep'
Final consonant deletion	/dɔ/ 'dog'; /mæti/ 'matches'
Voicing Changes	
Prevocalic voicing	/zup/ 'soup'; /ðʌm/ 'thumb'
Final consonant devoicing	/nus/ *or* [no:s] 'nose'
Manner Changes	
Stopping	/tu/ 'shoe'; /tʌm/ 'thumb'
Affrication	/tsop/ 'soap'; /fɪtʃɪŋ/ 'fishing'
Deaffrication	/ʒus/ 'juice'; /ʃɪn/ 'chin'
Place Changes	
Palatalization	/ʃop/ 'soap'
Depalatalization; fronting	/wɑts/ 'watch'; /fʌdz/ 'fudge'
Multiple Changes	
Stridency deletion[a]	/op/ 'soap'; /ɪ/ 'fish'

[a]Stridency deletion also includes instances of cluster reduction, final consonant deletion, stopping, and deaffrication that involve omissions of stridents or substitutions of nonstridents for the stridents, /f, v, s, z, ʃ, ʒ, tʃ, dʒ/.

the loss of distinction between such minimal pairs as 'sip'/'tip,' 'fat'/'pat,' 'thin'/'tin,' and 'ship'/'tip.'

As in the case of other phonological processes, there is some interest in determining whether a child with a stopping problem makes any distinction between the stops used in 'sip' and 'tip.' Does the stop used in 'sip' somehow sound less like the /t/ used in 'tip' and more like /s/? Two possible means have been proposed by which children could reduce the loss of distinction between fricatives and stops—spirantization during the stop closure and prolongation of frication noise after the stop release (Weismer, 1984). **Spirantization** is a release of air due to an incomplete stop closure. It shows on a spectrogram as fill preceding the release spike. Prolongation of frication noise after the stop release appears on a spectrogram as a much longer than usual period of fill (from 0 to 40 msec) following the release spike (Klatt, 1975; Zue, 1976).

Affrication involves the conversion of a fricative into an affricate, as in /tsop/ for 'soap' and /fɪtʃɪŋ/ for 'fishing' (Hodson & Paden, 1983). Use of this process results in the loss of distinction between minimal pairs like 'shop' and 'chop.'

Deaffrication is the reverse of affrication in that an affricate is converted to a fricative, as in /ʒus/ for 'juice' and /ʃu/ for 'chew' (Hodson & Paden, 1983). It appears that this process involves only the /tʃ/ and /dʒ/ affricates and the loss of distinction in minimal pairs like 'shoe' and 'chew,' as shown in Figure 8–11.

Palatalization, Depalatalization, and Fronting

Palatalization, depalatalization, and fronting are related in that they involve changes in place of articulation for fricatives and affricates. The change is between the alveolar and

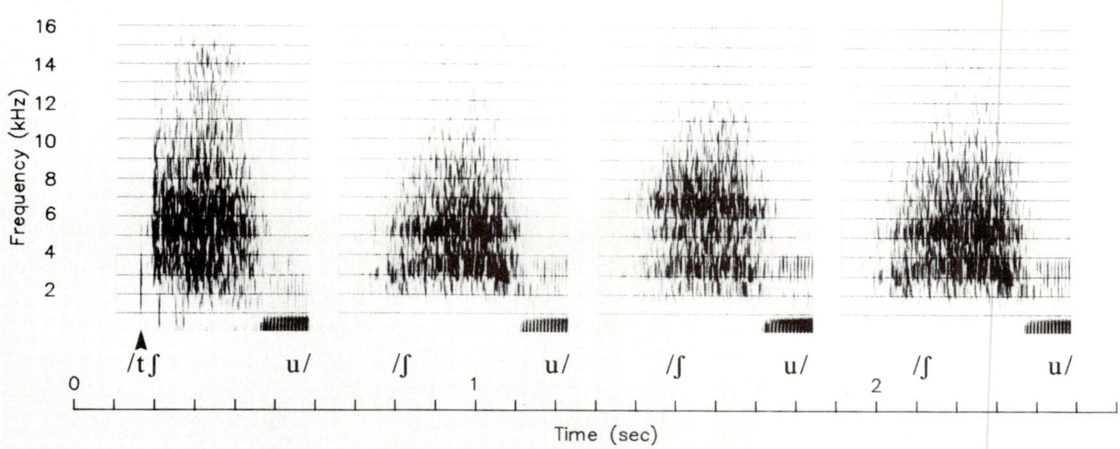

Figure 8–11
Spectrograms of a child's normal and deaffricated productions of 'chew' followed by a child's normal and deaffricated productions of 'shoe.' The arrow along the *x* axis indicates the release of the stop portion of /tʃ/. Since deaffrication does not affect /ʃ/, the two patterns of 'shoe' are similar. Part of the vowel was removed from each pattern to save space.

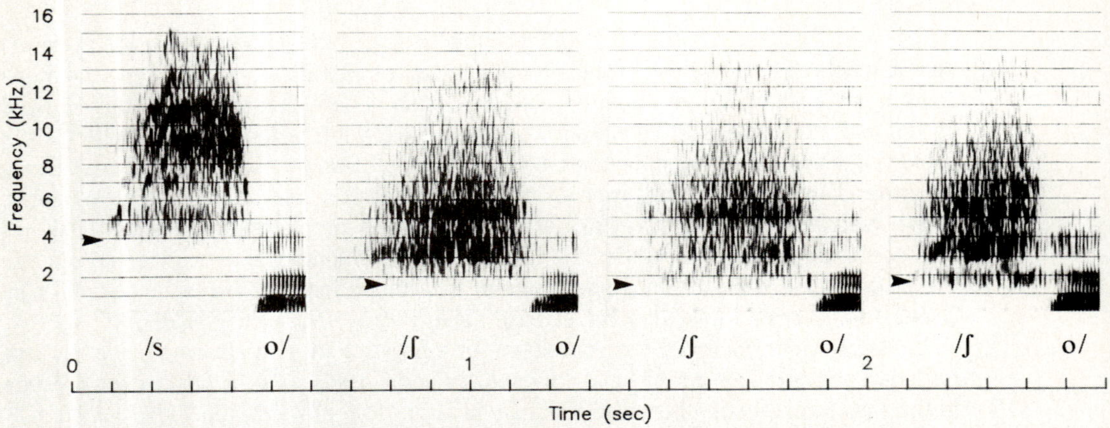

Figure 8–12
Spectrograms of a child's normal and palatalized productions of 'so' followed by a child's normal and palatalized productions of 'show.' Arrows along the *y* axis mark the lower border of relatively intense spectral energy for each fricative. Since palatalization does not affect /ʃ/, the two patterns of 'show' are similar. Part of the vowel was deleted from each pattern to save space.

palatal fricatives. **Palatalization** involves the substitution of the palatal for the alveolar fricative, as in /ʃo/ for 'sew' (Hodson & Paden, 1983). This substitution results in the loss of distinction in minimal pairs like 'sew' and 'show,' as shown in Figure 8–12.

Depalatalization is the reverse of palatalization, as in the pronunciation of 'watch' as /wɑts/ and 'shoes' as /suz/ (Hodson & Paden, 1983). These substitutions result in the loss of distinction in minimal pairs like 'cats' and 'catch' and 'sue' and 'shoe.' Fronting includes the same type of change as depalatalization. But depalatalization applies only to fricatives and affricates, while fronting also applies to the substitution of alveolar stops for velar stops (described in Chapter 6).

Stridency Deletion

Stridency is a term used by some phoneticians to describe sounds that are produced by forcing the airstream through a small opening. It is one of a number of distinctive features proposed by Chomsky and Halle (1968) in their set of binary features used to describe all English phonemes. According to their terminology, /f, v, s, z, ʃ, ʒ, tʃ, dʒ/ are **stridents** and /θ, ð/ are nonstridents. These terms are analogous to sibilant and nonsibilant in the classification of fricatives and affricates, except that /f, v/ are not sibilants. **Stridency deletion** is an umbrella term for a number of phonological processes that influence the strident sounds, including initial (or prevocalic) consonant deletion, final consonant deletion, cluster reduction, deaffrication, and stopping. Stridency deletion is a common symptom of disordered phonology (Hodson & Paden, 1983). Omissions occur for stridents as a function of initial consonant deletion, as in /op/

for 'soap,' final consonant deletion, as in /hɑʊ/ for 'house,' and cluster reduction, as in /tɑp/ for 'stop.' Substitutions occur for stridents as a function of stopping, as in /pɔɚk/ for 'fork,' and deaffrication, as in /tɛɚ/ for 'chair,' if Hodson and Paden's (1983) definition of deaffrication as including the replacement of an affricate by a stop is accepted.

GLOSSARY

Affrication. The conversion of a fricative into an affricate; a phonological process.

Deaffrication. The conversion of an affricate into a fricative; a phonological process.

Dentalized. Describes variants of /s, z, t, d, n/ produced in the context of /θ/ and /ð/ with apicodental tongue contact.

Dental lisp. A lisp in which /s/ and /z/ are produced with the tongue tip too close to the teeth.

Depalatalization. The substitution of alveolar for palatal fricatives; a phonological process.

Frontal lisp. A lisp in which /θ/ and /ð/ substitute for /s/ and /z/.

Labiodentalized. Describes /s/ and /z/ variants produced in the context of /f/ and /v/ with the lower lip intruding between the teeth; a lisp involving the use of such variants in other contexts.

Lateral lisp. A lisp in which air flows over one or both sides of the tongue during /s/ and /z/ production.

Lisping. An articulation disorder in which /s/ and /z/ are produced with deviant tongue positions, resulting in a loss of sibilant quality.

Omission. Deletion of a sound from a word; a type of misarticulation.

Palatalization. The substitution of palatal for alveolar fricatives; a phonological process.

Palatalized /h/. An /h/ variant produced when /j/ follows and frication noise occurs in the oral cavity.

Protruded lisp. Frontal lisp.

Retroflex lisp. A lisp in which /s/ and /z/ are produced from an apicopalatal position.

Spirantization. The release of air due to incomplete stop closure. Appears as fill prior to the release spike on a spectrogram.

Stopping. The substitution of stops for fricatives; a phonological process.

Stridency deletion. Any one of a number of phonological processes that result in the omission of or substitution for strident sounds, including prevocalic consonant deletion, final consonant deletion, cluster reduction, and stopping.

Strident. Describes sounds produced by forcing the airstream through a small opening; sibilant fricatives and affricates plus /f, v/.

Substitution. A misarticulation in which one phoneme replaces another.

REVIEW QUESTIONS

A. For each word in the left-hand column, choose a minimal pair contrast word from the right-hand column by inserting the appropriate letter.

1. batch ________	a. claws
2. loft ________	b. nose
3. noose ________	c. clothe
4. cloth ________	d. lost
5. mash ________	e. math
6. close (adj.) ____	f. news
7. safe ________	g. badge
8. node ________	h. save

****

Key: 1. g; 2. d; 3. f; 4. a; 5. e; 6. c; 7. h; 8. b

B. Indicate the word in which the following allophonic changes for fricatives may occur by inserting the appropriate letter: (a) labiodental to bilabial; (b) alveolar to labiodental; (c) alveolar to interdental; (d) voiceless to voiced; (e) unrounded to rounded.

1. vote ________	5. laughs ________
2. moths ________	6. moves ________
3. camphor ________	7. hole ________
4. behead ________	8. breathes ________

****

Key: 1. e; 2. c; 3. a; 4. d; 5. b; 6. b; 7. e; 8. c

C. Indicate the correct description of each type of lisp by inserting the appropriate letter.

1. Lateral lisp ________	a. [sˡ]
2. Frontal lisp ________	b. [s̢]
3. Retroflex lisp ________	c. /θ/
4. Dental lisp ________	d. [z̪]
5. Protruded lisp ________	

****

Key: 1. a; 2. c; 3. b; 4. d; 5. c

D. Indicate the type of phonological process represented by the following changes by inserting the correct letter.

1. /kæts/ for 'catch' ______
2. /bɛri/ for 'very' ______
3. /paɪ/ for 'spy' ______
4. /ʃip/ for 'cheap' ______
5. /tʃo/ for 'show' ______
6. /ʃus/ for 'shoes' ______
7. /vaɪn/ for 'fine' ______
8. /op/ for 'soap' ______

a. Affrication
b. Prevocalic voicing
c. Final consonant devoicing
d. Deaffrication
e. Stopping
f. Depalatalization
g. Palatalization
h. Stridency deletion
i. Cluster reduction

****

Key: 1. f; 2. e; 3. h *or* i; 4. d; 5. a; 6. c; 7. b; 8. h

LABORATORY ASSIGNMENT

Tape III, Side B
IIIB1: Normal and Abnormal /s, z/ Variants (Tape running time: 9:25; Elapsed time: 00:00–09:25)

a. Normal and Abnormal /s, z/ Variant Models

Listen to the normal and abnormal variants of /s, z/ produced in a /Cæp/ context by a child. If necessary, stop the tape at any time, rewind, and listen again.

1. /sæp/ (normal); /tæp/ (stopped); /θæp/ (protruded); [s̪æp] (dentalized); [sˡæp] (lateralized); /ʃæp/ (palatalized); /tsæp/ (affricated); /æp/ (omitted); /zæp/ (voiced)
2. /zæp/ (normal); /dæp/ (stopped); /ðæp/ (protruded); [z̪æp] (dentalized); [zˡæp] (lateralized); /ʒæp/ (palatalized); /dzæp/ (affricated); /æp/ (omitted); /sæp/ (devoiced)

b. Minimal Pair Contrast of Normal and Abnormal /s/ Variants

Listen to the minimal pairs produced by a child and indicate if the first (1) or second (2) one is a normal /s/.

1. ________ 2. ________ 3. ________ 4. ________ 5. ________

6. ________ 7. ________ 8. ________

****

Key: 1. 2; 2. 1; 3. 2; 4. 1; 5. 1; 6. 1; 7. 1; 8. 2

c. Minimal Pair Contrast of Normal and Abnormal /z/ Variants

Listen to the minimal pairs produced by a child and indicate if the first (1) or second (2) one is a normal /z/.

1. ________ 2. ________ 3. ________ 4. ________ 5. ________

6. ________ 7. ________ 8. ________

****

Key: 1. 1; 2. 2; 3. 1; 4. 2; 5. 2; 6. 2; 7. 2; 8. 2

d. Transcription of Normal and Abnormal /s, z/ Variants in Minimal Contrast Syllables

Transcribe each normal and abnormal /s, z/ variant as it is pronounced by a child in a minimal contrast context in prevocalic position.

1. ________ 2. ________ 3. ________ 4. ________ 5. ________

6. ________ 7. ________ 8. ________ 9. ________ 10. ________

11. ________ 12. ________

****

Consensus: 1. /z^{l}/ 2. /dz/ 3. [z̪] 4. /ð/ 5. [s^{l}] 6. /t/ 7. /ð/ 8. [s̪] 9. /θ/ 10. /ʃ/ 11. [z^{l}] 12. /ʒ/

Variants: 2. /ʤ/ 3. /z/ 4. [s^{l}] 12. /ʤ/

e. Transcription of Normal and Abnormal /s, z/ Variants in Minimal Contrast Syllables in Context

Transcribe each normal and abnormal /s, z/ variant as it is pronounced by a child in a minimal contrast context in a sentence.

1. ________ 2. ________ 3. ________ 4. ________ 5. ________

6. ________ 7. ________ 8. ________ 9. ________ 10. ________

****

Consensus: 1. [z^{l}] 2. /θ/ 3. /s/ 4. /ts/ 5. /ʒ/ 6. /z/ 7. /ð/ 8. [z^{l}] 9. /ʃ/ 10. /dz/

Variants: 2. [s̪] 3. [s̪] 4. /tʃ/ 5. [z^{l}] 7. [z̪] 10. /ʤ/

f. Transcription of Normal and Abnormal /s, z/ Variants in Words in Isolation

Transcribe each normal and abnormal /s, z/ variant as it is pronounced by a child in words in isolation.

1. soap ________ 2. zap ________ 3. zoo ________ 4. sick ________

5. sail ________ 6. zap ________ 7. supper ________ 8. Sunday ________

9. soak ________

****

Consensus: 2. /z/ 3. /ð/ 4. /t/ 5. /θ/ 6. [z̪] 7. [s^{l}] 8. /ts/ 9. /s/

Variants: 1. [s^{l}]; [s̪]; /ʃ/ 3. /θ/ 6. /z/ 7. /s/ 8. /tʃ/ 9. [s̪]

g. Transcription of Prevocalic Normal and Abnormal /s, z/ Variants in Words in Context

Transcribe each prevocalic /s, z/ variant as it is pronounced by a child in words in the following sentences: 'I can say ________ '; 'Say the word ________ '; ' ________ is the word.'

1. thigh ________ 2. sop ________ 3. sap ________ 4. zone ________

5. zipper ________ 6. zoom ________ 7. sit ________ 8. suit ________

9. sunny ________

****

Consensus: 1. /θ/ 2. /s/ 3. /t/ 4. /dz/ 5. [z^{l}] 6. /dz/ 7. /s/ 8. /ʃ/ 9. /ts/

Variants: 2. [s̪] 4. /z/ 7. [s̪] 9. /t/

h. Transcription of Intervocalic Normal and Abnormal /s, z/ Variants in Words in Context

Transcribe each intervocalic /s, z/ variant as it is pronounced by a child in words in the following sentences: 'I can say ________ '; 'Say the word ________ '; ' ________ is the word.'

1. lesson ________ 2. kissing ________ 3. racer ________ 4. reason ________

5. lizard ________ 6. messy ________ 7. icy ________ 8. aside ________

9. easy ________ 10. dozen ________

****

Consensus: 2. /ʃ/ 3. /s/ 4. /ð/ 5. /ʒ/ 6. /ts/ 7. /t/ 8. /s/
9. /d/ 10. [z^{l}]

Variants: 1. /s/; /θ/; [s̪] 2. [s̪] 6. /t/ 7. /ts/ 8. [s̪] 9. /dz/

i. Transcription of Postvocalic Normal and Abnormal /s, z/ Variants in Words in Context

Transcribe each postvocalic /s, z/ variant as it is pronounced by a child in words in the following sentences: 'I can say ________ '; 'Say the word ________ '; ' ________ is the word.'

1. peace ________ 2. loss ________ 3. puss ________ 4. bass ________

5. blouse ________ 6. face ________ 7. kiss ________ 8. loose ________

9. please ________ 10. bus ________

****

Consensus: 1. /s/ 2. /ð/ 3. [s^{l}] 4. /ʃ/ 5. /θ/ 6. [s̪] 7. /tʃ/ 8. /s/ 9. /z/ 10. /s/

Variants: 5. /ð/ 6. /s/ 7. /ts/ 8. [s^{l}] 9. [z̥]

IIIB2: Transcription of Complete Words with Vowels, Glides, Stops, and Fricatives

(Tape running time: 3:18; Elapsed time: 09:25–12:43)

The purpose of this section is to provide students with practice in transcribing complete words that include the sounds covered so far—vowels, glides, stops, and fricatives. Transcribe each word below as it is produced by a child, reversing the tape as needed to listen to an utterance again. After you have finished, check your transcriptions against the key.

1. bossy ________________ 14. bridge ________________

2. zoo ________________ 15. zipper ________________

3. father ________________ 16. waffle ________________

4. stop ________________ 17. soap ________________

5. racer ________________ 18. garage ________________

6. sugar ________________ 19. sweater ________________

7. shoe ________________ 20. feather ________________

8. zap ________________ 21. table ________________

9. fussy ________________ 22. loser ________________

10. thick ________________ 23. supper ________________

11. shoes ________________ 24. pass ________________

12. zap ________________ 25. silly ________________

13. sister ________________

****

Consensus: 1. /bɔθi/ 2. /ðu/ 3. /fɑðɚ/ 4. [s̪tɑp] 5. /resɚ/ 6. /ʃugɚ/ 7. /ʃu/ 8. [z̪æp] 9. /fʌsi/ 10. /θɪk/ 11. /ʃuʃ/ 12. /ðæp/ 13. /sɪstɚ/ 14. /brɪdʒ/ 15. [zˡɪpu] 16. /wɔfəl/ 17. /θop/ 18. /gəwɑʒ/ 19. [fwɛtɚ] 20. /bɛfə/ 21. /pebo/ 22. /luzɚ/ 23. [sˡʌpu] 24. [pæsˡ] 25. /θɪli/

Variants: 1. [bɑs̪i] 2. /θu/ 4. /stɑp/ 8. /zæp/ 10. /fɪk/ 12. [zˡæp] 15. [zˡɪpə] 16. [wɑfl̩] 18. /gwɑʒ/ 19. [pwɛrə] 20. [bɛɣ̥ə] 21. /bebo/ 23. [s̪ʌpu] 24. /pæθ/

IIIB3: Deaffricated and Depalatalized /tʃ, dʒ/ Variants (Tape running time: 3:06; Elapsed time: 12:43–15:49)

a. Normal and Abnormal /tʃ, dʒ/ Variant Models

Listen to the normal and abnormal variants of /tʃ, dʒ/ produced in /Co/ and /oC/ contexts by a child. If necessary, stop the tape at any time, rewind, and listen again.

1. /tʃo/ (normal); /ʃo/ (deaffricated); /otʃ/ (normal); /oʃ/ (deaffricated); /dʒo/ (normal); /ʒo/ (deaffricated); /odʒ/ (normal); /oʒ/ (deaffricated)
2. /tʃo/ (normal); /tso/ (depalatalized); /otʃ/ (normal); /ots/ (depalatalized); /dʒo/ (normal); /dzo/ (depalatalized); /odʒ/ (normal); /odz/ (depalatalized)

b. Minimal Pair Contrast of Normal and Abnormal /tʃ, dʒ/ Variants

Listen to the minimal pairs produced by a child and indicate if the first (1) or second (2) is an abnormal /tʃ/ or /dʒ/ variant.

1. ________ 2. ________ 3. ________ 4. ________ 5. ________

6. ________ 7. ________ 8. ________

****

Key: 1. 1; 2. 2; 3. 2; 4. 1; 5. 1; 6. 2; 7. 2; 8. 2

c. Transcription of Normal and Abnormal /tʃ, dʒ/ Variants in Words in Context

Transcribe each /tʃ, dʒ/ variant as it is pronounced by a child in words in the following sentences: 'I can say ________ '; 'Say the word ________ '; ' ________ is the word.'

1. chin ________ 2. watching ________ 3. catch ________

4. badge ________ 5. jeans ________ 6. bridge ________

7. chin ________ 8. watching ________ 9. catch ________

10. badge ________ 11. jeans ________ 12. bridge ________

****

Consensus: 1. /tʃ/ 2. /ts/ 3. /s/ 5. /ʒ/ 7. [s̺] 8. /tʃ/
9. /tʃ/ 10. /dʒ/ 11. /dʒ/ 12. /dʒ/

Variants: 4. [ʒ̥]; [z̥]; [z̺] 6. /ʤ/; /dz/; [dz̺] 7. /ʃ/

IIIB4: /f, v, θ, ð/ Errors: Labialization and Stopping (Tape running time: 4:27; Elapsed time: 15:49–20:16)

a. Normal and Abnormal /f, v, θ, ð/ Variant Models

Listen to the normal and abnormal variants of /f, v, θ, ð/ produced in /Cum/ and /muC/ contexts by a child. If necessary, stop the tape at any time, rewind, and listen again.

1. /fum/; /pum/; /vum/; /bum/; /muf/; /mup/; /muv/; /mub/
2. /θum/; /tum/; /fum/; /ðum/; /dum/; /vum/; /muθ/; /mut/; /muf/; /muð/; /mud/; /muv/

b. Minimal Pair Contrast of Normal and Abnormal /f, v/ Variants

Listen to the minimal pairs produced by a child and indicate if the first (1) or second (2) is an abnormal variant of /f/ or /v/.

1. ________ 2. ________ 3. ________ 4. ________

****

Key: 1. 2; 2. 2; 3. 1; 4. 2

c. Minimal Pair Contrast of Normal and Abnormal /θ, ð/ Variants

Listen to the minimal pairs produced by a child and indicate if the first (1) or second (2) is an abnormal variant of /θ/ or /ð/.

1. ________ 2. ________ 3. ________ 4. ________ 5. ________

6. ________ 7. ________ 8. ________

****

Key: 1. 2; 2. 1; 3. 1; 4. 2; 5. 1; 6. 1; 7. 1; 8. 1

d. Transcription of Normal and Abnormal /f, v/ Variants in Words in Context

Transcribe each /f, v/ variant as it is pronounced by a child in words in the following sentences: 'I can say ________ '; 'Say the word ________ '; ' ________ is the word.'

1. four ________ 2. laugh ________ 3. over ________ 4. four ________

5. laugh ________ 6. over ________

****

Consensus: 1. /f/ 2. /p/ 3. /v/ 4. /p/ 5. /f/ 6. /b/

Variants: None.

e. Transcription of Normal and Abnormal /θ, ð/ Variants in Words in Context

Transcribe each /θ, ð/ variant as it is pronounced by a child in words in the following sentences: 'I can say ________ '; 'Say the word ________ '; ' ________ is the word.'

1. thumb ________ 2. toothache ________ 3. father ________

4. that ________ 5. father ________ 6. toothache ________

7. thumb ________ 8. toothache ________ 9. father ________

10. that ________ 11. father ________ 12. toothache ________

****

Consensus: 1. /b/ 2. /θ/ 3. /t/ 4. /ð/ 6. /θ/ 7. /θ/ 8. /θ/
9. /ð/ 10. /ð/ 11. /ð/ 12. /f/

Variants: 1. /f/ 2. /f/ 5. /ð/; [v̥]; /t/

CHAPTER 9

Analysis of Nasals and Nasalization

In Chapter 5, the acoustic correlates of the physiologic events that differentiate nasals from other consonants were described. Nasals are characterized by formants that reflect the resonance of the glottal tone by the closed oral and open nasal cavities. The formants for nasals are relatively invariant in frequency compared to vowel formants because the nasal cavity does not have articulatory structures. Discontinuities between formants for nasals and for preceding and following vowels show the abrupt, radical change in the resonating systems for the two types of sounds—an open vocal cavity and closed nasal cavity for vowels and a closed vocal cavity and open nasal cavity for nasals. This chapter covers the differences in place of articulation for nasal phonemes of English and their allophones. Since nasal consonants are not generally subject to misarticulation, there is little to say about them in reference to articulatory and phonological disorders. Nasalization of vowels and nonnasal consonants, as well as denasalization of nasal consonants, however, are identified as speech problems, and they are dealt with in this chapter.

NASAL CONSONANTS AND ALLOPHONIC NASALIZATION

Figure 9–1 schematically shows the patterns of normal and abnormal nasalization that occur in American English. In normal production of vowels, glides, and oral consonants, the velopharyngeal mechanism closes off the nasal cavity so that no nasal resonance occurs and air, as it flows through the vocal tract, does not escape through the nose. The major difference between vowels and consonants is that the oral cavity is open for vowels and either blocked or constricted for consonants (see Figure 9–1). For nasal

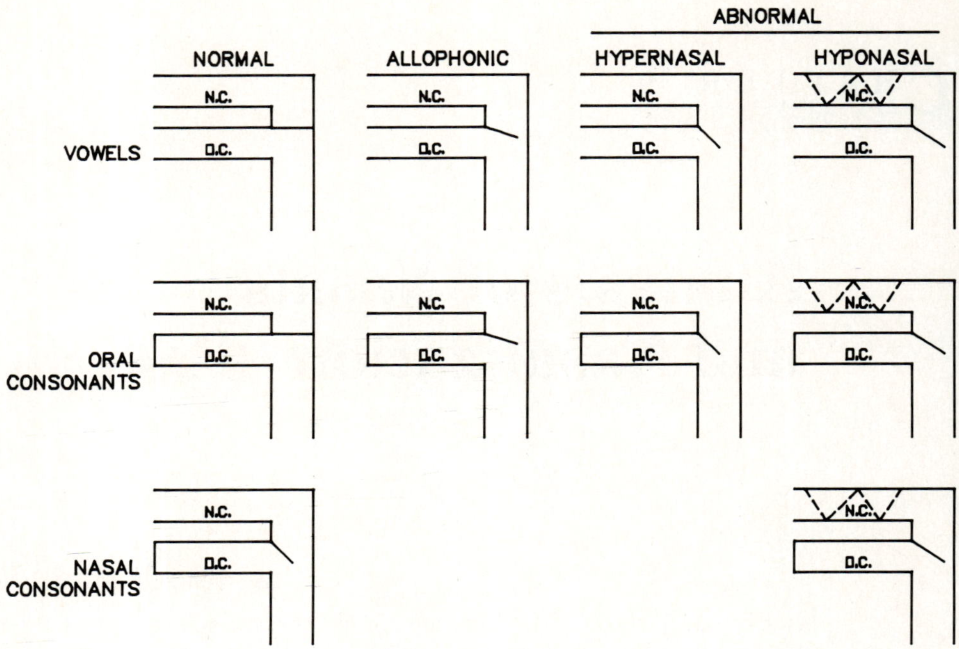

Figure 9–1
Schematic diagrams of patterns of oral cavity (O.C.) and nasal cavity (N.C.) modifications in normal, nasalized (hypernasal), and denasalized (hyponasal) sounds. A solid vertical line at the front of the oral cavity represents constriction or closure for the production of fricatives, stops, or nasals. Absence of this line indicates the relatively open cavity present in vowels, glides, and liquids. A solid line extending downward from the posterior upper surface of the oral cavity represents the velopharyngeal closure mechanism, usually closed for normal (oral) vowels and consonants and open for nasal consonants. A dashed line within the nasal cavity represents a blockage.

consonants the oral cavity is blocked, and the velopharyngeal mechanism is relaxed, so that the resonance system includes the nasal cavity.

Vowels, glides, fricatives, and stops in context with nasal consonants may have some nasalization, as shown by the slight opening of the velopharyngeal port for allophonic nasalization in Figure 9–1. Examples of words in which preceding or following nasals may produce nasalization in other sounds are given in Table 9–1. Although the influence of nasal consonants can extend over several sounds, it is greatest on adjacent sounds (Moll, 1962).The examples in Table 9–1 are restricted to adjacent sounds. Any vowel can become nasalized when preceded or followed by a nasal consonant. Nasalized vowels in English are allophones of their respective phonemes. The nasalization of vowels is a strong perceptual cue to the manner and place of production of adjacent nasal consonants (Ostreicher & Sharf, 1976; Kurowski & Blumstein, 1984; Repp, 1986; Ohde, 1988a). For normal speakers this cue is presumably redundant because the nasal consonants themselves provide adequate cues to manner of production. But it has been

Table 9–1
Examples of contextual nazalization of vowels, glides, stops, and fricatives.

	Context					
	Following			Preceding		
Sound Type	/m/	/n/	/ŋ/	/m/	/n/	/ŋ/
Vowel	my	knee	singer	aim	sign	song
Glide						
/j/	mute	new[a]	–	–	–	–
/w/	tramway	runway	gangway	–	–	–
/r/	emery[b]	inroad	stingray	army	darn	–
/l/	omelet[b]	only	wrongly	elm	illness	–
Stop						
Bilabial	dumbbell	henpeck	songbird	topmost	apnea	–
Alveolar	empty[c]	under	hangdog	boatman	jitney	–
Velar	pumpkin[c]	encase	anger	acme	acne	–
Fricative						
Labiodental	comfort	invert	songfest	caveman	deafness	–
Dental	something	anthem	strengthen	bathmat	ethnic	–
Alveolar	aims	answer	singsong	plasma	isn't	–
Palatal	gumshoe	mention	–	bushman	fishnet	–

[a]Pronounced /n j u/.
[b]Pronounced with two syllables.
[c]Pronounced without the adjacent /p/.

suggested that, for esophageal speakers, who tend to close the velopharyngeal port during nasal consonant production in order to build up intraoral air pressure, nasalization of adjacent vowels may be an important cue to manner (Miller & Hamlet, 1988).

Contextual or allophonic nasalizing is not as likely to occur for stops as for vowels since the air pressure buildup required for stops is incompatible with opening the velopharyngeal port. Any consonants that become nasalized in the context of nasal consonants are classified, like nasalized vowels, as allophones of their phonemes. For glides, nasalization can be expected when they follow nasals in 'mute,' 'omelet,' 'inroad,' and 'English,' and when they precede them in 'elm,' 'arm,' and 'barn.' Nasalization of stops can occur when they follow nasals in 'empire,' 'enter,' and 'bank,' and when they

Figure 9–2
Spectrograms of 'heat' (top panel), 'hat' (middle panel), and 'hoot' (bottom panel) produced by a normal child (left panels) and a child with a cleft palate (right panels). Arrows along the *y* axis (ordinate) indicate the approximate location of added or weakened formants in nasalized vowels.

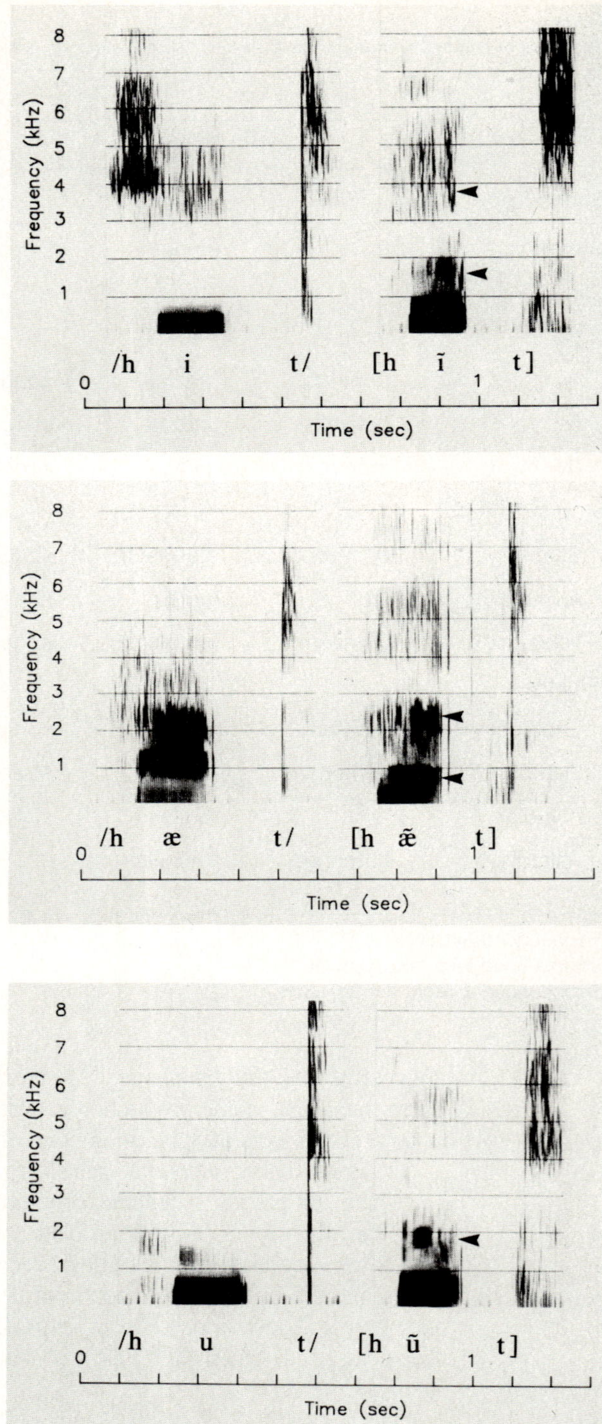

precede them in 'admiral' and 'acne.' Nasalization of fricatives can be expected when they follow nasals in 'comfort,' 'tenth,' and 'something,' and when they precede them in 'plasma' and 'isn't.'

Figure 9–1 also shows modifications for hypernasality and hyponasality. In hypernasality the velopharyngeal port is open more than is normal for contextual or allophonic nasality. Moreover, the port is open for sounds that are not adjacent to nasals as well as for those that are. In hyponasality, blockage in the nasal cavity inhibits the usual resonance of the open nasal cavity.

The spectrograms in figures 9–2 and 9–3 show how the open nasal cavity changes the resonances of vowels even though the tongue configurations do not change. By comparing the normal and nasalized vowels in these figures, you can see formants that are either added to or weakened in the nasalized versions. The acoustic cues to nasalization are rather complex (Dickson, 1962), but since speech and language pathologists have relatively little difficulty in perceiving nasality, they do not need to rely on acoustic analysis.

Nasalization may have various effects on other consonants. The open velopharyngeal port may make it impossible to build up sufficient air pressure for stops, and the sounds may be more like fricatives than stops. Even a small amount of escaping air can weaken the release pulse. Figures 9–4 and 9–5 include spectrograms of normal and cleft-palate productions by adults and children of stops in words so that you can observe the loss of energy that occurs with nasalization. This loss reduces the VOT for prevocalic stops and may result in the absence of postvocalic stops.

Nasalized fricatives are also weakened by the loss of airflow. This loss of energy may make the nonsibilant fricatives, /f, v, θ, ð/, imperceptible. The overwhelming

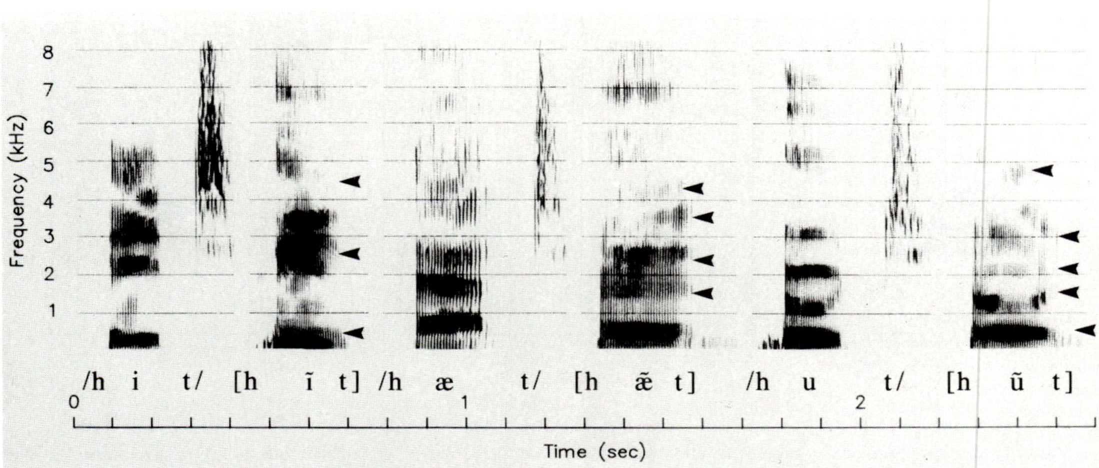

Figure 9–3
Spectrograms of normal and nasalized vowels produced by an adult male in 'heat,' 'hat,' and 'hoot.' Arrows along the *y* axis indicate the approximate location of added or weakened formants in the nasalized vowels.

effect for stops and fricatives may be a rush of air out of the nasal cavity. Figures 9–6 and 9–7 include spectrograms of nasal and nonnasal fricatives produced by a normal child, a child with a cleft palate, and an adult. You can observe the effect of nasalization on these sounds. Note the loss of frication energy, shown by its shortening or complete absence in the nasalized fricatives.

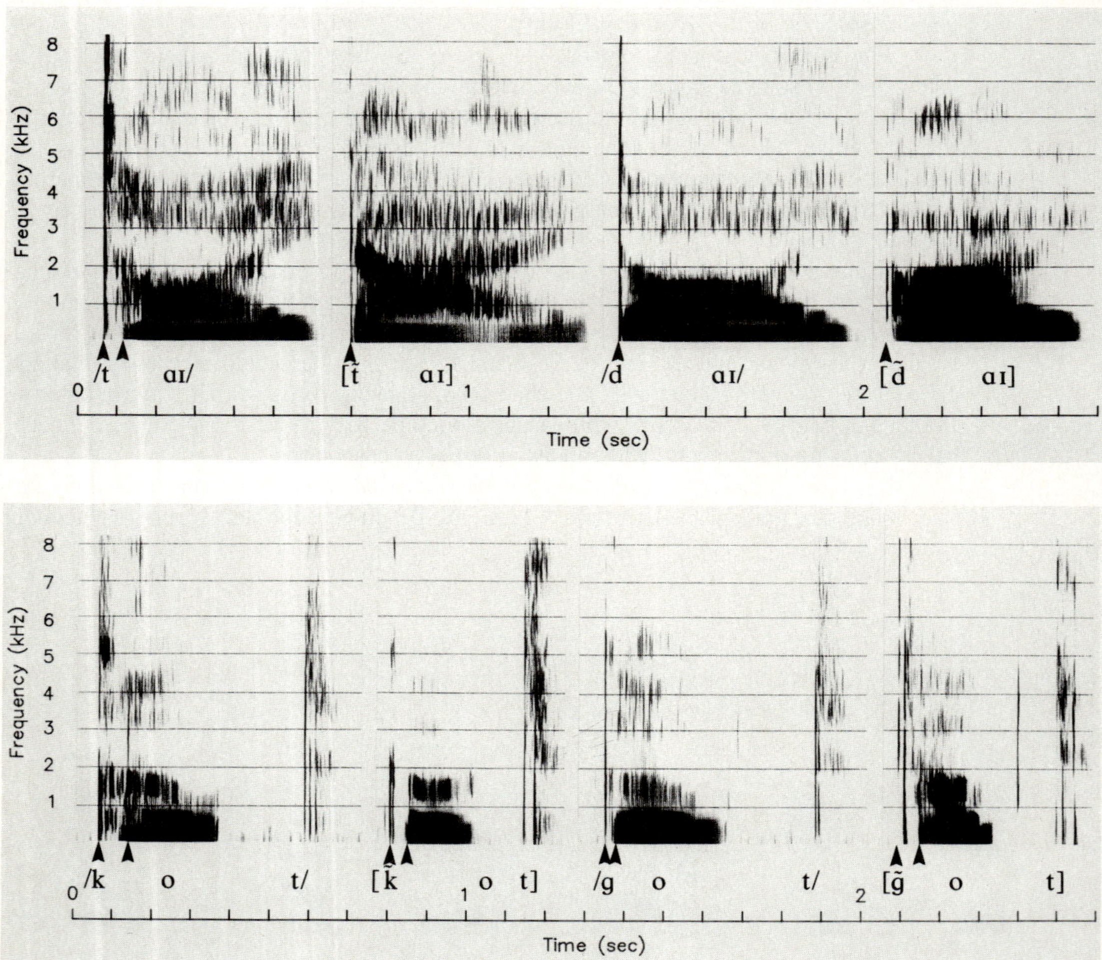

Figure 9–4
Spectrograms of stops produced by a normal child and nasalized stops produced by a child with a cleft palate saying 'tie' and 'die' (top panel) and 'coat' and 'goat' (bottom panel). Arrows along the *x* axis indicate the duration of voice onset time (VOT) for each initial stop; one arrow indicates a very short VOT. VOT durations are 64 msec for /tɑɪ/ and 16 msec for [t̃ɑɪ]; 24 msec for /dɑɪ/ and 16 msec for [d̃ɑɪ]; 80 msec for /kot/ and 40 msec for [k̃ot]; and 32 msec for /got/ and 48 msec for [g̃ot].

The other abnormal pattern of nasality (shown in Figure 9–1) is hyponasality, often referred to as **denasalization.** For this problem to occur, there must be (1) a blockage in the nasal cavity anterior to the velopharyngeal port, due to a very bad head cold, a sinus infection, a deviated septum, or a tumor, or (2) a blockage posterior to the velopharyngeal port, due to enlarged tonsils or adenoids. The major acoustic effect of

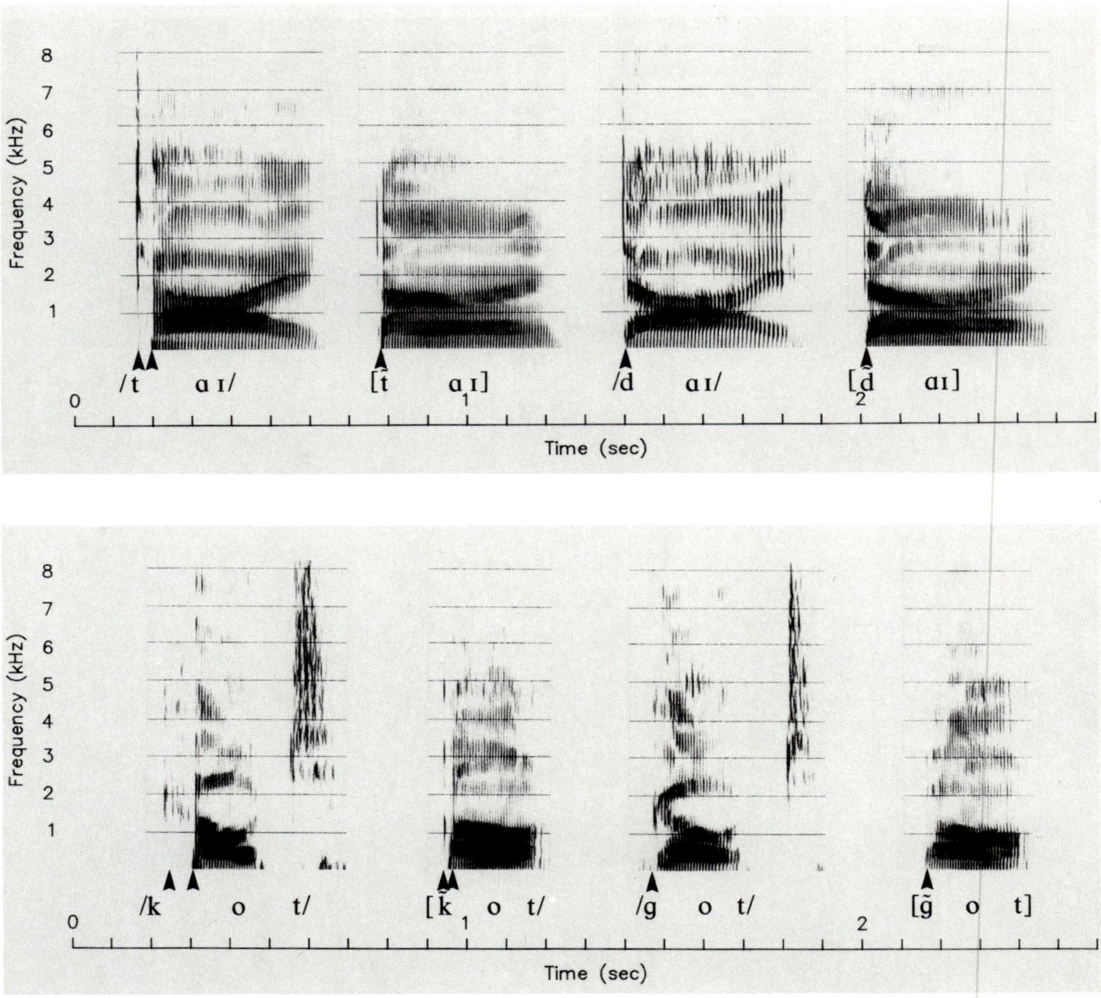

Figure 9–5
Spectrograms of normal and nasalized stops produced by an adult male saying 'tie' and 'die' (top panel) and 'coat' and 'goat' (bottom panel). Arrows along the *x* axis indicate the duration of voice onset time (VOT) for each initial stop consonant; one arrow indicates a very short VOT. These VOT durations are 44 msec for /tɑɪ/ and 16 msec for [t̃ɑɪ] ; 12 msec for /dɑɪ/ and 8 msec for [d̃ɑɪ]; 80 msec for /kot/ and 24 msec for [k̃ot]; and 20 msec for /got/ and 0 msec for [g̃ot].

the blockage is on sounds with nasal resonance, primarily the nasal consonants and secondarily those sounds with contextual nasalization. Hyponasality is often described as sounding like the speech of someone with a bad head cold. The major articulatory cue is that nasal consonants sound like stop consonants, which makes some normally distinct words homophonous. Examples are 'mom'/'bob,' 'noon'/'dude,' and 'sang'/'sag.' If you compare the diagram for nasal consonants with the one for hyponasal consonants in

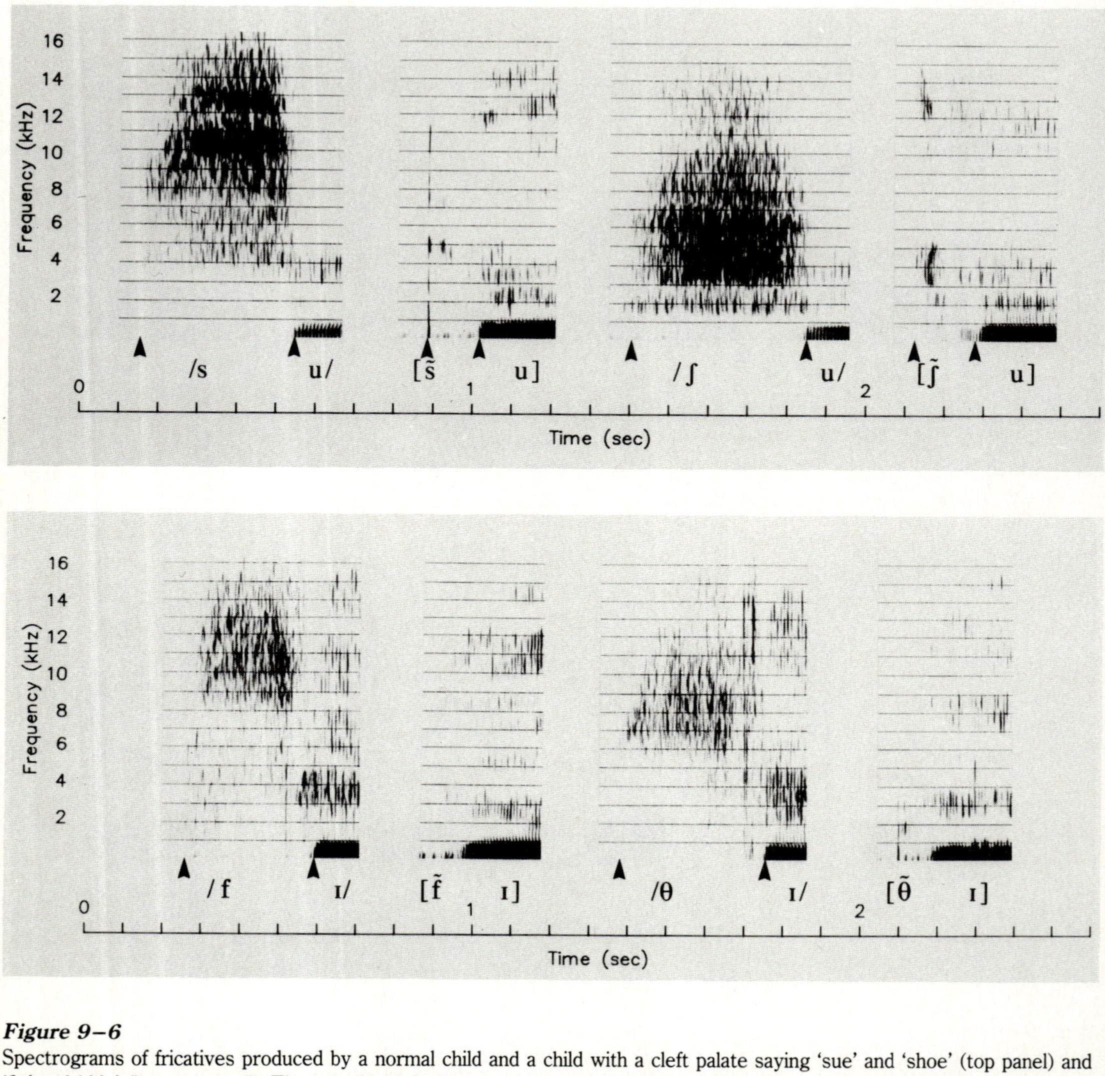

Figure 9–6

Spectrograms of fricatives produced by a normal child and a child with a cleft palate saying 'sue' and 'shoe' (top panel) and 'fin' and 'thin' (bottom panel). The vowel and final consonant have been truncated to save space. Arrows along the *x* axis indicate the onset and offset of frication energy for each fricative, unless it was too weak to identify. Frication durations are 391 msec for /su/ and 136 msec for [s̃u]; 455 msec for /ʃu/ and 168 msec for [ʃ̃u] (168 ms); 343 msec for /fɪn/ and 96 msec for [f̃ɪn]; and 375 msec for /θɪn/ and 88 msec for [θ̃ɪn].

Figure 9–1, you can see how obstruction of the nasal cavity changes the mechanism. Figures 9–8 and 9–9 are spectrograms of an adult and a child producing normal and hyponasalized versions of these words so that you can observe the acoustic effect. Note the loss of the nasal murmur in Figures 9–8 and 9–9, which results in voiced gaps similar to those characteristic of stop sounds.

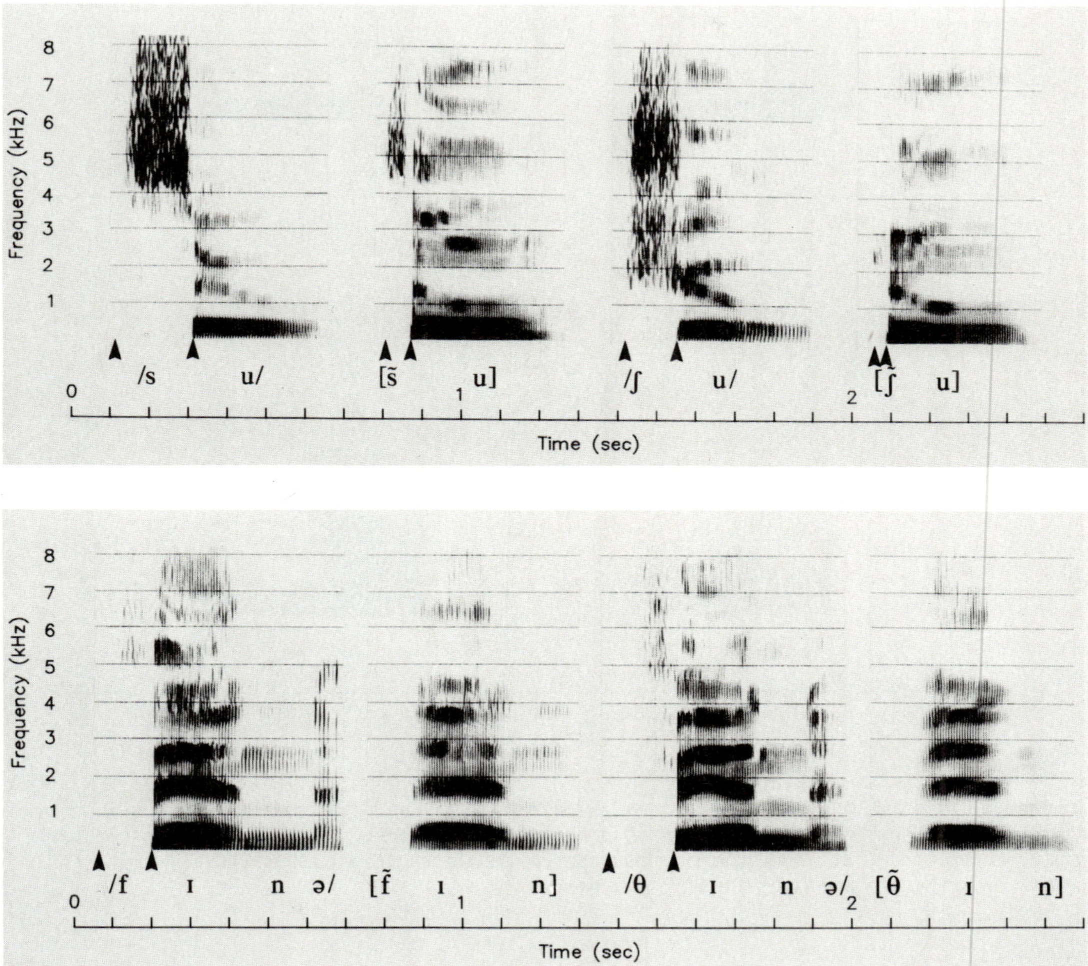

Figure 9–7
Spectrograms of normal and nasalized fricatives produced by an adult male saying 'sue' and 'shoe' (top panel) and 'fin' and 'thin' (bottom panel). Arrows along the *x* axis indicate the onset and offset of frication energy for each fricative, unless it was too weak to identify. Frication durations are 188 msec for /s u/ and 80 msec for [s̃ u]; 136 msec for /ʃ u/ and 52 msec for [ʃ̃ u]; 112 msec for /f ɪ n/ and 0 msec for [f̃ ɪ n]; and 160 msec for /θ ɪ n/ and 0 msec for [θ̃ ɪ n]. Final schwa indicates a release of the nasal consonant.

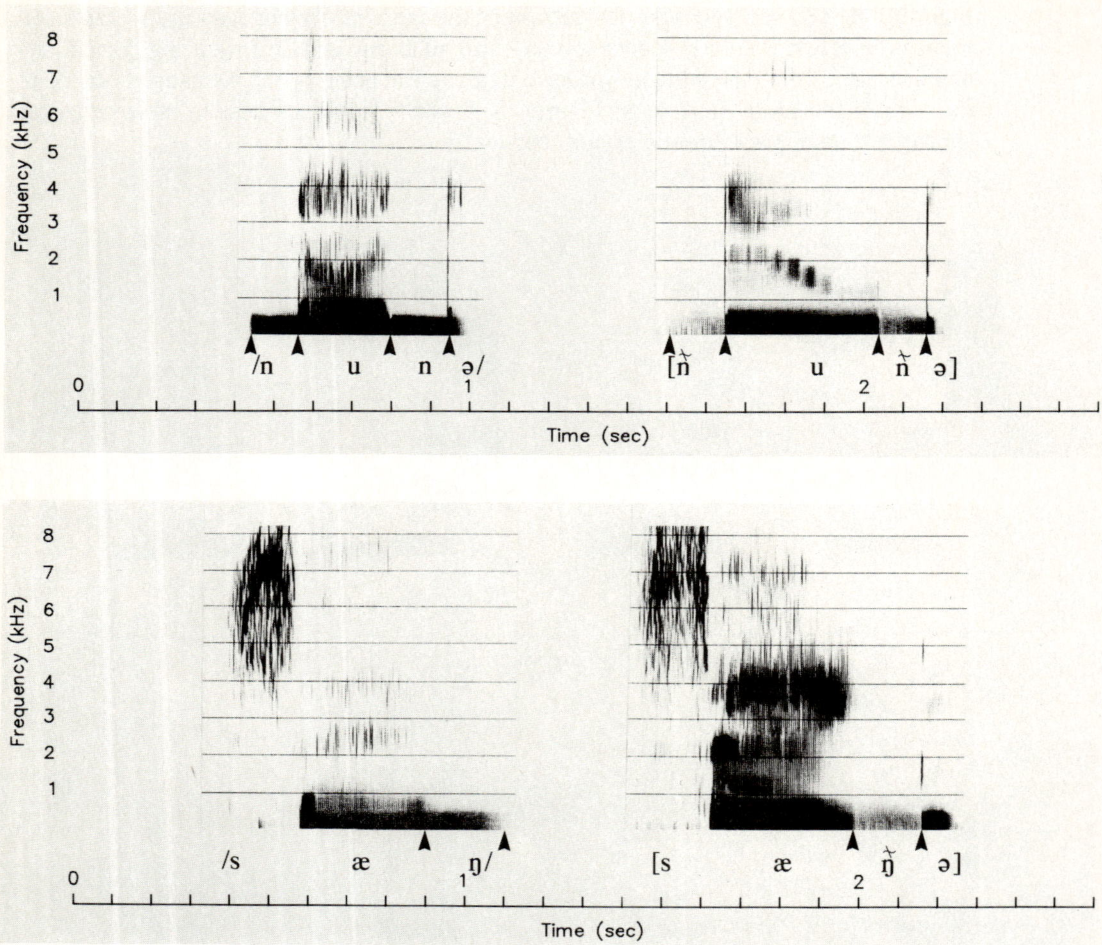

Figure 9–8

Spectrograms of normal and hyponasal (denasalized) nasal consonants produced by a child saying 'noon' (top panel) and 'sang' (bottom panel). Normal productions are in the left panels; hyponasal ones are in the right panels. Arrows along the x axis indicate the onset and offset of nasal murmur in the normal productions and pressure buildup in the hyponasal productions. Final schwa indicates a release of the nasal consonant.

ALLOPHONES OF THE NASAL CONSONANTS

Table 9–2 presents examples of allophonic variants of nasal consonants. When /m/ precedes /f/ or /v/, as in words like 'comfort,' 'camphor,' 'symphony,' and 'triumvirate,' its place of articulation changes from bilabial to labiodental in anticipation of the following

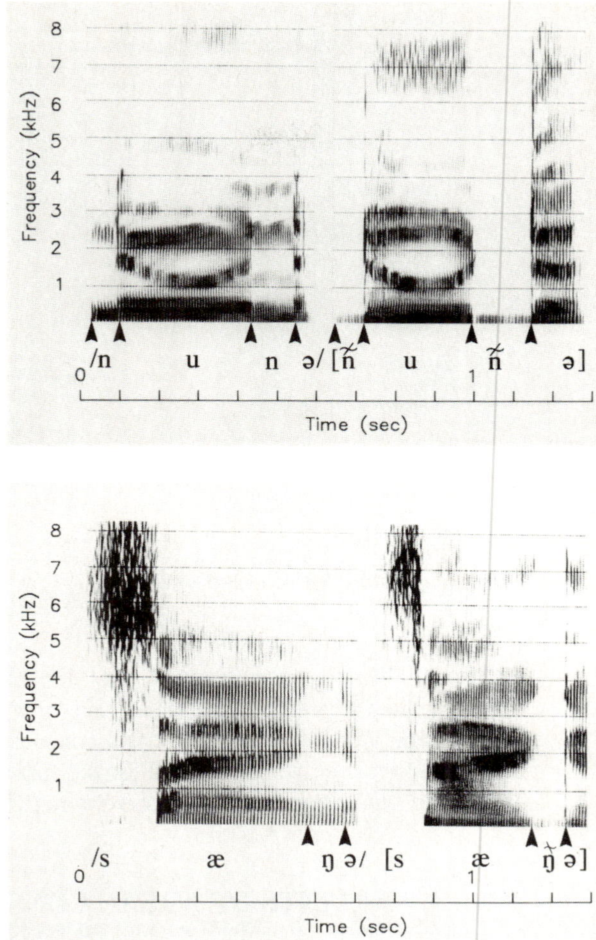

Figure 9–9
Spectrograms of normal and hyponasal (denasalized), nasal consonants produced by an adult male in 'noon' (top panel) and 'sang' (bottom panel). Arrows along the *x* axis indicate the onset and offset of nasal murmur in the normal productions and pressure buildup in the hyponasal productions. Final schwa indicates a release of the nasal consonant.

labiodental sounds. In discussing the allophonic variants of the labiodentals, it was noted that /f/ and /v/ might become bilabials under the influence of preceding /m/, as in 'comfort.' Although both changes are possible, it is much more likely that the nasal will change to a labiodental sound than vice versa.

When the alveolar nasal /n/ precedes /θ/, as in 'ninth,' 'tenth,' and 'month,' its place of articulation becomes dental or interdental in anticipation of the following interdental sounds. This type of change is not limited to single words, but also occurs in phrases like 'in the house' and 'on the mark,' in which /n/ precedes /ð/.

When the velar nasal /ŋ/ follows front vowels, as in 'sing' and 'sang,' its place of articulation changes to palatal under the influence of the preceding vowel. You can feel this shift in position when you say the minimal pairs 'sing' and 'song,' 'ring' and 'wrong,' 'bang' and 'bong.'

Table 9–2
Allophonic variants of the nasal consonants.

	Nasal		
Variant/Context	/m/	/n/	/ŋ/
Labiodental			
Before /f, v/	[ɱ] comfort	–	–
Bilabial			
Before /p, b, m/	–	[m] input	–
Dental			
Before /θ, ð/	–	[n̪] ninth	–
Palatal			
After front vowel	–	–	[ŋ⁺] sing
Rounded			
Before/after rounded vowel	[m̹] moo/ohm	[n̹] no/own	–

The nasal consonants /m/ and /n/ may become rounded when they precede rounded vowels, as in 'more' and 'new,' or when they follow rounded vowels, as in 'home' and 'tune.' During nasal consonant production in such words, the rounded lip position is either anticipated for the following vowel or carries over from the preceding one, but anticipatory effects are generally considered stronger than carryover effects.

ABNORMAL VARIANTS OF NASAL CONSONANTS AND NASALIZATION

Phonological Processes

Table 9–3 presents phonological processes that influence the production of nasal consonants and nasality. Nasal consonants that occur in prevocalic and postvocalic positions are sometimes omitted, as in /bi/ for 'bean' and /pɪk/ for 'pink.' Such omissions are classified as final consonant deletion and cluster reduction, respectively. A more complex example of nasal cluster reduction is [tɛ̃t] for 'tent,' where the nasal consonant is deleted while the nasalization of the preceding vowel persists, an example of nasal assimilation. These deletions are much more common for stops, fricatives, and affricates than they are for nasals.

Although velar nasal consonants are subject to the influence of deletion processes, they are more frequently influenced by fronting, as in /fɪʃɪn/ for 'fishing,' where /n/ replaces /ŋ/. Another place change that occurs for nasals is due to the influence of labial assimilation, as in /pɪm/ for 'pin.' In this change, the alveolar nasal becomes a bilabial under the influence of the initial bilabial stop consonant.

Table 9–3
Phonological processes that influence the production of nasal consonants and nasality.

Process	Change
Omissions	
Final consonant deletion	/bi/ for 'bean'
Cluster reduction	/pɪk/ for 'pink'; /tɛt/ for 'tent'
Manner Changes	
Nasal assimilation	[grĩ] for 'green'; /nʌ̃n/ for 'sun'
Denasalization	/mʌdi/ for 'money'
Vocalization (vowelization)	[mɪʔə] for 'mitten'
Place Changes	
Fronting	/fɪʃɪn/ for 'fishing'
Labial assimilation	/pɪm/ for 'pin'

The manner of production of vowels, nasals, and other consonants may be influenced by the phonological processes of nasal assimilation, denasalization, and vocalization. **Nasal assimilation** is a process that most often influences vowels but sometimes affects consonants as well (Hodson & Paden, 1983). Vowels may become nasalized in the context of nasal consonants, as in [grĩ] for 'green' and [nʌ̃n] for 'sun,' and nasal consonants may replace other consonants, as in [nʌ̃n] for 'sun' and /nʌnə/ for 'another.' In 'sun,' notice that /s/ changes to /n/ and the vowel becomes nasalized under the assimilative influence of the following /n/. In 'another,' /n/ replaces /ð/ under the assimilative influence of the preceding /n/. Hodson and Paden (1983) note the occurrence of a nasal emission of air for /s/ in 'smoke,' which is presumably due to the influence of the /m/ sound.

Denasalization is a process which causes the nasal consonants /m/ and /n/ to be changed into the stops /b/ and /d/. An example of this process is /mʌdi/ for 'money.' Changes may be classified as due to the influence of a process if there is no evidence of a blockage in the nasal cavity. The denasalization process is not very common.

Vocalization, or vowelization, which frequently influences the liquid sounds, may also influence nasal consonants, though much less frequently. Edwards and Shriberg (1983) give [mɪʔə] for 'mitten' as an example of this process. Although they classify vocalization as a place-changing process, we believe that manner-changing is a more appropriate classification of it.

Articulatory Disorders of Nasalization

Nasal consonants are few in number and generally cause no serious production problems. The most severe form of nasality disorder is hypernasality, which affects vowels and nonnasal consonants. The seriousness of hypernasality ranges from the severe effects of organic velopharyngeal insufficiency characteristic of cleft-palate speakers to the mild effects of functional velopharyngeal port inactivity characteristic of speakers with a "nasal twang." Generally, phonetics texts tend to focus on the functional rather than the organic problem, describing the behavior as a general basis of articulation in some American dialects (Heffner, 1952), a faulty usage when the nasalization of vowels is excessive (Bronstein, 1960), or an undesirable voice quality (Calvert, 1980).

Figure 9–10 contains a spectrogram of the sentence 'See the dog barking on the porch' as spoken by an individual with a "nasal twang" that results in excessive nasalization of vowels. For comparison, a spectrogram of a speaker with normal nasal quality is also shown. Note that the nasalized vowels are characterized by a loss of energy concentration in F_2 and F_3 as compared with normal vowels. The stops and fricatives,

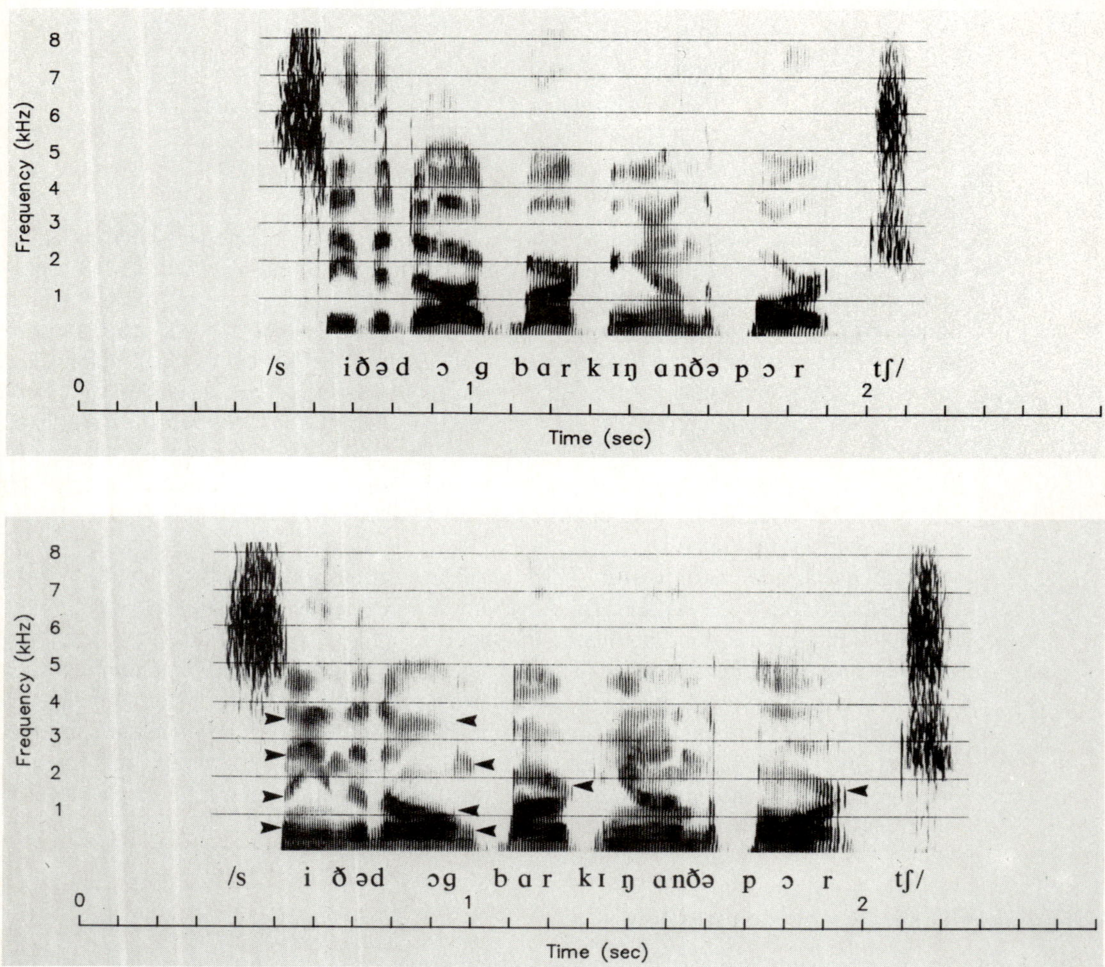

Figure 9–10
Spectrograms of 'See the dog barking on the porch' for an adult producing normal (top panel) and "nasal twang" (bottom panel) versions. Arrows along the *y* axis indicate weakened or missing formants in the nasalized version. See the text for a comparison of acoustic features in these productions.

however, are unchanged by the addition of nasal resonance, presumably because the velopharyngeal port is sufficiently closed during their production to prevent consonant deterioration.

Although nasalization of vowels is generally easy to perceive, it does not have a great effect on speech intelligibility. But inadequate velopharyngeal port closure for consonant production, as may happen with cleft-palate speakers, greatly reduces intelligibility. The acoustic effects of such nasality are shown by the spectrograms in Figure 9–11. Note the loss of energy in the formants of the nasalized utterance as compared with the normal one. Note also that the loss of air pressure through the nasal

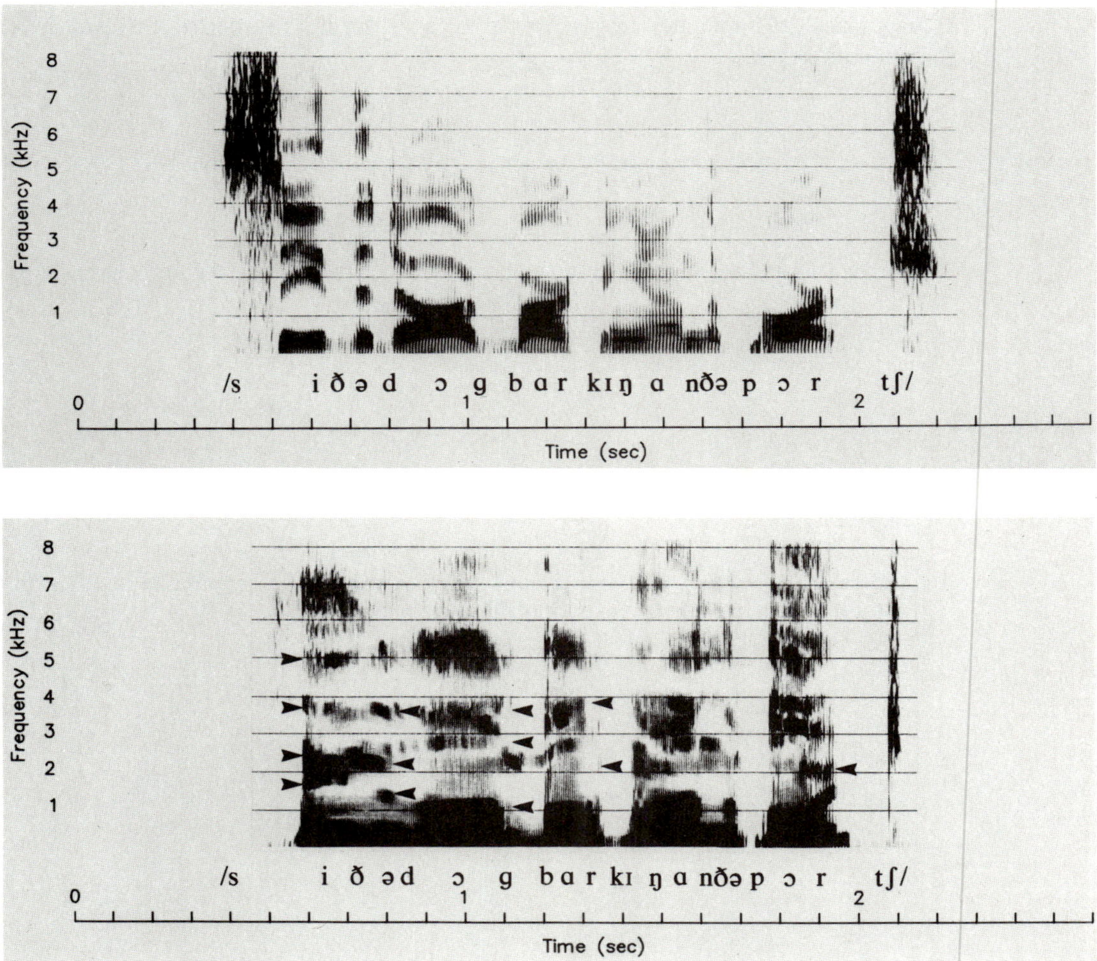

Figure 9–11
Spectrograms of 'See the dog barking on the porch' for an adult producing normal (top panel) and hypernasalized (bottom panel) versions. Arrows along the *y* axis indicate weakened or missing formants in the nasalized version. See the text for a comparison of acoustic features in these productions.

cavity during the stop closure is evident from the shortened or missing stop gaps for the /d/ and /g/ of 'dog,' the /b/ and /k/ of 'barking,' and the /p/ and /tʃ/ of 'porch.' The weakness of consonants is also manifested in the fricatives. Frication energy for the /s/ of 'see' and the /tʃ/ of 'porch' is lacking in Figure 9–11.

Hypernasality can be transcribed with the nasal diacritic over the symbol for the vowels and consonants so produced. Methods were presented in Chapter 6 for indicating the variations in stop production that occur in cleft-palate speech, including the use of dorsopharyngeal and glottal stop replacements.

In Chapter 6 the perceptual effects of hyponasality were discussed; primarily, they involved the conversion of /m/ to /b/ , /n/ to /d/, and /ŋ/ to /g/. Although hyponasality theoretically influences vowels, it is not clear that any changes can be perceived. Hyponasality can be notated by placing the hyponasality diacritic above the symbols for the affected vowels.

GLOSSARY

Denasalization. The substitution of /b/ for /m/, /d/ for /n/, and /g/ for /ŋ/; a phonological process.

Nasal assimilation. Acquisition by a nonnasal consonant of the nasal feature of a nasal consonant in the same context; a phonological process.

REVIEW QUESTIONS

A. Indicate the context that would most likely result in contextual nasalization for the following sounds by inserting the appropriate letter.

1. /l/ ______	a. dismal
2. /r/ ______	b. no
3. /j/ ______	c. gangway
4. /w/ ______	d. attention
5. /o/ ______	e. palm
6. /s/ ______	f. farm
7. /z/ ______	g. music
8. /f/ ______	h. dance
9. /θ/ ______	i. camphor
10. /ʃ/ ______	j. ethnic

****

Key: 1. e; 2. f; 3. g; 4. c; 5. b; 6. h; 7. a; 8. i; 9. j; 10. d

B. Indicate the allophone that would occur in the following contexts by inserting the appropriate letter.

1. in the pan ________ a. [m̓]
2. comfortable ________ b. [ɱ]
3. note ________ c. [n̓]
4. comb ________ d. [n̪]
5. anthem ________ e. [ŋ$^{+}$]
6. king ________

****

Key: 1. d; 2. b; 3. c; 4. a; 5. d; 6. e

C. Indicate the phonological processes illustrated by the examples by inserting the appropriate letter.

1. Final consonant deletion ________ a. /nʌn/ for 'son'
2. Cluster reduction ________ b. /bub/ for 'boom'
3. Nasal assimilation ________ c. /bi/ for 'bean'
4. Denasalization ________ d. [bʌʔə] for 'button'
5. Vocalization ________ e. /hæd/ for 'hand'
6. Fronting ________ f. /rʌnɪn/ for 'running'
7. Labial assimilation ________ g. /pæm/ for 'pan'

****

Key: 1. c; 2. e; 3. a; 4. b; 5. d; 6. f; 7. g

LABORATORY ASSIGNMENT

Tape III, Side B
IIIB5: Nasal Consonants (Tape running time: 3:47; Elapsed time: 20:16–24:03)

a. Nasal Consonant Models

Listen to the nasal consonants as they are produced in /Cæ t/ and /t æ C/ contexts by an adult and a child. If necessary, stop the tape at any time, rewind, and listen again.

1. Adult: /m æ t/; /n æ t/; /t æ m/; /t æ n/; /t æ ŋ/
2. Child repeats above.

b. Transcription of Nasals in Minimal Contrast Syllables

Transcribe each nasal as it is pronounced by an adult and a child in a minimal contrast context.

1. ________ 2. ________ 3. ________ 4. ________ 5. ________

6. ________ 7. ________ 8. ________ 9. ________ 10. ________

****

Consensus: 1. /n/ 2. /m/ 3. /m/ 4. /ŋ/ 5. /n/ 6. /n/ 7. /ŋ/ 8. /m/ 9. /n/ 10. /m/

Variants: 8. /n/ 9. /m/

c. Transcription of Nasals in Minimal Contrast Syllables in a Sentence

Transcribe each nasal consonant as it is pronounced by an adult and a child in a minimal contrast context.

1. ________ 2. ________ 3. ________ 4. ________ 5. ________

6. ________ 7. ________ 8. ________ 9. ________ 10. ________

****

Consensus: 1. /m/ 2. /m/ 3. /n/ 4. /ŋ/ 5. /n/ 6. /n/ 7. /m/ 8. /n/ 9. /m/ 10. /ŋ/

Variants: None.

d. Transcription of Nasals in Words in Context

Transcribe each nasal consonant as it is pronounced by an adult and a child in words in the following sentences: 'I can say ________ '; 'Say the word ________ '; '________ is the word.'

1. neat ________ 2. comb ________ 3. mother ________ 4. sing ________

5. can ________ 6. long ________ 7. meat ________ 8. lawn ________

9. sin ________ 10. cone ________

****

Consensus: 1. /n/ 2. /m/ 3. /m/ 4. /ŋ/ 5. /n/ 6. /ŋ/ 7. /m/ 8. /n/ 9. /n/ 10. /n/

Variants: None.

IIIB6: Normal and Abnormal Nasal Variants (Tape running time: 3:08; Elapsed time: 24:03–27:11)

The purpose of this section is to train students to identify the difference between normal and abnormal variants of /n, ŋ/ according to features of place and manner.

a. Normal and Abnormal /n/ Variant Models

Listen to the normal and abnormal variants of /n, ŋ/ as they are pronounced for you in a minimal contrast context by an adult and a child.

1. Adult: /bɪʃɪŋ/ (normal); /bɪʃɪn/ (fronted)
2. Child repeats above.

3. Adult: /pun/ (normal); /pum/ (labialized)
4. Child repeats above.
5. Adult: /rin/ (normal); /ri/ (deleted); [rĩ] (deleted and nasalized)
6. Child repeats above.
7. Adult: /sʌni/ (normal); /sʌdi/ (denasalized)
8. Child repeats above.

b. Minimal Pair Contrast of Normal and Abnormal /n/ Variants

Listen to the minimal pairs produced by an adult and a child and indicate if the first (1) or second (2) is normal /n/.

1. ________ 2. ________ 3. ________ 4. ________ 5. ________
6. ________

****

Key: 1. 2; 2. 2; 3. 2; 4. 1; 5. 1; 6. 1

c. Minimal Pair Contrast of Normal and Abnormal /ŋ/ Variants

Listen to the minimal pairs produced by an adult and a child and indicate if the first (1) or second (2) is normal /ŋ/.

1. ________ 2. ________ 3. ________ 4. ________

****

Key: 1. 2; 2. 1; 3. 1; 4. 2

d. Transcription of Normal and Abnormal /n, ŋ/ Variants in Words in Context

Transcribe each /n, ŋ/ variant as it is pronounced by an adult and a child in words in the following sentences: 'I can say ________'; 'Say the word ________'; '________ is the word.'

1. pan ________ 2. falling ________ 3. funny ________ 4. brain ________
5. nap ________ 6. brain ________ 7. pan ________ 8. falling ________
9. funny ________ 10. brain ________ 11. nap ________ 12. brain ________

****

Consensus: 1. /n/ 2. /ŋ/ 3. /d/ 4. /0/ 5. /n/ 6. /n/ 7. /n/ 8. /n/
9. /n/ 10. /n/ 11. /m/ 12. /0/

Variants: 3. [n͊]

Tape IV, Side A
IVA1: Nasalized Vowels and Consonants (Tape running time: 2:56; Elapsed time: 00:00–02:56)

The purpose of this section is to train students to identify the difference between normal and nasalized vowels and consonants.

a. Nasalized Vowel and Consonant Models

Listen to the vowels and consonants as they are pronounced normally and nasalized in a minimal contrast context by an adult and a child.

1. Adult: /s i l/ (normal); [s ĩ l] (nasalized); /s æ l/ (normal); [s æ̃ l] (nasalized); /l i s/ (normal); [l ĩ s] (nasalized); /l æ s/ (normal); [l æ̃ s] (nasalized)
2. Child repeats above.

b. Minimal Pair Contrast of Normal and Nasalized Sounds

Listen to the minimal pairs produced by an adult and a child and indicate if the first (1) or second (2) is normal.

1. ________ 2. ________ 3. ________ 4. ________ 5. ________

6. ________ 7. ________ 8. ________

****

Key: 1. 1; 2. 2; 3. 2; 4. 1; 5. 2; 6. 1; 7. 1; 8. 1

c. Transcription of Normal and Nasalized Sounds in Words in Context

Indicate if the nonnasal vowels and consonants are normal or nasalized in the words pronounced by an adult and a child in the following sentences: 'I can say ________ '; 'Say the word ________ '; '________ is the word.'

1. seal ____________________
2. chair ____________________
3. seal ____________________
4. soap ____________________
5. fussy ____________________
6. peace ____________________
7. thumb ____________________
8. throw ____________________
9. father ____________________
10. mother ____________________

****

Key: 1. nasal; 2. normal; 3. normal; 4. nasal; 5. nasal; 6. nasal; 7. normal; 8. nasal; 9. normal; 10. nasal

IVA2: Transcription of Complete Words with Vowels, Glides, Stops, Fricatives, and Nasals (Tape running time: 3:25; Elapsed time: 02:56–06:21)

The purpose of this section is to provide students with practice in transcribing complete words that include the sounds covered so far—vowels, glides, stops, fricatives, and nasals. Transcribe each word below as it is produced by a child, reversing the tape as needed to listen to an utterance again. After you have finished all the words, check your transcriptions against the key.

1. bounce ____________
2. thank you ____________
3. buzzing ____________
4. foreign ____________
5. lawn ____________
6. coins ____________
7. spoon ____________
8. lamb ____________
9. fishing ____________
10. mother ____________
11. sing ____________
12. kissing ____________
13. send ____________
14. penny ____________
15. towns ____________
16. string ____________
17. Santa ____________
18. raising ____________
19. sign ____________
20. fishing ____________
21. merry ____________
22. string ____________
23. reason ____________
24. Santa ____________
25. lamb ____________

****

Consensus: 1. /bɑʊnts/ 3. /bʌdzɪŋ/ 4. /fɔrən/ 5. /jɔn/ 6. /kɔɪnz/ 7. /pum/ 8. /læm/ 9. /fɪtsɪn/ 10. /mʌfə/ 11. /θɪŋ/ 12. /kɪʃɪŋ/ 14. /pɪni/ 15. /tɑʊnz/ 16. /nek/ 17. /nænə/ 19. /θɑɪn/ 20. /fɪʃɪŋ/ 21. /mɛwi/ 22. /strɪŋ/ 23. /riðən/ 24. /sæntə/ 25. /næm/

Variants: 1. /baʊns/ 2. /fæŋkju/; [p⁼æŋkju]; /dæŋkju/ 3. [bʌdz̪i] 4. /forən/ 5. /jɑn/ 6. /pɔɪnz/ 9. [fɪtʃṇ] 12. [kɪʃŋ] 13. /tɛt/; [tɛ̃t]; [tɛ:t] 15. [taʊnz̥] 16. [nĩk] 18. /ˈrezɪg/; /rezɪŋk/; /rezɪk/ 20. [fɪʃŋ̍] 23. /riðə/

CHAPTER 10

Coarticulation and Assimilation

Although much of the discussion in the preceding chapters has focused on the analysis of individual sounds, it should be clear that speech is not made up of sound segments joined together like beads on a string. In describing the phonemes of each class of sounds, emphasis was placed on the importance of contextual influence. For example, allophones of stops, nasals, and fricatives that are produced with lip rounding in the context of rounded vowels were described, as well as vowels that are nasalized in the context of nasal consonants. Until now, however, there has been no discussion of the nature of the articulatory system operation that is responsible for such contextual modifications, of the types of modifications that occur in normal and abnormal speech, or of the importance to clinical phonetics of understanding the basis for these modifications.

COARTICULATORY BASIS FOR ASSIMILATION

Coarticulation is a concept that has become increasingly important in the study of phonetics. Basic to this concept is the assumption that speech involves a complex articulatory system with a number of interacting components that are responsible for the production of certain **properties.** It is not clear what the specific properties involved are, or how their productive components interact, but there has been conjecture about the general configuration of the system. Figure 10–1 is a schematic diagram of a coarticulatory system of speech production. For the sake of simplification, a limited number of components is assumed for achieving the following articulatory gestures: (1) voicing—constricting the vocal folds; (2) nasalizing—opening the velopharyngeal port;

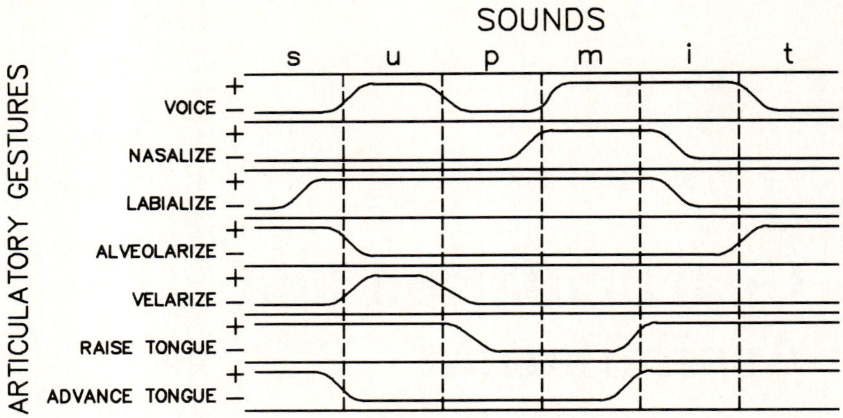

Figure 10–1
Schematic diagram of the coarticulatory process during the production of 'soup meat' /s u p m i t/. Curves between the levels of the + and − signs indicate activation and deactivation of the articulatory gestures that produce the sound features noted. Vertical dashed lines indicate hypothetical boundaries for the sounds in the utterance.

(3) labializing—creating a bilabial constriction; (4) alveolarizing—creating an apico-alveolar constriction; (5) velarizing—creating a dorsovelar constriction; (6) raising and lowering the body of the tongue; and (7) advancing and retracting the body of the tongue. Such articulatory mechanisms are assumed to be responsible for producing the various properties of the sounds of English. **Articulatory gestures** are the movements of the articulators that result from the opposing muscle forces acting upon them during speech production (Hoffman, Schuckers, & Daniloff, 1989).

Viewed from the perspective of Figure 10–1, speech is a function of a number of semi-independent articulatory systems that are continually changing from an active (+) to an inactive (−) state. At a given point in time, the coexistence of certain states leads to a particular speech sound. For example, absence of voicing, nasalizing, labializing, and velarizing plus presence of alveolarizing are steady-state specifications for the /s/ sound in an utterance like 'soup meat' in Figure 10–1. Of particular interest is that the on-off states of the articulatory gestures, as shown in the model, are not instantaneous. Certain properties may extend beyond the hypothesized boundaries of more than one sound. What is most important is that certain properties may be anticipated or carried over into the production of sounds which do not normally include them. For example, observe the "nasalize" articulatory gesture during the /p/ and /i/ sounds and the "labialize" articulatory gesture during the /s/ and /i/ sounds. The spreading to other sounds of properties not normally characteristic of them is a consequence of coarticulation as it is currently understood. Unfortunately, our understanding of what is responsible for coarticulation is incomplete. Possible explanations include anticipatory changes made by a system that scans ahead during speech production, limitations on the responsiveness of articulatory structures in shifting between sounds, and learned phonological patterns of a language. Whatever mechanisms account for coarticulation, it presumably underlies changes in the pronunciation of words and utterances that are recognized as examples of assimilation.

Not all phoneticians agree on the relationship between coarticulation and assimilation. The process of sound change and the changes that occur have been described as arising from coarticulation (Shriberg & Kent, 1982) and from assimilation (Bronstein, 1960). Coarticulation may be viewed as the basis for assimilation (Tiffany & Carrell, 1977; Calvert, 1980). Or assimilation and coarticulation may be considered as two different forms of a sound change process of accommodation (MacKay, 1987). The lack of clear understanding or agreement about the processes responsible for sound changes is related to unresolved differences about the nature of motor control of speech. Some researchers assume that articulation is regulated much the same way that movement of the limbs is governed (Kelso, Saltzman, & Tuller, 1986). Others assume that articulation is determined to some extent by phonetic representation in the central nervous system, which may be influenced by language-specific experience (Smith & McLean-Muse, 1986, 1987; Flege, 1988). There are indications that speech production skills continue to develop until at least ten or eleven years of age (Smith & McLean-Muse, 1986).

Despite the uncertainty about the nature of motor control, speech and language pathologists should be aware of contextual sound changes and the complexity of the system that produces them. The first implication of this awareness is that rehabilitation for articulation disorders must include training to produce sounds in context, because otherwise the necessary dynamics for normal production will not be mastered. Second, research on motor control suggests that the central phonetic representation of the dynamics of speech sounds may be refined slowly as a result of experience in hearing and speaking (Smith & McLean-Muse, 1986). Thus, training to produce sounds correctly in context may require practice in perception as well as production.

In order to describe assimilations that occur in normal and abnormal speech, different terms are used to specify the direction, extent, and degree of influence that one sound exerts over another (see Table 10–1). *Direction of influence* refers to whether a sound influences a preceding one, as when the /f/ of 'comfort' changes /m/ to a labiodental sound (referred to as regressive, anticipatory, or **right-to-left assimilation**), or a sound influences a following sound, as when the /m/ in 'comfort' changes /f/ to a bilabial sound (referred to as progressive, perseverative, or **left-to-right assimilation**).

Extent of influence refers to whether the effect of a sound is only on a preceding or following sound, as when /m/ and /f/ influence each other in 'comfort,' or whether it extends beyond the preceding or following one, as when the /n/ of 'pin' changes to /m/ under the influence of /p/. Influence only on a preceding or following sound is **contiguous assimilation;** influence stretching beyond adjacent sounds is **noncontiguous assimilation.**

Degree of influence refers to whether a sound changes to become exactly like another one, as when /t/ changes to /k/ in 'take,' or whether a sound takes on a feature of another sound, as when /d/ takes on the place feature of the /k/ sound in 'duck' and becomes /g/. The first is **complete assimilation;** the second is **partial assimilation.**

Table 10–1
Characteristics of assimilation changes.

Direction of Influence

Regressive; anticipatory; right-to-left

Later sound influences earlier one: adult–/m/ and /f/ in [kʌɱfɚt] for 'comfort'; child–/t/ and /b/ in /bebu/ for 'table'

Progressive; perseverative; left-to-right

Earlier sound influences later one: adult–/m/ and /f/ in [kʌmɸɚt] for 'comfort'; child–/p/ and /n/ in /pɪm/ for 'pin'

Extent of Influence

Contiguous

Effect is between adjacent sounds: adult–/m/ and /f/ in [kʌɱfɚt] *or* [kʌmɸɚt] for 'comfort'; child–/s/ and /w/ in /fwit/ for 'sweet'

Noncontiguous

Effect is between nonadjacent sounds: adult–no examples; child–/p/ and /n/ in /pɪm/ for 'pin'

Degree of Influence

Partial

One sound takes on at least one but not all features of another sound: adult–/t/ and /θ/ in [et̪θ] for 'eighth'; child–/d/ and /k/ in /gʌk/ for 'duck'

Complete

All features of another sound are taken on: adult–/s/ and /ʃ/ in [hɔrʃ:u] for 'horseshoe'; child–/t/ and /k/ in /kek/ for 'take'

ASSIMILATIONS IN NORMAL SPEECH

In normal speech, assimilations may involve features of place, voicing, and manner of production. Some of the changes are fairly widespread in English speech; others are limited to just one or two words. Some changes are so deeply embedded in normal speech that most speakers are not aware of the discrepancy between spelling and pronunication they entail. It should be noted that assimilations occur more frequently in casual than in formal speech. Sample assimilations are presented in Table 10–2 along with indications of the direction and degree of the assimilation influence.

Labial Assimilation

Labial assimilations occur in just a few words in English when the alveolar nasal /n/ becomes a bilabial nasal /m/ in the context of a following bilabial consonant, /p, b, m/, as in 'input' and 'inbred.' In 'grandma' and 'grandpa,' the change involves prior deletion

Table 10–2
Assimilations that occur in normal speech production, with indications of direction of influence (RE = regressive; PR = progressive) and degree of influence (# = complete; ” = partial). Note that > means “changes to”; C = consonant; V = vowel; hyphens indicate incomplete transcriptions of examples. All examples are of contiguous assimilation.

Assimilation Type	Context	Example	Direction	Degree
Place Changes				
Labial assimilation				
/n/ > /m/	/-nm-/	grandma[a]	RE	”
	/-np-/	grandpa		
	/-nb-/	inbred		
/f/ > [ɸ]	/-mf-/	comfort, camphor	PR	”
Labiodental assimilation				
/m/ > [ɱ]	/-mf-/	comfort, camphor	RE	”
Dental assimilation				
/t/ > [t̪]	/-tθ-/	eighth	RE	”
	/-tð/	hit the mark		
/d/ > [d̪]	/-dθ/	width, breadth	RE	”
	/-dð/	led the way		
/n/ > [n̪]	/-nθ/	month, tenth	RE	”
	/-nð/	on the top		
[ŋ$^{+}$] > [n̪]	/-nθ/	strength, length	RE	”
/l/ > [l̪]	/-lθ/	health, wealth	RE	”
	/-lð-/	all the way		
/s/ > [s̪]	/-sθ-/	aesthetic	RE	”
	/-sð-/	pass the salt		
/z/ > [z̪]	/-zð-/	has the time, goes there	RE	”
Palatal/velar assimilation				
/n/ > /ŋ/ *or* [ŋ$^{+}$]	/-ng-/	congress	RE	”
	/-nk/	think, bank		
/k/ > [k^{+}]	/kV-/	key, kill	RE	”
	/-Vk/	sick, sack	PR	”
/g/ > [g^{+}]	/gV-/	gate, give	RE	”
	/-Vg/	bag, big, tag	PR	”
/s/ > /ʃ/	/-sʃ-/	horseshoe, horseshow	RE	#
	/-stʃ-/	mischief, question	RE	”
Voicing Changes				
Voicing assimilation				
/θ/ > /ð/	/-VθV-/	northern, worthy	RE & PR	”
/t/ > [ɾ]	/-VtV-/	batter, battle, later	RE & PR	”
/s/ > /z/	/-bsV-/	absorb	RE & PR	”

continued

Table 10–2 continued

Assimilation Type	Context	Example	Direction	Degree
Devoicing assimilation				
/w/ > [w̥]	/t w-/	twice, twin	PR	”
	/k w-/	quick, quack		
/r/ > [r̥]	/t r-/	trick, train	PR	”
	/k r-/	crack, creek		
	/p r-/	pray, proud		
/l/ > [l̥]	/k l-/	click, close	PR	”
	/p l-/	play, plow		
/j/ > [j̥]	/k j-/	cue, cute	PR	”
	/p j-/	pew, compute		
/z/ > /s/	/-z t-/	used to[b]	RE	”
/v/ > /f/	/-v t-/	have to[b]		
/d/ > /t/	/-Cd/	guessed, laughed[b]	PR	”
Manner Changes				
Nasal assimilation				
/V/ > [Ṽ]	/CV/	may, new	PR	”
	/VC/	lamb, pan, sing	RE	”
Lip rounding assimilation				
/C/ > [C̹]	/CV/	two, do, sew	RE	”
	/VC/	oak, push, suit	PR	”

[a]'Grandma' may be considered a case of complete assimilation.
[b]Some phoneticians consider these changes to be the result of morphophonemic rules rather than assimilation.

of /d/ so that /n/ and /m/ are contiguous in 'grandma' and /n/ and /p/ in 'grandpa.' In words like 'comfort,' 'comfortable,' and 'camphor,' /f/ may become a bilabial under the influence of the preceding /m/.

Labiodental Assimilation

Although a left-to-right assimilation may occur in a word like 'comfort,' it is more likely that a right-to-left, labiodental, assimilation will occur. In this case, the /m/ becomes a labiodental sound. This same change occurs in words like 'comfortable' and 'camphor.'

Dental Assimilation

Dental assimilation was referred to when the allophones of /t, d, n, l, s, z/ were discussed. It occurs: (1) when /θ/ precedes /n/, as in 'ethnic,' or precedes /l/, as in 'athlete,' 'Catholic,' and 'decathlon'; or (2) when /θ/ follows /t/, as in 'eighth,' /d/, as in 'width' and 'breadth,' /n/ as in 'month,' 'ninth,' and 'tenth,' /l/ as in 'health,' 'wealth,' and 'stealth,' and /s/ as in 'aesthetic.' In each case, the alveolar sound changes to a dental one. The stops in 'eighth' and 'width' often are deleted so that these words are pronounced as /eθ/ and /wɪθ/. Preceding alveolar consonants may become dental consonants under the influence of /ð/ in 'the' in phrases like 'hit the mark,' 'on the top,' and 'all the way.'

In 'length' and 'strength,' /ŋ/ becomes dental when followed by /θ/. Like some other assimilations, this one does not occur in the pronunciation of all speakers of English. It is common, however, and not just in the speech of poorly educated people.

Palatal/Velar Assimilation

Bilabial and alveolar sounds can assimilate to palatal or velar sounds, and palatal sounds can become velar. The change from the bilabial nasal /m/ to the velar nasal /ŋ/ occurs in 'pumpkin' as it is pronounced in a few dialects of English. This change involves the deletion of the second /p/ sound so that the /k/ influences the preceding /m/ directly, resulting in /pʌŋkɪn/. Interestingly, this same change does not occur in the only analogously structured word in English, 'bumpkin.'

In words where /s/ is followed by /ʃ/ or /tʃ/, the alveolar fricative changes to a palatal one. This assimilation occurs in words like 'horseshoe' and phrases like 'horse show,' in which the final /s/ in 'horse' assimilates to the initial /ʃ/ in 'shoe' or 'show,' yielding an /-ʃʃ-/ or /-ʃ:-/ sequence. In words like 'mischief,' 'gesture,' and 'question,' the fricative sequence changes from /-stʃ-/ to /-ʃtʃ-/. The /s/ changes to /ʃ/ in the first syllable of each word under the influence of /ʃ/ or of /tʃ/ in the second syllable.

A very common change in this category is from apico-alveolar to dorsopalatal nasal in the context of front vowels, as in 'handkerchief' or to dorsovelar nasal in the context of back vowels, as in 'congress.' In 'handkerchief,' the /d/ is deleted so that the /n/ is influenced by the following /k/. In 'congress,' /n/ is influenced by the following /g/. Analogous changes occur in many words, such as 'anchor,' 'bank,' 'thank,' and 'anger.' These assimilations occur in anticipation of the adjacent stops /k/ and /g/, and they produce a change from alveolar to palatal nasal following a front vowel, as in 'sing,' or to velar nasal following a back vowel, as in 'song' (Bronstein, 1960; Tiffany & Carrell, 1977; Calvert, 1980). An equally common assimilation occurs for the nominally velar stop sounds /k/ and /g/ when they are produced in the context of front vowels; dorsopalatal variants occur in such contexts, as in 'key' and 'gay.'

Voicing Assimilation

In describing the allophones of the /t/ and /d/ phonemes, we mentioned the loss of voicing distinction between these sounds in the intervocalic positions of minimal pairs like 'bitter'/'bidder.' This allophone of /t/ is an example of voicing assimilation in intervocalic context. The alveolar voiceless stop has presumably taken on the voicing feature of the preceding and/or following vowel. This assimilation does not occur for the voiceless bilabial and velar stops. A limited change of this type occurs for the voiceless fricative /θ/ in 'north,' 'south,' and 'worth,' which becomes /ð/ in 'northern,' 'southern,' and 'worthy' because of the voicing of the preceding and/or following vowels (Bronstein, 1960).

A change in voicing occurs for /s/ in a /-bs V-/ context, where it is preceded and followed by voiced sounds. In this context, /s/ may take on the voicing feature of the vowel and/or /b/ and be pronounced /z/, as in 'absurd.'

Devoicing Assimilation

In discussing the allophones of /w/, /r/, /l/, and /j/, it was mentioned that a change occurs when these sounds are produced following voiceless stops and fricatives. In these contexts, the glides take on the voiceless feature, at least for the part of their production that immediately follows the voiceless consonant. This type of assimilation occurs for /w/ in words like 'twice' and 'sweet,' for /r/ in words like 'trick' and 'shrub,' for /l/ in words like 'clock' and 'fly,' and for /j/ in words like 'cute' and 'few.'

A very common assimilation process occurs for /d/ in the *-ed* tense ending in words like 'guessed,' 'lacked,' 'laughed,' and 'passed' (Bronstein, 1960). In these words, /d/ has taken on the voiceless feature of the preceding voiceless consonant. When the preceding consonant is voiced, as is the case in words like 'lagged,' the /d/ remains voiced. Compare your productions of 'lacked' and 'lagged,' listening for the contrast of /t/ and /d/. Now compare your productions of 'guessed' and 'guest' and of 'passed' and 'past.' Although the spellings lead one to assume that these pairs differ in the voicing of their final consonants, they are actually pronounced alike.

Devoicing occurs for /z/ in 'used to' and for /v/ in 'have to' (Bronstein, 1960). In the case of 'used to,' the /d/ is first deleted, so that the /z/ is adjacent to the /t/. These types of changes are not universal, since they do not occur in the analogous cases of 'used two,' 'have two,' or 'love to.'

Nasal Assimilation

In describing the allophones of vowels and glides, it was mentioned that these sounds become nasalized in the context of nasal consonants. Vowels and glides are subject to nasal assimilation when preceded or followed by nasal consonants, as in 'may,' 'new,' 'own,' 'earn,' 'arm,' 'elm,' 'onion,' and 'inward.'

Lip Rounding Assimilation

In describing the allophones of stops, fricatives, glides, and nasal consonants, it was mentioned that these sounds become somewhat rounded in the context of rounded vowels. Consonants are subject to rounding assimilation when followed by rounded vowels, as in 'two,' 'sew,' 'new,' 'foe,' 'go,' and 'row,' or when preceded by rounded vowels, as in 'own,' 'oat,' 'oak,' and 'ooze.' Rounding appears to be greater in consonants preceding rounded vowels than in those following them.

Before going on to describe the assimilations that occur in children's speech, it is interesting to note the characteristics of those that occur in adult speech. Most of the changes by far are regressive. Major exceptions are in voicing and manner. All changes are contiguous, and few are complete, that is, in few does one sound take on all the features of another sound.

PHONOLOGICAL PROCESSES OF ASSIMILATION

Among the many processes that occur during normal and abnormal speech development are those that can be explained in terms of assimilation (Ingram, 1976). For example, a child who pronounces 'table' as /bebu/ and 'pin' as /pɪm/ could be diagnosed as substituting /b/ for /t/ and /m/ for /n. But if this child pronounces /t/ correctly in words like 'two' and /n/ correctly in words like 'new,' such a diagnosis would be open to question, especially if the substitutions occurred only in the context of labial consonants. Given this evidence, one would conclude that bilabial assimilation was operating, not substitution. Children's assimilation processes are not the same as those of adult language.

Table 10–3 presents definitions of the most common assimilation processes. Examples of these assimilations are presented in Table 10–4 along with indications of

Table 10–3
Phonological processes of assimilation.

Type of Assimilation	Change
Place Changes	
Labial	Nonlabial consonant takes on labial feature in context of labial consonants /p, b, f, v, m, w/
Alveolar	Nonalveolar consonant takes on alveolar feature in context of alveolar consonants /t, d, s, z/
Palatal	Nonpalatal consonant takes on palatal feature in context of palatal consonants /ʃ, ʒ/
Velar	Nonvelar consonant takes on velar feature in context of velar consonants /k, g, ŋ/
Voicing Changes	
Prevocalic consonant voicing	Voiceless prevocalic stop or fricative takes on voicing feature of following vowel
Final consonant devoicing	Voiced postvocalic stop or fricative takes on voiceless feature of following silence
Manner Changes	
Nasal	Nonnasal consonant takes on nasal feature in context of nasal consonants /m, n, ŋ/

Table 10–4
Examples of children's assimilation process changes and other processes (in parentheses) that are confused with them (> means "changes to"). Direction of influence (RE = regressive; PR = progressive), contiguity of influence (+C = contiguous; −C = noncontiguous), and degree of influence (# = complete; " = partial) are also shown; dashes are used for nonassimilation processes.

Type of Change	Example	Direction	Contiguity	Degree
Place Changes				
Labial assimilation				
/n/ > /m/	/pum/ for 'spoon'	PR	−C	"
/d/ > /b/	/bɛb/ for 'bed'	PR	−C	#
/t/ > /p/	/pebo/ for 'table'	RE	−C	"
/t/ > /b/	/bap/ for 'stop'	RE	−C	"
/k/ > /p/	/pʌp/ for 'cup'	RE	−C	#
/t/ > /f/	/fwi/ for 'tree'	RE	+C	"
/s/ > /f/	/fpun/ for 'spoon'; /fwɛtɚ/ for 'sweater'	RE	+C	"
/s/ > /p/	/pup/ for 'soup'	RE	−C	#
/θ/ > /w/	/wʌm/ for 'thumb'	RE	−C	"
/θ/ > /f/	/fʌm/ for 'thumb'	RE	−C	"
/ð/ > /v/	/fɛvɚ/ for 'feather'	PR	−C	"
(Labialization)				
/θ/ > /f/	/fɪk/ for 'thick'; /fɪŋk/ for 'think'	–	–	–
Alveolar assimilation				
/b/ > /d/	/dɛd/ for 'bed'	RE	−C	#
/g/ > /d/	/dɔd/ for 'dog'; /dɔdi/ for 'doggie'	PR	−C	#
/j/ > /l/	/lɛlo/ for 'yellow'	RE	−C	#
(Apicalization)				
/p/ > /t/	/taɪ/ for 'pie'	–	–	–
/b/ > /d/	/di/ for 'bee'; /do/ for 'bow'	–	–	–
/f/ > /s/	/sɔr/ for 'four'; /sud/ for 'food'	–	–	–
/θ/ > /s/	/sʌm/ for 'thumb'	–	–	–
/ð/ > /z/	/fɛzɚ/ for 'feather'	–	–	–
(Fronting)				
/k/ > /t/	/ti/ for 'key'; /taʊ/ for 'cow'	–	–	–
/g/ > /d/	/do/ for 'go'	–	–	–
/ŋ/ > /n/	/bɪtʃɪn/ for 'fishing'	–	–	–
/k/ > /p/[a]	/paʊ/ for 'cow'	–	–	–
(Depalatalization)				
/ʃ/ > /s/	/su/ for 'shoe'; /fɪsɪŋ/ for 'fishing'	–	–	–
/tʃ/ > /ts/	/mæts/ for 'match'	–	–	–
/ʒ/ > /z/	/mɛzɚ/ for 'measure'	–	–	–
/dʒ/ > /dz/	/dzʌmp/ for 'jump'; /brɪdz/ for 'bridge'	–	–	–
Palatal assimilation				
/z/ > /ʃ/	/ʃuʃ/ for 'shoes'	PR	−C	#
/f/ > /ʃ/	/ʃɪʃ/ for 'fish'	RE	−C	#
/s/ > /ʃ/	/ʃu/ for 'sue'	RE	+C	"

Table 10–4 continued

Type of Change		Example	Direction	Contiguity	Degree
Velar assimilation					
	/t/ > /k/	/kok/ for 'coat'	PR	−C	#
		/gek/ for 'gate'	PR	−C	”
		/kek/ for 'take'	RE	−C	#
		/kwɪŋ/ for 'string'	RE	−C	”
	/tʃ/ > /k/	/kɪkən/ for 'chicken'	RE	−C	#
	/p/ > /k/	/skwɪŋ/ for 'spring'	RE	−C	”
	/d/ > /g/	/gɔg/ for 'dog'; /gɔgi/ for 'doggie'	RE	−C	#
		/gʌk/ for 'duck'	RE	−C	”
	/t/ > /g/	/gɑɪgu/ for 'tiger'	RE	−C	#
(Backing)					
	/t/ > /k/	/kɑp/ for 'top'; /ku/ for 'two'[b]	–	–	–
	/f/, /v/ > /k/	/kɑɪk/ for 'five'	–	–	–
	/d/ > /g/	/gu/ for 'do'[b]	–	–	–
	/s/ > /h/	/hop/ for 'soap'	–	–	–
(Palatalization)					
	/s/ > /ʃ/	/ʃu/ for 'sue'[c]; /ʃɪp/ for 'sip'	–	–	–
Voicing Changes					
Prevocalic voicing					
	/t/ > /d/	/dʌb/ for 'tub'	RE	+C	”
	/tʃ/ > /d/	/dɪkən/ for 'chicken'	RE	+C	”
	/p/ > /b/	/bepɚ/ for 'paper'	RE	+C	”
Postvocalic devoicing					
	/d/ > /t/	/bɛt/ for 'bed'; /bit/ for 'bead'	RE	+C	”
	/dʒ/ > /tʃ/	/petʃ/ for 'page'	RE	+C	”
	/g/ > /k/	/dɔk/ for 'dog'	RE	+C	”
	/z/ > /s/	/gos/ for 'goes'; /nos/ for 'nose'	RE	+C	”
Manner Changes					
Nasal assimilation					
	/l/ > /n/	/næm/ for 'lamb'	RE	−C	”
		/mɛn/ for 'smell'	PR	−C	”
	/t/ > /n/	/nɪŋ/ for 'string'	RE	−C	”
	/k/ > /n/	/nʌno/ for 'candle'; /næni/ for 'candy'	RE	−C	#
	/s/ > /n/	/nænə/ for 'Santa'; /nʌn/ for 'sun'	RE	−C	#
	/f/ > /n/	/nʌn/ for 'fun'	RE	−C	#
	/θ/ > /n/	/nʌm/ for 'thumb'	RE	−C	”
	/ð/ > /n/	/nʌnə/ for 'another'	PR	−C	#
	/i/ > [ĩ]	[grĩ] for 'green'[d]	RE	+C	”

[a]This is an infrequent change (Hodson & Paden, 1983).
[b]This change is also considered velar assimilation.
[c]This change is also considered to be palatal assimilation.
[d]Some phoneticians do not consider this to be an assimilation.

the direction, contiguity, and degree of the assimilation. Also included in Table 10–4 are examples of changes produced by other processes that are often confused with assimilation changes (Ingram, 1976; Lund & Duchan, 1978; Weiner, 1979; Shriberg & Kwiatkowski, 1980; Hodson & Paden, 1981; Elbert & Gierut, 1986; Khan & Lewis, 1986).

Labial Assimilation

Consonants may take on the labial feature in the context of the labial consonants, /p, b, m, f, v/. This change may be regressive in words like 'table,' in which the sound changed, /t/, precedes the bilabial, /b/, or progressive in words like 'pin,' in which the sound changed, /n/, follows the bilabial, /p/. Influence is usually noncontiguous, extending across a vowel in most examples, and even stretching across syllable boundaries in the case of /pebo/ for 'table.' Generally the assimilation is partial, except for /bɛb/ for 'bed,' /pʌp/ for 'cup,' and /pup/ for 'soup.'

It is important not to confuse labial assimilation with labialization. Children may use a labial for another consonant when there is no labial consonant in the context, as in /fɪk/ for 'thick.' If a child substitutes labial consonants for others only in the context of labial consonants, the problem is labial assimilation. If the child substitutes labial consonants even when there are none in the context, the problem is **labialization.**

Alveolar Assimilation

In **alveolar assimilation,** consonants take on the alveolar feature in the context of the alveolar consonants, /t, d, s, z/. The change may be regressive, as in /dɛd/ for 'bed,' or progressive, as in /dɔd/ for 'dog.' All the examples reflect noncontiguous and complete assimilation. It is important not to confuse alveolar assimilation with apicalization, fronting, or depalatalization (see Table 10–4). **Apicalization** involves the substitution of alveolar consonants for labial and dental consonants when there are no alveolar consonants in the context. Fronting involves the substitution of alveolar consonants for palatal and velar consonants when there are no alveolar consonants in the context. **Depalatalization** involves the substitution of alveolar for palatal fricatives in contexts with no alveolar consonants.

Palatal Assimilation

Palatal assimilation involves the substitution of palatal fricatives for other fricatives in the context of palatal fricatives. The assimilation may be progressive, as in /ʃuʃ/ for 'shoes,' or regressive, as in /ʃɪʃ/ for 'fish.' Both cases reflect noncontiguous and complete assimilation. The example of /ʃu/ for 'sue' is a possibly contiguous but partial assimilation involving the back vowel /u/. The assimilation is palatal because /s/ assumes the palatal feature of /u/ and becomes /ʃ/. It is partial because the change does not involve the other features of /u/. Some phoneticians question the validity of such examples as exemplifying palatal assimilation, since there is no palatal fricative in the context. According to their classification system, /ʃu/ for 'sue' is an example of palatalization. Palatalization involves the substitution of palatal fricatives for other fricatives when there are no palatal fricatives in the context. Although it is generally agreed that /ʃu/ for 'sue' is an example of a phonological process, it is not clear whether the change is an example of palatalization or palatal assimilation.

Velar Assimilation

Velar assimilation refers to the substitution of velar consonants for other consonants in the context of the velar consonants, /k, g, ŋ/. Most of these changes are regressive, as in /kek/ for 'take,' but there are cases of progressive change, as in /kok/ for 'coat.' All the examples reflect noncontiguous assimilation with the exception of /ku/ for 'two,' but this type of change is not accepted by all phoneticians as reflecting velar assimilation. About half of the changes are complete, as in /kek/ for 'take,' and half are partial, as in /gʌk/ for 'duck.' Velar assimilation should not be confused with backing. **Backing** involves the substitution of back consonants, including velars, when there are no velar consonants in the context, as in /kæn/ for 'tan.'

Prevocalic Consonant Voicing

Although assimilation does not appear in the name of this process, it is considered an assimilation process under the assumption that a voiceless consonant is influenced by the following vowel and becomes voiced. All these changes are, by definition, regressive, contiguous, and partial, since a vowel is exerting an influence over a preceding consonant.

Postvocalic Consonant Devoicing

This is also an assimilation process, even though the name does not clearly reflect that fact. It is assumed that the final consonant takes on the absence of voicing that characterizes the following silence. All the examples of this process are, by definition, regressive, contiguous, and partial, since the silence at the end of the word presumably exerts an influence over the preceding consonant.

Nasal Assimilation

Nasal assimilation involves the acquisition of the nasal feature by a nonnasal consonant in the context of a nasal consonant. Most changes are regressive and noncontiguous, as in /nʌm/ for 'thumb.' Exceptions are /nʌnə/ for 'another,' which is a progressive change, and [grĩ] for 'green,' which is a contiguous change. The form [grĩ] is not generally accepted as an example of nasal assimilation because it involves a nasalization of the vowel by the following nasal consonant before it is deleted. In all the other examples a nasal consonant replaces a nonnasal one. In some cases, assimilation is complete, as in /nʌn/ for 'fun'; in others, assimilation is partial, as in /nʌm/ for 'thumb.'

There are noticeable differences between the assimilations that occur in adult speech and those that occur in child speech, as is evident by comparing the examples in tables 10–2 and 10–4. For both, regressive changes appear to be more common than progressive ones. All the assimilations are contiguous in adult speech, while those in child speech are overwhelmingly noncontiguous. Moreover, complete assimilations are rare in adult speech but relatively common in child speech. Although all assimilations tend to simplify transitions between the different articulatory states that characterize different sounds, those in child speech appear to be more pervasive than those in adult speech. It is important to note assimilation processes in children's speech for clinical phonetics because of the potential of assimilation for explaining the nature of misarticulations. The basis for sound substitutions that appear to reflect contextual influences may differ from the basis for those that do not. Such a differentiation could be important for the development of better diagnosis and rehabilitation procedures than are possible without such phonological specificity.

GLOSSARY

Alveolar assimilation. The acquisition by one consonant of the alveolar feature of an alveolar consonant in the same context; a phonological process.

Apicalization. The substitution of alveolar for labial and dental consonants in contexts with no alveolar consonants; a phonological process.

Articulatory gesture. Any of a number of constrictions or movements by the articulators that contribute to the production of speech sounds.

Backing. The substitution of back for front consonants in contexts with no back consonants; a phonological process.

Coarticulation. The articulatory processes through which one sound influences the production of others in the same context.

Complete assimilation. Change of one sound totally to another sound.

Contiguous assimilation. Influence of one sound on an immediately preceding or following sound.

Depalatalization. The substitution of alveolar for palatal fricatives in contexts with no alveolar consonants; a phonological process.

Labialization. The substitution of labial for other consonants, particularly labiodentals for interdentals, in contexts with no labial consonants; a phonological process.

Left-to-right assimilation. Influence of one sound on the production of a following sound; also called perseverative assimilation and progressive assimilation.

Noncontiguous assimilation. The influence of one sound on sounds other than those that immediately precede or follow it.

Palatal assimilation. The acquisition by one consonant of the palatal feature of a palatal consonant in the same context; a phonological process.

Partial assimilation. Change of at least one but not all the features of one sound to those of another.

Property. An articulatory characteristic of a speech sound.

Right-to-left assimilation. Influence of one sound on a preceding sound; also called anticipatory assimilation and regressive assimilation.

REVIEW QUESTIONS

A. Indicate the context in which the assimilative changes would occur by inserting the appropriate letter.

1. Alveolar to dental /l/ ________	a. sitter
2. Alveolar to labial ________	b. grandpa
3. Alveolar to velar ________	c. strength
4. Alveolar to palatal ________	d. sink
5. Intervocalic voicing ________	e. soup
6. Lip rounding ________	f. conquer
7. Alveolar to dental /n/ ________	g. stealthy
8. Palatal to dental /n/ ________	h. seventh
9. Alveolar to dental /d/ ________	i. add them up

****

Key: 1. g; 2. b; 3. f; 4. d; 5. a; 6. e; 7. h; 8. c; 9. i

B. Indicate the phonological process of assimilation represented by the examples by inserting the appropriate letter.

1. Labial ________	a. /gek/ for 'bake'
2. Alveolar ________	b. /nʌm/ for 'gum'
3. Velar ________	c. /wes/ for 'weighs'
4. Prevocalic consonant voicing ________	d. /gɪti/ for 'kitty'
5. Devoicing final consonant ________	e. /dæd/ for 'bad'
6. Nasal ________	f. /bʌbəl/ for 'double'

****

Key: 1. f; 2. e; 3. a; 4. d; 5. c; 6. b

C. Indicate whether the following are examples of assimilation changes by inserting Y for yes and N for no.

1. /fʌm/ for 'thumb' ______
2. /dɔd/ for 'dog' ______
3. /dʌb/ for 'tub' ______
4. /gos/ for 'goes' ______
5. /ʃɪʃ/ for 'fish' ______
6. /kek/ for 'take' ______
7. /næm/ for 'lamb' ______
8. /hop/ for 'soap' ______
9. /do/ for 'go' ______
10. /gɔg/ for 'dog' ______
11. /gu/ for 'do' ______

****

Key: 1. Y; 2. Y; 3. Y; 4. Y; 5. Y; 6. Y; 7. Y; 8. N; 9. N; 10. Y; 11. N

D. Indicate the direction (REGressive or PROgressive), contiguity (CONtiguous or NONcontiguous), and degree (COMplete or PARtial) of assimilation represented in the following examples by checking the appropriate columns.

	REG	PRO	CON	NON	COM	PAR
1. /fʌm/ for 'thumb'	______	______	______	______	______	______
2. /dɔd/ for 'dog'	______	______	______	______	______	______
3. /ʃuʃ/ for 'shoes'	______	______	______	______	______	______
4. /gʌk/ for 'duck'	______	______	______	______	______	______
5. /bepɚ/ for 'paper'	______	______	______	______	______	______
6. /dɔk/ for 'dog'	______	______	______	______	______	______
7. /nʌm/ for 'thumb'	______	______	______	______	______	______
8. /nænə/ for 'Santa'	______	______	______	______	______	______
9. /pum/ for 'spoon'	______	______	______	______	______	______
10. /gek/ for 'gate'	______	______	______	______	______	______

****

Key: 1. REG/NON/PAR; 2. PRO/NON/COM; 3. PRO/NON/COM; 4. REG/NON/PAR; 5. REG/CON/PAR; 6. REG/CON/PAR; 7. REG/NON/PAR; 8. REG/NON/COM; 9. PRO/NON/PAR; 10. PRO/NON/PAR

LABORATORY ASSIGNMENT

Tape IV, Side A
IVA3: Assimilations in Adult and Child Speech (Tape running time: 9:14; Elapsed time: 06:21–15:35)

The purpose of this section is to provide students with transcription practice for assimilations that occur in the speech of adults and children.

a. Assimilations in Adult Speech Production

Listen to the words as they are pronounced by an adult and transcribe the entire utterance, making sure to note any phonetic modifications that occur as a result of assimilation. In this subsection and subsequent ones, stop the tape if necessary, rewind, and listen again.

1. grandpa ____________________
2. question ____________________
3. passed ____________________
4. husband ____________________
5. have to ____________________
6. batter ____________________
7. congress ____________________
8. southern ____________________
9. length ____________________
10. husband ____________________
11. batter ____________________
12. have to ____________________
13. length ____________________
14. has the time ____________________

****

Consensus: 1. /græmpə/ 2. /kwɛʃtʃən/ 3. /pæst/ 4. /hʌzbənd/ 5. /hæftu/ 6. /bærɚ/ 7. /kaŋgrəs/ 8. /sʌðɚn/ 9. /lɛŋθ/ 10. /hʌsbənd/ 11. /bætɚ/ 12. /hævtu/ 13. [lɛŋ̪θ] 14. /hæzðətaɪm/

Variants: 7. /kaŋgrɪs/

b. Labial Assimilations and Labialization

Listen to the words as they are pronounced by a child and transcribe the entire utterance, making sure to note any phonological process changes.

1. spoon ____________________
2. feather ____________________
3. thumb ____________________
4. table ____________________
5. stop ____________________
6. tree ____________________
7. feather ____________________
8. sweater ____________________
9. thick ____________________
10. table ____________________
11. thank you ____________________
12. thumb ____________________

****

Consensus: 1. /pum/ 2. /bɛfə/ 3. /θʌm/ 4. /pebo/ 5. /bap/ 6. /fwi/ 7. /fɛðɚ/ 8. /fwɛtə/ 9. /θɪk/ 10. /tebəl/ 12. /fʌm/

Variants: 1. /pu/ 7. /θɛðɚ/ 11. /fæŋkju/; /dæŋkju/; /bæŋkju/

c. Alveolar Assimilations, Fronting, and Apicalization

Listen to the words as they are pronounced by a child and transcribe the entire utterance, making sure to note any phonological process changes.

1. doggie ____________________
2. thumb ____________________
3. yellow ____________________
4. feather ____________________
5. doggie ____________________
6. thumb ____________________
7. feather ____________________
8. thumb ____________________
9. pie ____________________
10. yellow ____________________
11. fishing ____________________
12. cow ____________________

****

Consensus: 1. /dɔdi/ 2. /θʌm/ 3. /lɛlo/ 4. /fɛðɚ/ 5. /dɔgi/ 6. /sʌm/ 7. /fɛðɚ/ 8. /sʌm/ 9. /taɪ/ 10. /jɛlo/ 11. /fɪtsɪn/ 12. /taʊ/

Variants: 1. /dadi/ 5. /dagi/

d. Palatal and Velar Assimilations and Backing

Listen to the words as they are pronounced by a child and transcribe the entire utterance, making sure to note any phonological process changes.

1. dog ____________________ 2. coat ____________________

3. shoes ____________________ 4. tan ____________________

5. dog ____________________ 6. soap ____________________

7. shoes ____________________ 8. soap ____________________

****

Consensus: 1. /dɔg/ 2. /kok/ 3. /ʃuz/ 4. /kæt/ 5. /gɔg/ 7. /ʃuʃ/ 8. /sop/

Variants: 4. [kæ̃t] 6. /hop/; /ho/; /pop/

e. Palatalization and Depalatalization

Listen to the words as they are pronounced by a child and transcribe the entire utterance, making sure to note any phonological process changes.

1. match ____________________ 2. shoe ____________________

3. fishing ____________________ 4. bridge ____________________

5. match ____________________ 6. fishing ____________________

7. shoe ____________________ 8. bridge ____________________

****

Consensus: 1. /mætʃ/ 2. /ʃu/ 3. /fɪʃɪŋ/ 4. /brɪdz/ 5. /mæts/ 6. /fɪsɪŋ/ 7. /su/ 8. /brɪdʒ/

Variants: None.

f. Voicing and Manner Changes

Listen to the words as they are pronounced by a child and transcribe the entire utterance, making sure to note any phonological process changes.

1. dog ____________________ 2. paper ____________________

3. nose ____________________ 4. string ____________________

5. lamb ____________________ 6. Santa ____________________

7. nose ____________________ 8. thumb ____________________

9. lamb ____________________ 10. string ____________________

11. Santa ____________________ 12. dog ____________________

****

Consensus: 1. /dɔg/ 2. /bepə/ 3. /noz/ 4. /nek/ 5. /næp/ 6. /sæntə/ 7. /nos/ 8. /nʌp/ 9. /læm/ 10. /strɪŋ/ 11. /nænə/ 12. /dɔk/

Variants: 2. /bebə/ 4. [nĩk] 5. [læ:p] 7. /nʌs/

CHAPTER 11

Suprasegmental Analysis of Speech

Previous chapters focused on describing the properties of the phonemes of American English, the sound segments that are the basic units in the analysis of meaningful distinctions in speech. This aspect of the study of phonetics is referred to as **segmental** phonetics or segmental phonology. Intonation, tempo, stress, juncture, and rhythm are aspects of speech production that transcend the limits of individual phonemes, and they are collectively referred to as **suprasegmental** (Lehiste, 1970; Shriberg & Kent, 1982) or nonsegmental (Tiffany & Carrell, 1977; Crystal, 1982) phonetics or phonology. These suprasegmental features cannot be described with reference to a single sound segment but require consideration of effects over at least a syllable or of segments in different parts of an utterance. Some phoneticians use the term *prosody* to cover this aspect of phonetic and phonological analysis (Crystal, 1982). No matter what term is used, a complete understanding of the characteristics of normal and abnormal speech requires an analysis of intonation, tempo, stress, juncture, and rhythm.

INTONATION

Intonation is the systematic variation in the pitch of the voice that produces meaningful differences in units of speech comparable to phrases, clauses, and sentences. **Pitch** is the perception of frequency. In discussing intonation, pitch is the perception of the fundamental frequency—the frequency of vocal fold vibration. Crystal (1982) has identified five functional roles for the intonation system in English: (1) grammatical, (2) semantic, (3) attitudinal or emotional, (4) social, and (5) psychological. Traditionally the analysis of intonation has focused primarily on the grammatical, semantic, and emotional roles, as is done in this chapter. The following examples, however, should help to indicate the multiple roles of intonation in linguistic contrasts: (1) attitudinal or emotional—the surprise in the statement of a northern Florida resident saying 'I saw snow on the ground this morning,' compared with the same statement made matter-of-factly by a northern Michigan resident; (2) semantic—the same words said as a statement, 'You brought the money,' and as a question, 'You brought the money?' (3) grammatical—the implication of only one brother in stating 'My brother, who's abroad, wrote me a letter' and of more than one brother in stating 'My brother who's abroad wrote me a letter'; (4) social—the use of statements, identical in words, which suggest that a response is or is not expected; and (5) psychological—the use of varying emphasis on lexical items in statements so that they are easier or more difficult to recall (Crystal, 1982).

The variations in intonation noted so far involve changes in pitch that incorporate changes in stress and duration. Since it is based on variations in f_0, the perception of pitch variations is necessarily relative. Otherwise, it would not be possible for meaningful changes in pitch to be interpreted in the same way when spoken by male, female, and child speakers, whose mean fundamental frequencies are between 120 and 130 Hz, between 190 and 225 Hz, and about 265 Hz, respectively (Tiffany & Carrell, 1977; Cruttenden, 1986). If, for example, a fixed rather than a relative high pitch were indicative of a question, the intonation system would not be functional. Figures 11–1, 11–2, and 11–3 show spectrographic tracings of f_0 variations for a child, an adult female, and an adult male saying 'The answer is yes' as a complete statement, as an incomplete statement, and as a question. Notice that terminal f_0 for each speaker increases for the question, decreases for the complete statement, and is constant for the incomplete statement. Also notice that the overall level of the fundamental frequency decreases as follows: child, female adult, and male adult.

Units of Intonation

In listening to the flow of speech, it is possible to identify syllables that have greater prominence than others. For example, in the utterance 'I came, I saw, I conquered,' one can contrast the prominence of 'came,' 'saw,' and the first syllable of 'conquered' with the lack of prominence of 'I' and the second syllable of 'conquered.' This placement of maximum prominence on certain syllables is referred to as **tonicity** since it involves the placement of the **tonic accent**, the accent or primary stress of the tone sequence. The location of the tonic accent is reflected primarily by higher pitch, accompanied by longer duration and greater loudness.

The identification of the tonic accents in a flow of speech helps to define **intonation contours** or **pitch contours**, also known as **tone-units** (Crystal, 1982), breath groups (MacKay, 1987), or tone groups (Ladefoged, 1975). A pitch contour is a unit of speech which includes a syllable or syllables with a tonic accent and an associated group of unaccented syllables across which meaningful patterns of pitch change occur. The utterance 'I came, I saw, I conquered' is made up of three pitch contours, 'I came,' 'I saw,' and 'I conquered,' with the tonic accent falling on the second syllable of each

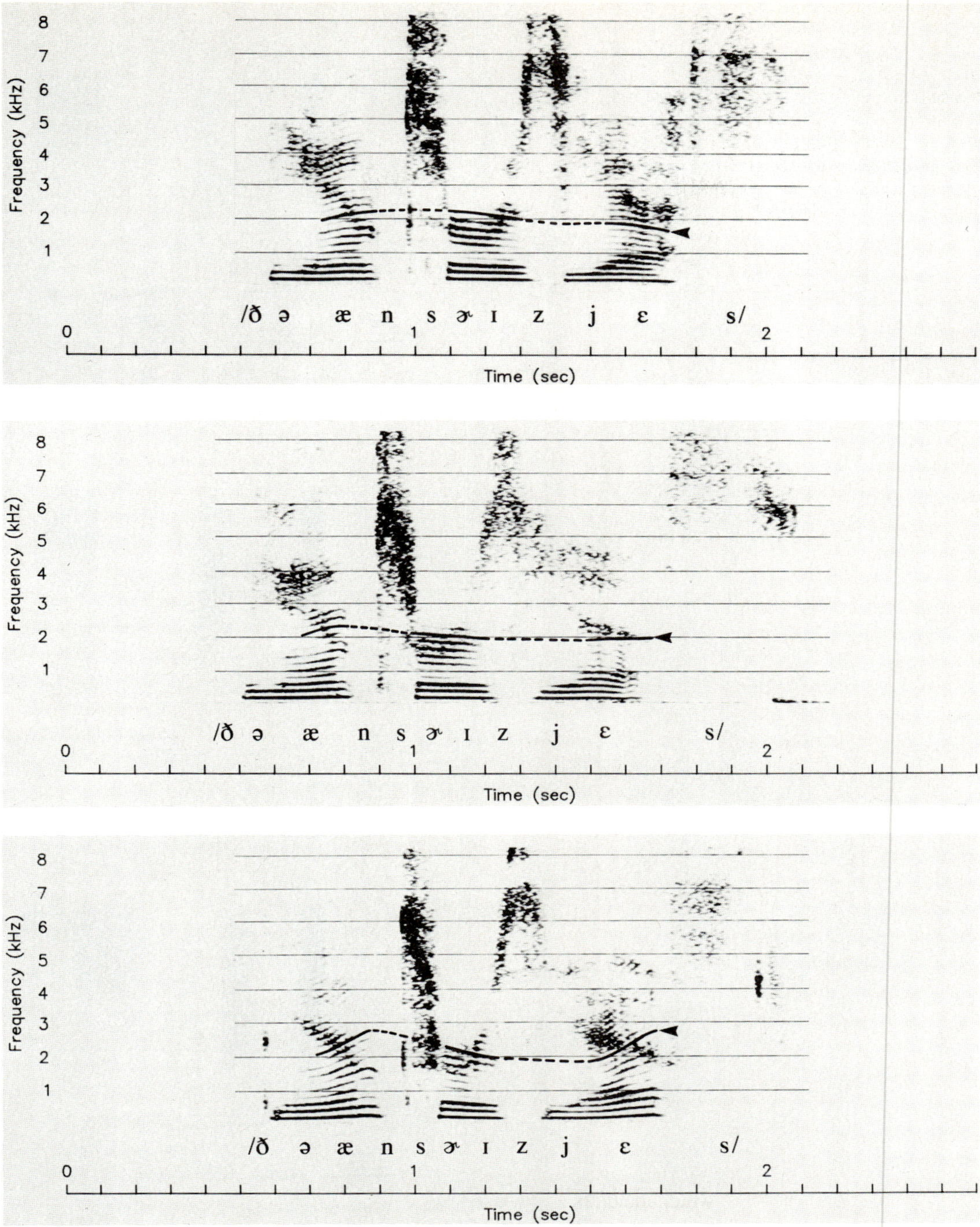

Figure 11–1

Tracings of the tenth harmonic from narrow band spectrograms of a child saying 'The answer is yes' as a statement (top panel), an incomplete statement (middle panel), and a question (bottom panel). Arrows along the *y* axis (ordinate) indicate the approximate location of the terminal frequency of the tenth harmonic.

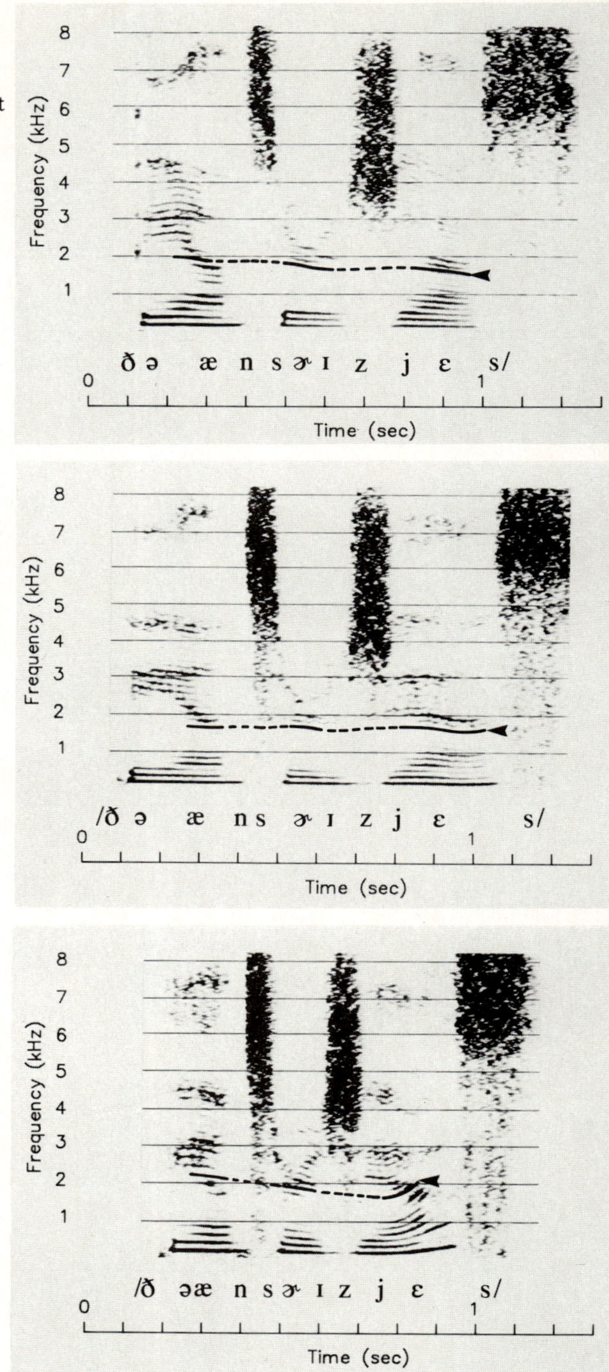

Figure 11–2
Tracings of the tenth harmonic from narrow band spectrograms of an adult female saying 'The answer is yes' as a statement (top panel), an incomplete statement (middle panel), and a question (bottom panel). Arrows along the *y* axis indicate the approximate location of the terminal frequency of the tenth harmonic.

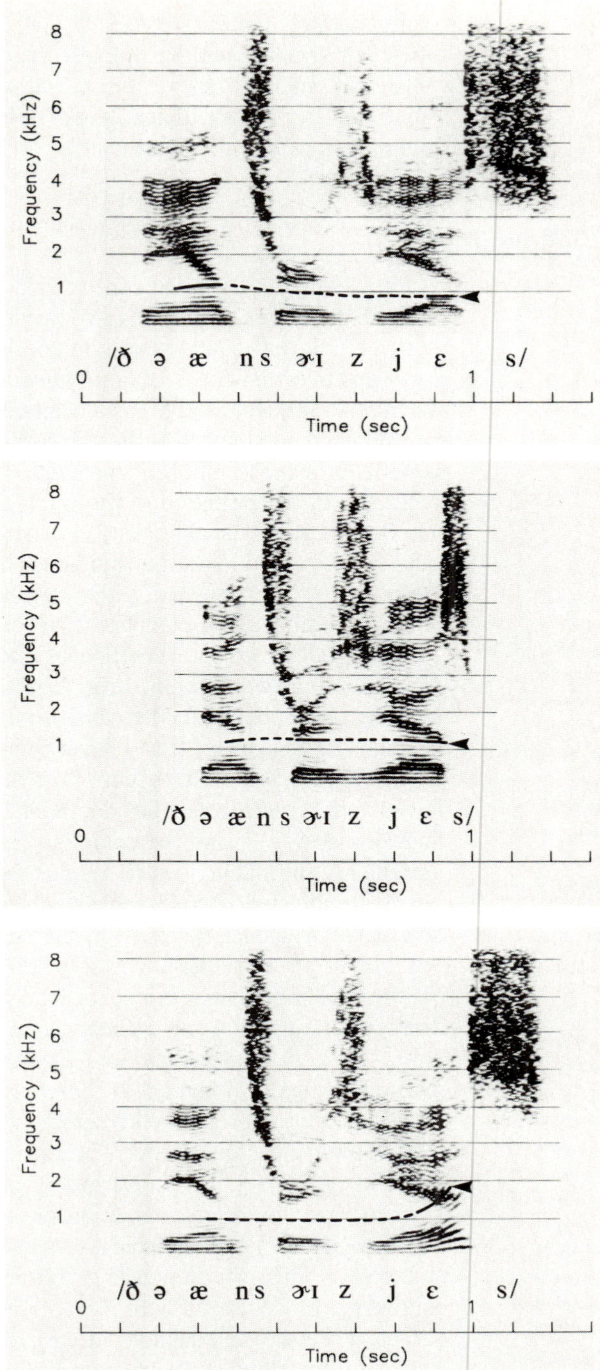

Figure 11–3
Tracings of the tenth harmonic from narrow band spectrograms of an adult male saying 'The answer is yes' as a statement (top panel), an incomplete statement (middle panel), and a question (bottom panel). Arrows along the *y* axis indicate the approximate location of the terminal frequency of the tenth harmonic.

contour. Pitch contours are usually associated with clauses or sentences, but they may also be associated with incomplete speech patterns, including one-word responses like 'yes' or items in a series like the fruits in the statement 'I bought apples, oranges, and bananas.' In these examples, 'yes,' 'I bought apples,' 'oranges,' and 'and bananas' are all identifiable as pitch contours.

Contour Types

Having identified the pitch contour and the tonic accent, the pitch variations that make such observations possible can be described. The utterance 'The answer is yes' spoken in three different contexts can be used as an example (1) of acquiescence to a request for a positive response; (2) as a question put to someone to determine if he is acquiescing to a request; and (3) as a hesitant acquiescence to a request which is followed by a qualifying 'but.' In each of these utterances the tonic accent occurs on 'yes.' When 'yes' is spoken in these different manners, meaningful differences can be identified by the contrasts in the direction of the pitch changes, as shown in figures 11–1, 11–2, and 11–3. The pitch usually falls [\] on complete statements, rises [/] on questions requiring a yes-or-no answer, and is usually level [—] on incomplete statements. These tones form the nucleus of pitch contours, and they may be used as a basis for the analysis of simple and complex variations in intonation.

In addition to the direction of pitch changes, their relative levels can be noted. Using a four-level system, level 2 is the average pitch, or the level on which most syllables are spoken. In the case of our examples, level 2 would normally be used in saying 'The answer is.' Level 3 is a higher pitch associated with the emphasis placed on a syllable or syllables, as occurs in saying 'yes' in each of the examples. Level 1 is the lowest pitch, and it can be identified by contrasting the incomplete statement 'The answer is yes . . .' and the complete statement 'The answer is yes.' In the incomplete statement, the pitch rises to level 3 on 'yes,' falls to level 2, and ends there. In the complete one, the pitch rises to level 3 on 'yes,' falls to level 2, and then finally falls to level 1. This final fall to level 1 is characteristic of terminations of complete statements.

In order to describe level 4, one more example is needed. Assume that the statement 'The answer is yes' is made by someone after being questioned about the strength of a previous acquiescence. In response, this individual might produce a very emphatic 'yes' tinged with some anger and annoyance, so that the tonic accent is marked by a rise to level 4, higher than for a routine statement.

Table 11–1 presents the common types of pitch contours of American English and methods for indicating them. The three main types are identified as falling [\], rising [/], and level [—]. Variations are given for each. As the name implies, the **falling contour** involves a fall in pitch on the tonic syllable either from level 3 [31#] or level 4 [41#]. The [#] symbol indicates that the pitch falls at the end rather than leveling off at level 1. This is called falling terminal juncture or falling external juncture. Both contours are associated with statements, but the low falling contour is more matter-of-fact, while the high falling contour is emotionally emphatic. The **rise-fall contour** is similar to the falling contour, except that it starts at level 2 and rises to level 3 [231#] or level 4 [241#] before falling off. These patterns are both more emphatic than the

Table 11–1
Common types of American English intonation patterns. Contour levels ([1] = lowest; [2] = average; [3] = high; [4] = highest), and terminal or external junctures ([#] = falling; [||] = rising; [|] = level) are shown in brackets. Implications of the variations for meaning appear in the right-hand column.

Pattern and Contour	Implications
Falling [\\]	
Low [31#]	Neutral, matter-of-fact statement
High [41#]	Emotional statement
Rise-Fall [/\\]	
Low [231#][a]	Definite statement
High [241#]	Emotional definite statement
Rising [/]	
Low [23||][b]	Question or incomplete statement
High [24||]	Question expressing surprise or incredulity
Fall-Rise [\\/] [323||]	Warning or cautionary statement
Level [—]	
Low [232	]	Incomplete statement; bored
High [23	]	Incomplete statement; enthusiastic

[a]This pattern is commonly used on questions beginning with *what, where, when, why, which, who,* and *how.*
[b]This pattern is commonly used on questions requiring a yes-or-no response, like 'Are you going?'

falling contours, and the high rise-fall has more of an emotional overlay than the low rise-fall. Saying 'I want breakfast now' with a [231#] contour and the tonic accent on 'now' would simply be a request to eat soon, but the same utterance with a [241#] contour and the tonic accent on 'now' is a response to the suggestion that it would be better to wait until later to eat.

The rise-fall contour, [/\\] or [231#], is also commonly used on questions that begin with *who, what, where, why, which, when,* and *how* (wh- questions). Thus, these questions do not usually differ in intonation from statements. You can hear this similarity by listening to your own productions of 'I am doing nothing' and 'Why am I doing nothing?'

The low **rising contour** goes from level 2 to level 3 and rises slightly at the end; the high rising contour goes from level 2 to level 4 and rises slightly at the end. The [||] symbol indicates the upward termination of a contour. This is called a rising terminal juncture or a rising external juncture. These contours are generally used for questions that require a yes-or-no answer, like 'Aren't you doing anything?' The low rising contour occurs for most questions of this type; the high rising contour would occur if the question involved disbelief or surprise. In the example given here, the surprise could be that the individual being questioned is not doing anything. The low rising contour may also occur on such incomplete utterances as all the items in a series except the last. For example, in the sentence 'I want red, white, and blue stripes,' 'I want red' and 'white' each might have a [23||] contour and 'and blue stripes' would have a [231#] contour.

The **fall-rise contour**, [\/] or [323||], is similar to the rising contour except that it involves an initial fall from level 3 to level 2 before rising again to level 3. Like all contours that end with a rising pitch, the fall-rise implies uncertainty (Jones, 1956) or doubt (Ladefoged, 1975), but it may also imply a warning or caution (Crystal, 1982). This contour might occur on an utterance like 'I think so' spoken with a good deal of self-doubt or on an utterance like 'He's a fool' spoken as a caution.

As indicated in Table 11–1, the **level contour** [—] may rise from level 2 to level 3 and end there [23 |] or may return to level 2 and end there [232 |]. Level contour indicates that the pitch does not fall at the end but stays at level 2 or 3. The level contour might occur in a dependent clause, as in 'When the rains came, [232 |] people moved to high ground' [231#], or in a series of items, as in 'I took courses in English, [232 |] history, [232 |] and economics' [231#]. The [|] symbol indicates a leveling off of pitch at the end of a contour rather than a fall [#] or a rise [||]. This is called a level terminal juncture or a level external juncture. According to Crystal (1982), this level pattern lends an attitude of routineness or boredom to a statement, as in 'He's a fool,' spoken as though there may be more negatives to come. Utterances like 'He's a fool' can be spoken with a rise-fall [231#] or a level [232 |] contour. The rise-fall contour is the expected pattern for a routine statement of fact; the level contour provides a shade of emotional implication to the statement. This emotional shading also applies to the level contour that ends at level 3 rather than level 2, indicating enthusiasm in the incomplete pattern. The distinction might occur in a statement like 'When the results came in, [23 |] I had won $5,000' [231#], as compared with 'When the results came in, [232 |] I had lost $5,000' [231#]. Not all phoneticians agree on the contours used in incomplete statements. For example, Ladefoged (1975) uses the rising pattern for such utterances.

Crystal (1982) reports the following frequencies of occurrence for contours in adult conversations: falling, 51.2%; rising, 20.8%; fall-rise, 8.5%; rise-fall, 5.2%; level, 4.9%. The other 9.4% is distributed between the rise-plus-fall and the fall-plus-rise patterns, which are similar to the rise-fall and fall-rise patterns, except that the patterns are spread across two tonically stressed syllables. According to Ladefoged (1975), the fall-rise contour is much more common than the rise-fall contour.

There is no information on how often the various intonation contours are used by children. But there is evidence to indicate that children use intonation purposively and grammatically on single-word utterances by 18 months (Galligan, 1987). This usage includes rising contours and fall-rise contours for asking questions and falling contours, rise-fall contours, and level contours for responding to wh- questions.

TEMPO

Tempo of speech may be defined as the perception of the rate of speech production. Speaking rate can be measured in syllables per second or in words per minute, but syllables are a better measure because they are more nearly standard in length. Whatever measure is used, differences in speaking rate reflect changes in the duration of the sounds produced and the pauses between them, both of which shorten as speaking rate increases and lengthen as speaking rate decreases. For this reason, speech tempo is described here in terms of speaking rate, sound and syllable duration, and pause duration and location.

Speaking Rate

During speech production, the mean speaking rate is between 3.7 and 6.5 syllables per second, but it is possible for adults to speed up to about 7.0 syllables per second or slow down to about 2.9 syllables per second (Tiffany & Carrell, 1977; Calvert, 1980; Smith, Sugarman, & Long, 1983; Smith, Wasowicz, & Preston, 1987). Not only do older children have faster rates than younger children, but adults have faster rates than children (Kent & Forner, 1980; Smith et al., 1983). The adult normal rate of four syllables per second is about the speed required to say 'Jack be nimble, Jack be quick, Jack jumped over the candlestick' in four seconds. Slower and faster fluctuations within speakers are probably no greater than from 15% to 20% of the mean rate (Tiffany & Carrell, 1977; Smith et al., 1983). Speaking rates are about 70% of the adult rate for 5-year-olds, about 77% for 7-year-olds, and about 93% for 9-year-olds; but both children and adults can increase their normal speaking rates by about 15% (Smith et al., 1983; Smith et al., 1987). This seems to imply that children can speak as rapidly as adults if they are pushed to do so. Even though they can speak faster, under normal conditions children and adults choose an "optimal" rate that may be between 70% and 80% of their maximum speaking rate (Lindblom, 1983; Smith et al., 1987).

When speaking rate becomes either too fast or too slow, the production of speech sounds changes. Figures 11–4 and 11–5 show spectrograms of child and adult speakers saying the sentence 'The sky is falling' at normal, rapid, and slow rates. At abnormally fast rates—above 8.0 syllables per second—the separate positions for different sounds cannot be achieved, and pauses are omitted. At abnormally slow rates—below 2.0 syllables per second—speech sounds and pauses are prolonged to three or four times their normal duration. As indicated in Figure 11–6 and Table 11–2, data from a number of studies of speaking and reading rates can be used as a basis for judging speech rate. In general, rates for spontaneous or extemporaneous speech are slower than those for reading or sentence repetition. The exceptionally slow reading rate of 2.0 syllables per second or less and the exceptionally fast reading rate of 7.0 syllables per second or greater are characteristic of severe apractic and severe parkinsonian dysarthric speakers, respectively. Slow spontaneous speech (2.0–2.9 syllables per second) is characteristic of preschool children, slow reading rate (4.0–4.9) is characteristic of 5-year-olds, and average reading rate (5.0–5.9) is characteristic of 9-year-olds.

Duration of Sounds and Syllables

When the rate of speech production is increased above normal, the duration of sounds and syllables generally becomes very short. They may be completely omitted. The [>] symbol may be used to indicate unusual shortening of individual sounds and the /0/

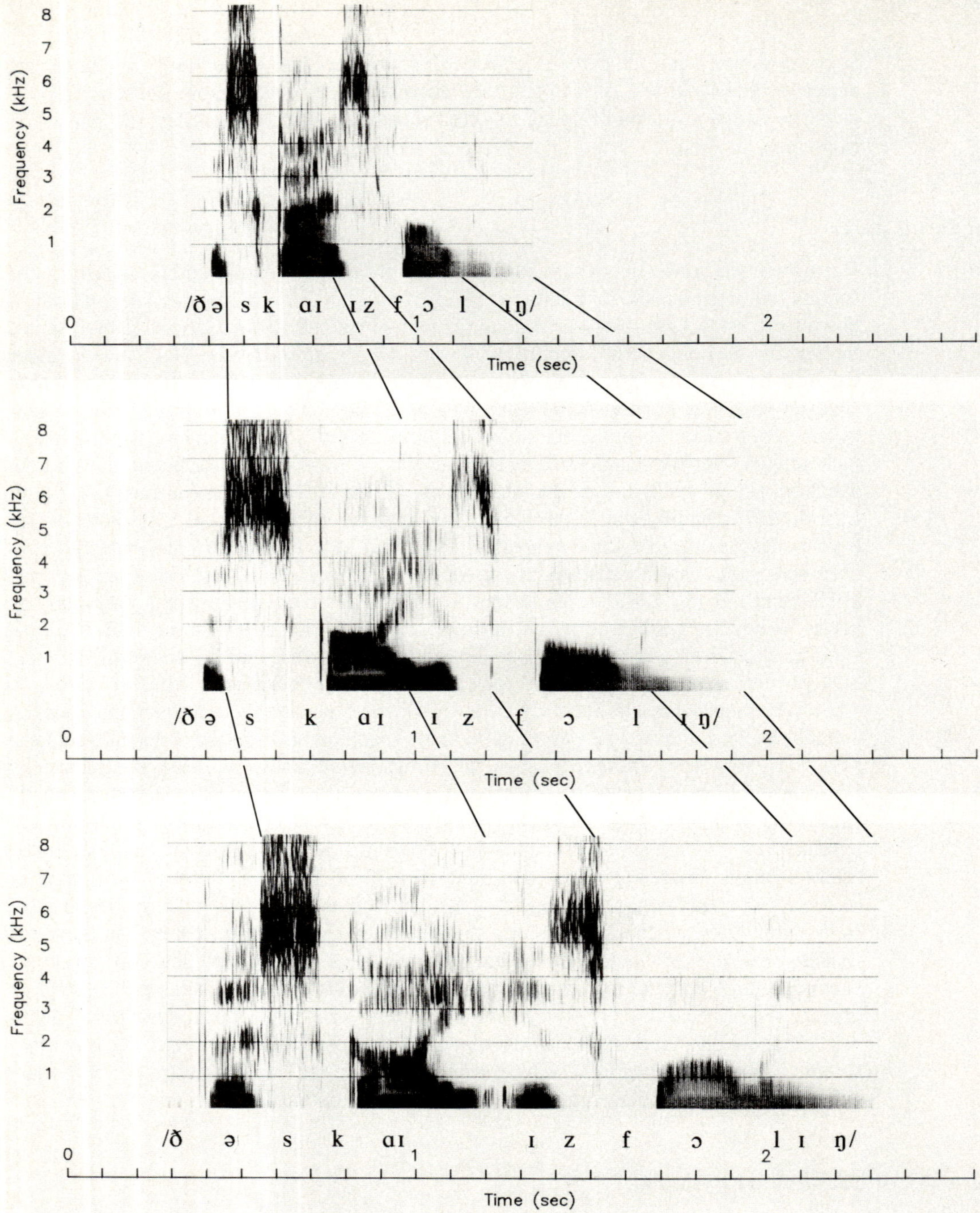

Figure 11–4

Spectrograms of a child saying 'The sky is falling' at very fast (top panel), normal (middle panel), and very slow (bottom panel) speaking rates. The speaking rates are 5.6 syllables per second for the very fast, 3.4 syllables per second for the normal, and 2.6 syllables per second for the very slow productions.

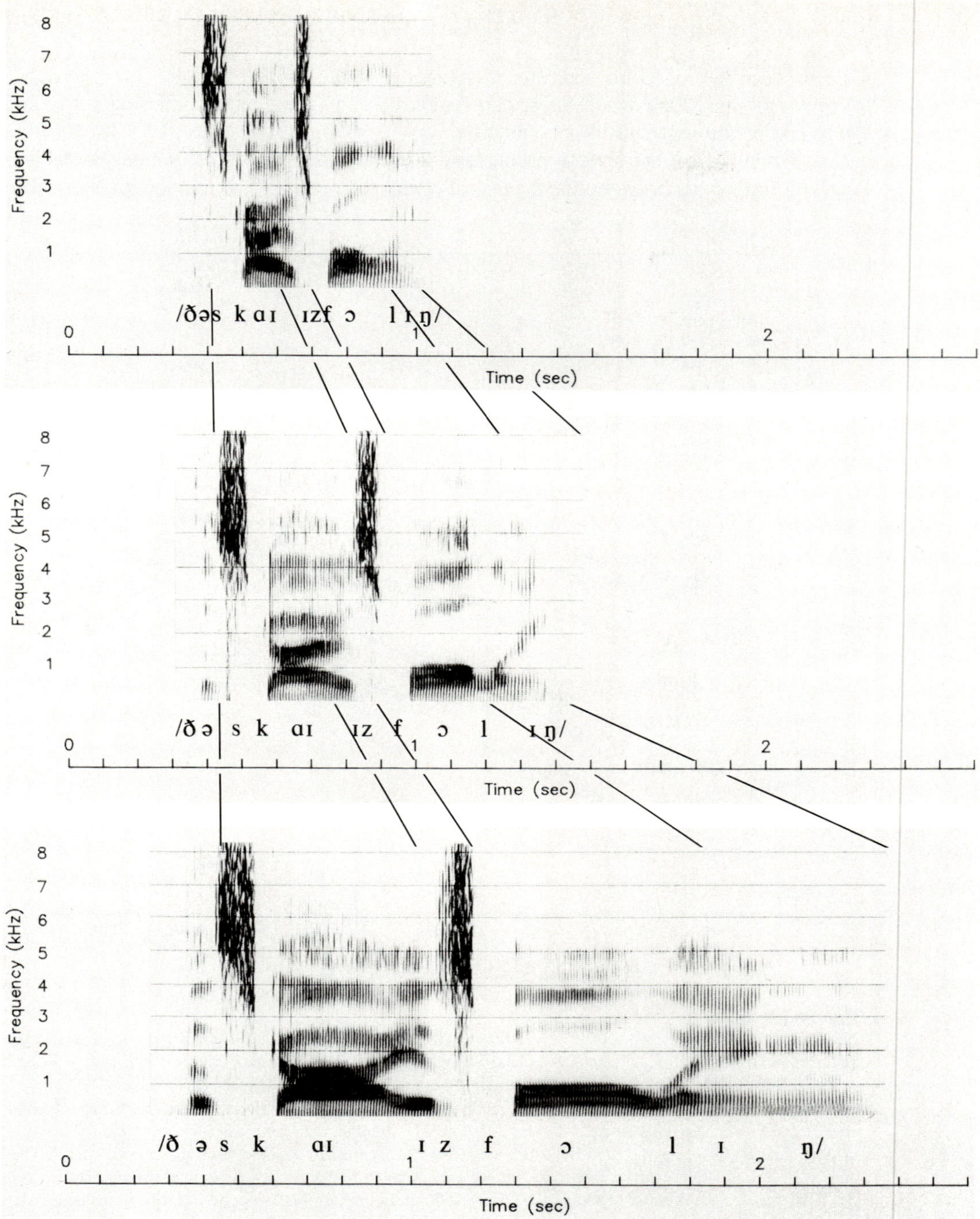

Figure 11–5
Spectrograms of an adult male saying 'The sky is falling' at very fast (top panel), normal (middle panel), and very slow (bottom panel) speaking rates. The speaking rates are 8.4 syllables per second for the very fast, 4.8 syllables per second for the normal, and 2.6 syllables per second for the very slow productions.

symbol can be used to indicate a sound omission. For example, [s>əprɑɪz], /s0prɑɪz/, and /00prɑɪz/ transcriptions indicate shortening of /s/, omission of /ə/, and omission of the first syllable of 'surprise.'

When the rate of speech production is reduced below normal, sounds, syllables, and the transitions between them generally become very long. It may be impractical to

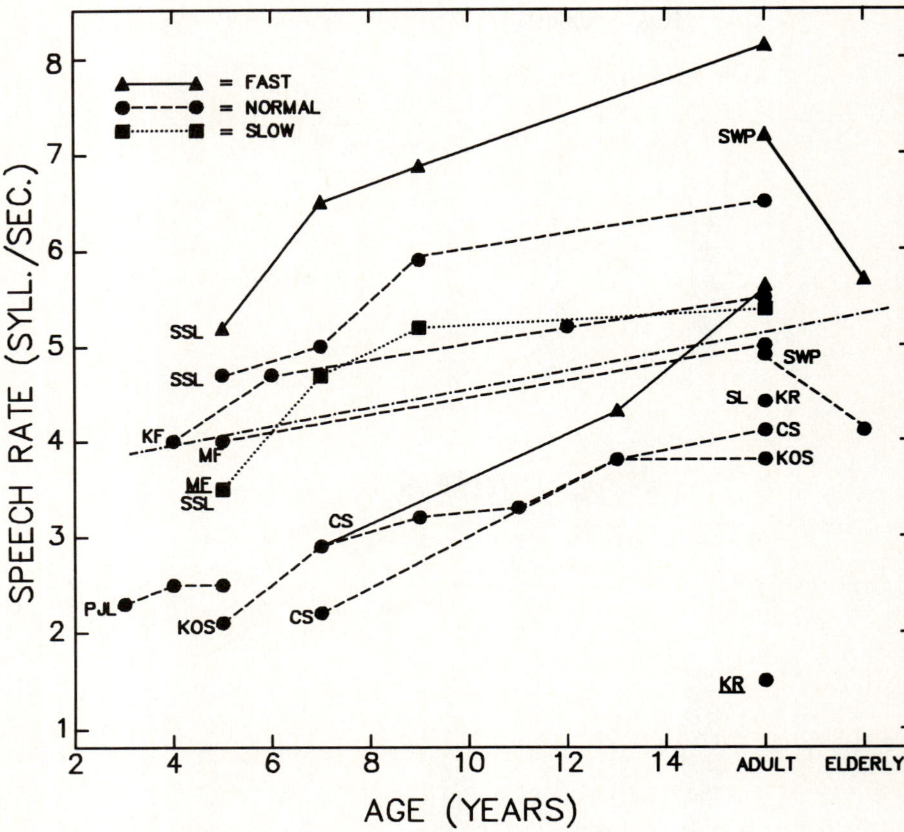

Figure 11–6
Speech rate (in syllables per second) for different age groups derived from the following studies of children and adults: CS = Chermak & Schneiderman (1986); KF = Kent & Forner (1980); KR = Kent & Rosenbek (1982); KOS = Kowal, O'Connell, & Sabin (1975); MF = Meyers & Freeman (1985); PJL = Pindzola, Jenkins, & Lokken (1989); SL = Sharf & Lehman (1984); SSL = Smith, Sugarman, & Long (1983); SWP = Smith, Wasowicz, & Preston (1987). *MF* denotes data from the Meyers & Freeman study for child stutterers, and *KR* indicates data from the Kent & Rosenbek study for apraxic adults. The lines connecting data points for individual studies are intended to reflect developmental trends. The dot-dash line separates most of the studies that used reading or sentence repetition tasks from those that used spontaneous or extemporaneous speech tasks (KOS, MF, PJL, & SL). Most studies required only normal or conversational speech rates, but a few also required fast and/or slow speech rates (CS, SSL, & SWP).

Table 11–2
Values, models, and approximate speaking rates[a] in syllables per second for judging tempo of reading/sentence repetition and spontaneous/extemporaneous speaking. See also Figure 11–6.

Tempo	Model	Syllables/Second
Exceptionally slow reading	Severe apractic	1.0–1.9
Slow spontaneous speech	Preschool child	2.0–2.9
Average spontaneous speech	Adult	3.0–3.9
Fast spontaneous/Slow reading	Adult/5-year-old child	4.0–4.9
Average reading	9-year-old child	5.0–5.9
Fast reading	Adult	6.0–6.9
Exceptionally fast reading	Parkinsonian dysarthric	7.0–

[a]Rates are approximations based on data from studies by Chermak & Schneiderman (1986), Kent & Forner (1980), Kent & Rosenbek (1982), Kowal, O'Connell, & Sabin (1975), Meyers & Freeman (1985), Pindzola, Jenkins, & Lokken (1989), Sharf & Lehman (1984), Smith, Sugarman, & Long (1983), and Smith, Wasowicz, & Preston (1987).

note prolongation of each sound with very slow speech, since all sounds are affected. In such a case it may be sufficient to note the abnormally slow rate and make the general observation that sounds and syllables are prolonged.

Pause Duration and Location

A natural consequence of changes in speaking rate is the change in the duration of pauses, lengthening with decreased rate and shortening with increased rate. Two different transitions between units of speech are examined below: (1) the transition between syllables in the same word or between adjacent words and (2) the transition between syllables that mark the boundaries between intonation contours.

Intersyllabic Transitions: Internal Juncture

The transition between syllables within a word or between adjacent words is referred to as **internal juncture**. Normally this type of transition does not involve a pause, but it does involve the marking of boundaries so that distinctions can be made between minimal pairs. Table 11–3 shows that 'night rate' and 'nitrate' can be described with the same sequence of phonemes, /nɑɪtret/. But these utterances can be differentiated for a number of reasons, including the following: (1) the first /t/ is unaspirated in 'night rate' and aspirated in 'nitrate,' (2) the /r/ is voiced in 'night rate' and devoiced in 'nitrate,' and (3) the intensity of the voice decreases with the first /t/ in 'night rate' and increases with the first /t/ in 'nitrate.' These differences are shown in the spectrograms in figures 11–7 and 11–8. The transition between syllables is referred to as **close internal juncture** in 'nitrate' /nɑɪtret/ and as **open internal juncture** in 'night rate' [nɑɪt+ret]. The phonemic distinction between these two utterances is indicated by the [+] symbol

Table 11–3
Examples of internal juncture contrasts produced by shifts between close and open juncture and shifts in open juncture position ([+] indicates juncture boundary).

Pattern A	Pattern B
Shifts between Close and Open Juncture	
nitrate /naɪtret/	night rate [naɪt+ret]
syntax /sɪntæks/	sin tax [sɪn+tæks]
a name /ənem/	an aim [ən+em]
Shifts in Open Juncture Position	
that's tough [ðæts+tʌf]	that stuff [ðæt+stʌf]
seem able [sim+ebəl]	see Mabel [si+mebəl]
its praise [ɪts+prez]	it sprays [ɪt+sprez]
grade A [gred+e]	gray day [gre+de]
keeps ticking [kips+tɪkɪŋ]	keep sticking [kip+stɪkɪŋ]

where the open internal juncture occurs; this symbol differs in position from the superscript plus sign used to indicate tongue advancement (see Figure B–1).

Included in Table 11–3 are examples of minimal pairs that are distinguished by the location of the open internal juncture. For example, the phoneme sequence /naɪtret/ can be pronounced as 'nitrate' /naɪtret/ or as 'night rate' [naɪt+ret], and the phoneme sequence /ɪtsprez/ can be pronounced as 'it sprays' [ɪt+sprez] or 'its praise' [ɪts+prez]. The location of the boundary in these utterances is determined by phonetic differences in the sounds that mark the boundary, including (1) postvocalic /t/, which is unaspirated in 'night rate' and 'it sprays' and aspirated in 'nitrate' or released with frication in 'its praise,' (2) /p/, which is unaspirated in 'it sprays' or released with frication in 'its praise,' and (3) /s/, which is longer in 'its praise' than in 'it sprays.' These differences are shown in the spectrograms in figures 11–7 and 11–8.

During normal speech production, the intervals between syllables within words and between words are very brief or nonexistent. Open internal juncture intervals are usually brief even at syllable boundaries, but apractic speakers tend to produce relatively long silent intervals between syllables, a practice which has been labeled **syllable segregation** (Kent & Rosenbek, 1982). Such speakers have very low speaking rates, between 1.0 and 3.0 syllables per second. Their intersyllabic intervals are two to six times longer than normal. The [++] symbol can be used for extended intervals due to syllable segregation, and the [+] symbol can be used for those due to open internal juncture.

Since syllable segregation may be pervasive, it may be redundant to indicate each instance of intersyllabic interval prolongation. If that is the case, note the abnormally slow rate of speaking and the general pattern of syllable segregation on the transcriptions of speakers with this problem.

Intercontour Transitions: Terminal or External Juncture

The basic units of intonation, variously called intonation contours, pitch contours, tone-units, or tone groups, are generally separated by pauses, or **terminal or external**

juncture. For example, in the sequence of sentences, 'He came home. I saw him,' a pause occurs between the intonation contours represented by the two sentences. Also, in the sentence, 'When the rains came, the people moved,' a pause occurs between the intonation contours represented by the two clauses. The use of pauses to mark the boundaries between intonation contours can be noted by using the juncture symbols shown in Table 11–3.

In some systems for transcribing intonation, a distinction is made between the duration of pauses marking juncture with the general expectation that they are longer between two sentences than they are between two clauses. Such distinctions are

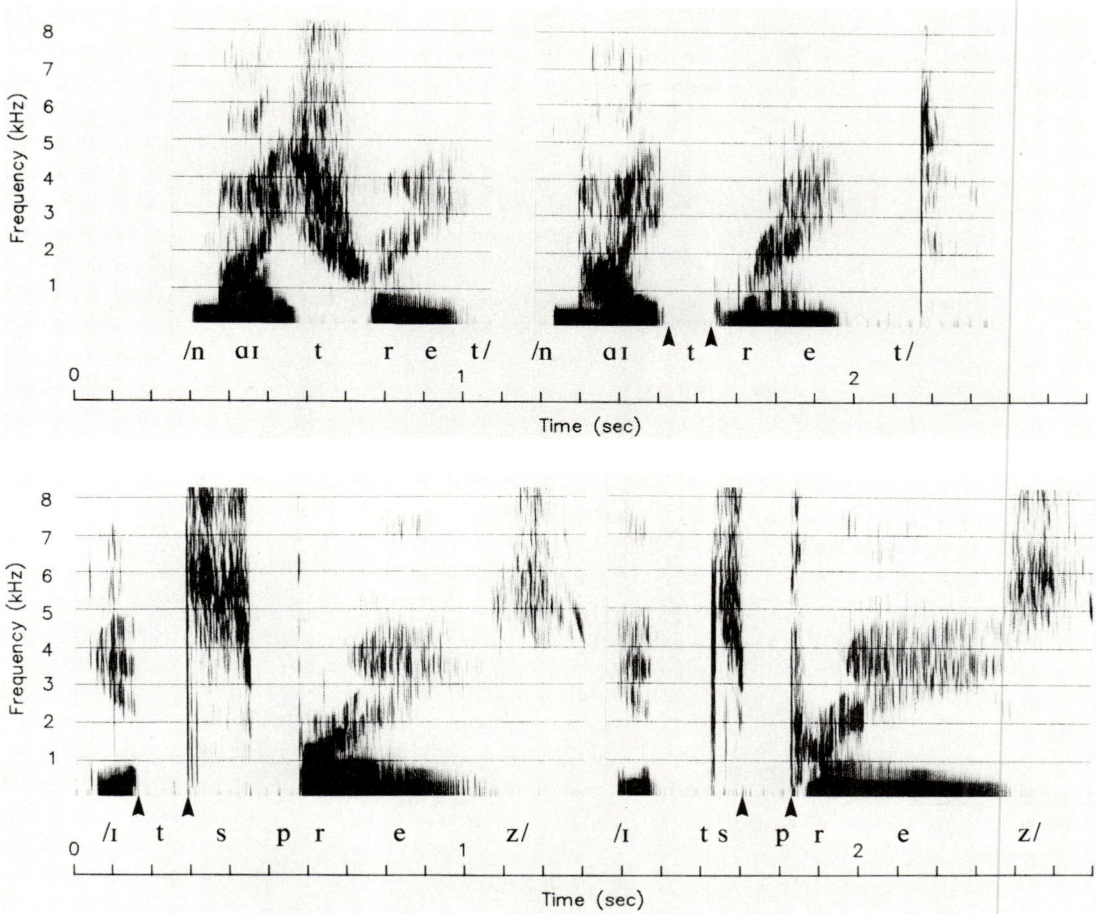

Figure 11–7
Spectrograms of a child's productions of 'nitrate' (close juncture) and 'night rate' (open juncture) in the upper panel and of 'it sprays' (open juncture) and 'its praise' (open juncture) in the lower panel. Arrows along the x axis indicate the approximate location of the open juncture. Note the frication energy that occurs in 'nitrate' at about the same location where the stop gap marks the open juncture in 'night rate.'

probably best differentiated by the intonation contours themselves, which fall for sentences and are level or rising for dependent clauses.

There does appear to be some need for noting variation in juncture in the utterances made by children during the process of bringing independent lexical items into syntactic or semantic relationship (Crystal, 1982). At an early stage of development, marked by one-word utterances, a sequence like 'Daddy#eat#' might appear in which the two words formed separate intonation contours. At a later stage, marked by the use of two-word utterances, the same sequence of phonemes might occur as one intonation contour, 'Daddy+eat#.' Unfortunately, children may use different length pauses be-

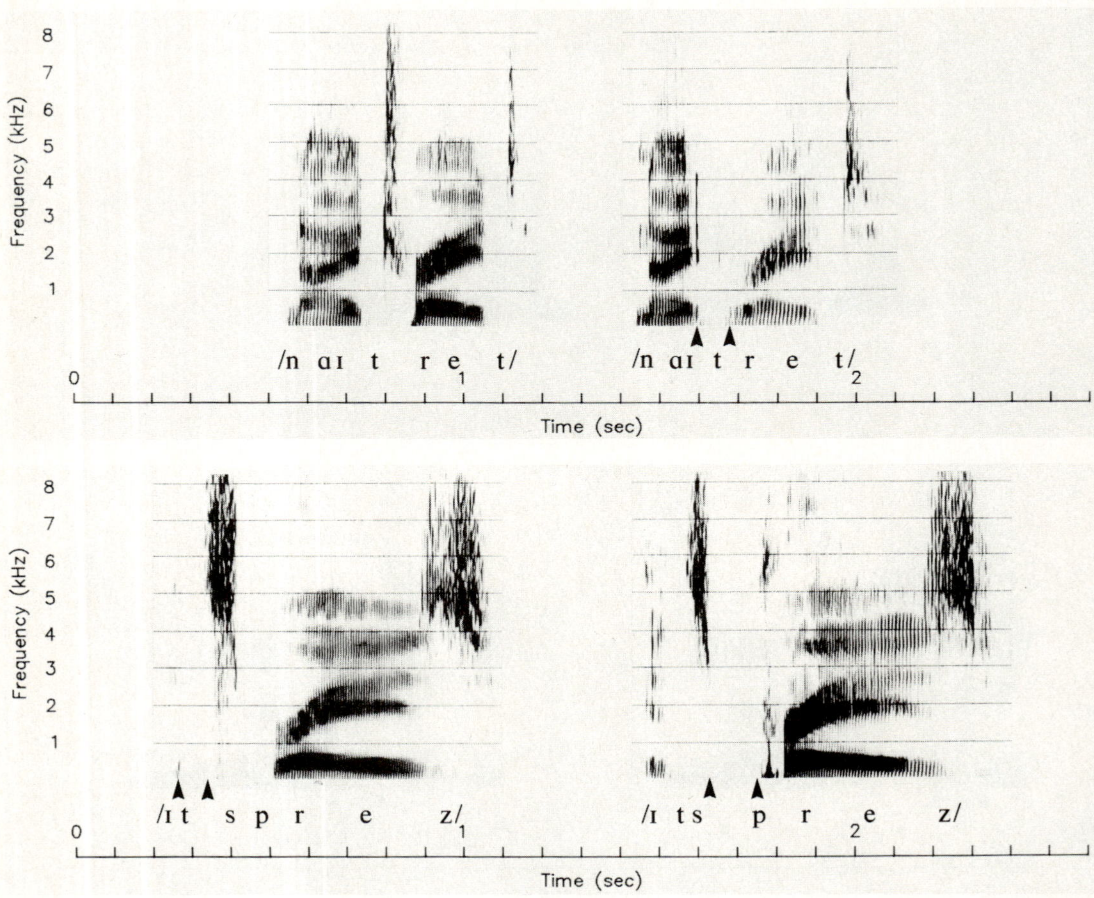

Figure 11–8
Spectrograms of an adult male's productions of 'nitrate' (close juncture) and 'night rate' (open juncture) in the upper panel and of 'it sprays' (open juncture) and 'its praise' (open juncture) in the lower panel. Arrows along the *x* axis indicate the approximate location of the open juncture. Note that the frication energy for /s/ in 'it sprays' is longer than it is in 'its praise.'

tween words so that it is difficult to decide if one or two sentences was intended. This may be particularly troublesome if the two words are nouns, like 'Daddy car,' rather than a noun and a verb like 'Daddy eat.'

STRESS

Stress is the relative prominence or emphasis placed on syllables in words or in larger units of speech like phrases and sentences. For example, the noun 'content' is usually pronounced with greater stress on the first than on the second syllable, while the adjective 'content' is usually given greater stress on the second syllable. Although there is general agreement about the stress pattern of words, there is disagreement about the basis for this differentiation. One can expect stressed syllables to have higher fundamental frequency, longer duration, and greater intensity than unstressed syllables, but there are exceptions to such generalizations (Lehiste, 1970; Ladefoged, 1975).

Within a phrase or sentence, the location of the greatest stress depends on the meaning intended. The adjective 'content' usually receives greatest stress in the sentence 'I am content,' but not in the sentence 'I am not content,' in which the greatest stress is on 'not.'

Figures 11–9 and 11–10 are spectrograms of productions by a child and an adult of the noun and verb forms of 'impact' with primary stress on the first and second syllables, respectively. The spectrograms indicate the duration, intensity, and fundamental frequency of the vowels in each syllable. Values for these parameters in the stressed syllable should exceed those in the unstressed syllable of 'impact.' As you can see in figures 11–9 and 11–10, this is not always the case. The evidence contradicts the expectation that duration is longer, intensity greater, and fundamental frequency higher in the stressed syllable than in the unstressed syllable, as follows: (1) 'im' is not longer than 'pact' in the child's or the adult's noun productions; (2) 'im' is not greater in intensity than 'pact' in the adult's noun production; (3) 'pact' is not higher in fundamental frequency than 'im' in the child's verb production. Despite such contradictory acoustic evidence, listeners would have no difficulty in differentiating the stress patterns of 'impact.' Since low vowels like /æ/ in the second syllable of 'impact' are innately longer, more intense, and lower in fundamental frequency than high vowels like /ɪ/ in the first syllable of 'impact,' listeners must in some way allow for these distinctions by making relative rather than absolute judgments of parameter differences for stress perception (Cruttenden, 1986). As indicated in figures 11–9 and 11–10, the following acoustic characteristics may differentiate the noun and verb forms of 'impact': (1) the first syllable is longer for the noun than it is for the verb; (2) the intensity of the first syllable is greater for the noun than for the verb; (3) the fundamental frequency decreases between the first and second syllables of the noun and increases between the first and second syllables of the verb for the adult.

In addition to the lack of unequivocal acoustic evidence to support stress differentiation, there is disagreement among phoneticians as to the number of different levels of stress and where the stress marks should be placed. Some describe only two

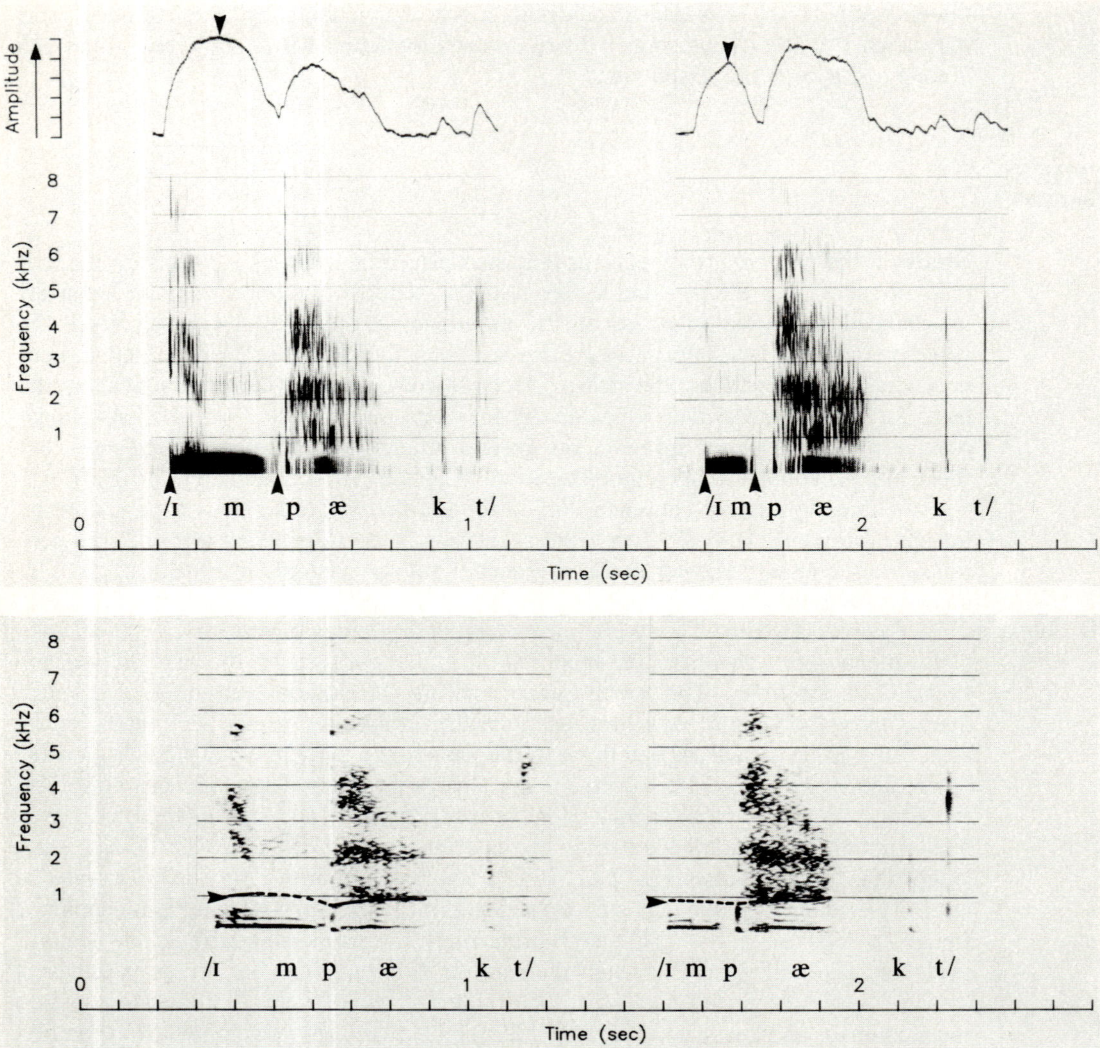

Figure 11–9
Spectrograms showing syllable duration, intensity, and fundamental frequency (f_0) of noun and verb forms of 'impact' produced by a child. These productions illustrate duration and intensity relationships between, from left to right, the noun 'impact' and the verb 'impact' (top panel), and f_0 relationships between, from left to right, the noun 'impact' and the verb 'impact' (bottom panel). In the top panel, arrows along the x axis of the wide band spectrogram indicate the duration of the first syllable in the noun (279 msec) and the verb (128 msec), and arrows along the abscissa of the amplitude display indicate the peak amplitude of the first syllable. In the bottom panel, tracings of the fifth harmonic from narrow band analyses indicate that f_0 (as reflected by tracings of the fifth harmonic) decreases from the first to second syllable of the noun and increases from the first to second syllable of the verb. The arrow along the y axis indicates the onset of the fifth harmonic.

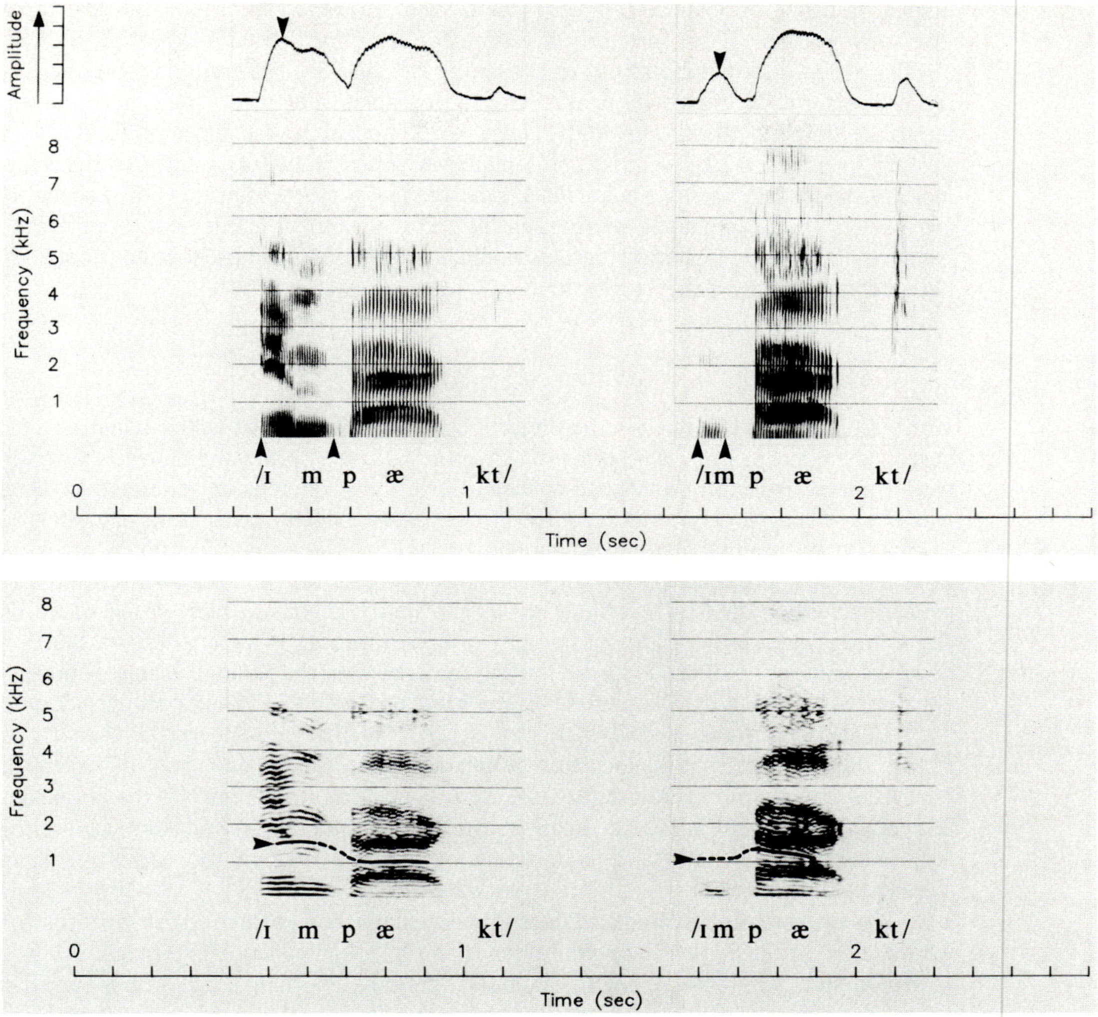

Figure 11–10
Spectrograms showing syllable duration, intensity, and fundamental frequency (f_0) of noun and verb forms of 'impact' produced by an adult male. These productions illustrate duration and intensity relationships between, from left to right, the noun 'impact' and the verb 'impact' (top panel), and f_0 relationships between, from left to right, the noun 'impact' and the verb 'impact' (bottom panel). In the top panel, arrows along the *x* axis of the wide band spectrogram indicate the duration of the first syllable in the noun (176 msec) and the verb (72 msec), and arrows along the abscissa of the amplitude display indicate the peak amplitude of the first syllable. In the bottom panel, tracings of the tenth harmonic from narrow band analyses indicate that f_0 (as reflected by tracings of the tenth harmonic) decreases from the first to second syllable of the noun and increases from the first to second syllable of the verb. An arrow along the *y* axis indicates the onset of the tenth harmonic.

levels, presence or absence of stress (Ladefoged, 1975), while others describe three levels (Bronstein, 1960; Shriberg & Kent, 1982) or four levels (Tiffany & Carrell, 1977). Some prefer placing stress marks before the syllable, while others prefer placing them directly over the vowel in the stressed syllables. For most practical purposes, including those of clinical phonetics, three levels appear to be sufficient. IPA uses a system in which a high-set mark [ˈ] indicates primary stress, a low-set mark [ˌ] indicates secondary stress, and no mark indicates tertiary or weak stress. Stress marks are placed at the beginning of the syllable. This system is somewhat troublesome because of the need to identify syllable boundaries, but it should present no problem in determining which syllable is affected.

Word Stress

Word stress serves two functions in English. One is to differentiate certain minimal pairs, such as the noun 'protest,' with primary stress on the first syllable, and the verb 'protest,' with primary stress on the second syllable. Since the phonemes or segments for both words are identical, /protɛst/, but the stress patterns differ, stress is usually referred to as a suprasegmental feature or phoneme of speech. The second function of stress is to provide an appropriate pattern of pronunciation for all words of English. Putting the primary stress on the first syllable of words like 'heavy,' on the second syllable of words like 'tomato,' and on the third syllable of words like 'education' is a necessary function of the pronunciation of such words. Putting the stress on the wrong syllable or putting equal stress on each syllable results in abnormal or foreign-sounding pronunciation.

In learning which syllables to stress, children may depend on at least three factors: (1) differences in the acoustic properties of stressed and unstressed syllables; (2) syntactic and grammatical differences associated with stress; and (3) the phonological classification of syllables according to their weight (strength) as heavy (strong) or light (weak). The limitations of using acoustic properties as cues to word stress have already been discussed.

Grammatical and syntactic differentiation establishes certain stress patterns for words. For example, the compound noun 'hotdog,' meaning frankfurter, has primary stress on 'hot,' whereas the adjectival phrase 'hot dog,' meaning a dog who is hot, has primary stress on 'dog,' or perhaps equal stress on 'hot' and 'dog.' Also, primary stress shifts systematically from the first to the second to the third syllable on grammatically related words like 'diplomat,' 'diplomacy,' 'diplomatic,' and 'telegraph,' 'telegraphy,' 'telegraphic.'

It has been proposed that a major phonological factor influencing stress placement is the weight (strength) of a syllable (Chomsky & Halle, 1968; Hyman, 1975; Sloat, Taylor, & Hoard, 1978). **Heavy (strong) syllables** are those which (1) include long (tense) vowels or diphthongs, as in the first syllable of 'tuba,' 'broken,' and 'baby,' or in the second syllable of 'away,' 'believe,' and 'suppose,' or (2) include short (lax) vowels terminated by a consonant, as in the first syllable of 'bunny,' 'penny,' and 'zipper,' or the second syllable of 'elect,' 'attack,' and 'arrest.' **Light (weak) syllables** are those which include short (lax) vowels not terminated by a consonant, as in the first syllable of 'away,' 'believe,' and 'suppose,' or in the second syllable of 'tuba,' 'broken,' and 'baby.' Heavy (strong) syllables receive primary stress.

Unlike some other languages, English words are not predictably stressed on a particular syllable. Therefore, it is not possible to provide a set of rules that leads automatically to the correct assignment of stress for even the most commonly used words. There have been a number of attempts to generate such rules—but with the acknowledgment that a large number of exceptions exist (Cruttenden, 1986; Hogg & McCully, 1987). The approach taken here is to show the various patterns of stress in English for the most common words.

Two-Syllable Word Stress Patterns

Table 11–4 presents comparisons of stress patterns for two-syllable words and compound nouns. The first comparison is between the [ˌ= ˈ=] and [ˈ= ˌ=] stress patterns (the equal sign represents a syllable), as exemplified by the pronunciations of 'white house,' and 'White House.' As indicated in Table 11–4, 'white house' refers to any house that is white; 'White House' refers to the home of the President. There are a number

Table 11–4
Examples of contrasts in common stress patterns for two-syllable words, compound nouns, and noun phrases ([ˈ] indicates primary stress; [ˌ] indicates secondary stress; [=] indicates a syllable).

Pattern A	Pattern B
[ˈ=ˌ=][a]	[ˌ=ˈ=]
White House (President's house)	white house (any white house)
redhot (a frankfurter)	red hot (extremely warm)
greenhouse (a house for plants)	green house (any green house)
blackbird (a bird species)	black bird (any black bird) Other words: untie, misspell, northwest, uphold
[ˈ=ˌ=][a]	[ˈ==][b]
mailman, snowman, he-man, ragman, con man, fat man, sandman	fireman, human, woman, horseman, gunman, foreman, simple, table, basket, capture
[ˈ=ˌ=][a]	[=ˈ=][c]
Nouns: recess, content, reject, suspect, produce, subject	Verbs: recess, content, reject, suspect, produce, subject, invest Other words: until, mistake, upon, abrupt, campaign, severe, police

[a]This pattern also occurs commonly in spondee words like 'greyhound,' 'railroad,' 'baseball,' 'hothouse,' 'horseshoe,' and 'pathway.'
[b]This pattern also occurs commonly in words where the accented syllable precedes unstressed suffixes like '-ing,' '-er,' '-est,' '-y,' and '-ly,' as in 'baking,' 'faster,' 'fastest,' 'windy,' and 'poorly.'
[c]This pattern also occurs commonly in words where the accented syllable follows unstressed prefixes like 'a-,' 'be-,' 're-,' 'de-,' 'ad-,' 'ex-,' and 'pre-,' as in 'around,' 'believe,' 'report,' 'detain,' 'admire,' 'explain,' and 'pretend.'

of contrasts of this nature in which the noun phrase carries a specific meaning and the compound noun carries a more general meaning, such as the following: 'redhot,' meaning a frankfurter and 'red hot,' meaning extremely warm. Other examples of compound nouns and noun phrase contrasts are presented in Table 11–4. In each pair, the phonemes are the same, but the stress patterns are different. There are some words other than noun phrases that tend to have the [ˌ = ˈ =] stress pattern. This pattern may occur in words that include bound prefixes, as in 'untie' and 'misspell' or in compound words, as in 'uphold' and 'northwest.'

It should be noted that spondee words used in hearing tests are described as being pronounced with primary stress on both syllables. These compound words are made up of free morphemes like those in 'greyhound,' 'hothouse,' 'horseshoe,' and 'pathway.' Such words are likely to be pronounced normally with a [ˈ = ˌ =] pattern.

The second comparison in Table 11–4 is between the [ˈ = ˌ =] and [ˈ = =] stress patterns, as exemplified by the pronunciations of 'mailman' and 'fireman.' Both words have primary stress on the first syllable. The second syllable of 'mailman,' however, has relatively greater stress than the second syllable of 'fireman.' One consequence of this difference in stress is that 'man' is pronounced /mæn/ in 'mailman' and /mən/ in 'fireman.' A frequent occurrence among vowels when the syllables they are in become relatively unstressed is a loss of quality and transformation into the schwa vowel /ə/. You can observe this difference in stress and vowel quality in other pairs like 'con man' and 'gunman' and all the other comparisons involving the '-man' suffix presented in Table 11–4. Of course, the [ˈ = =] stress pattern is not restricted to words ending in '-man.' It also fits words like 'simple,' 'table,' 'basket,' and 'mother,' as well as words ending in '-ing,' '-er,' '-y,' and '-ly' suffixes like 'baking,' 'faster,' 'windy,' and 'poorly.'

The third comparison in Table 11–4 is between the [ˈ = ˌ =] and [= ˈ =] stress patterns, as exemplified by the pronunciations of 'recess,' the noun, and 'recess,' the verb. It is clear that primary stress falls on the first syllable of the noun and on the second syllable of the verb. The first syllable of the verb 'recess' is relatively weak, as you can tell by comparing its vowel with that in the first syllable of the noun. In the noun the /i/ quality is maintained, but in the verb the vowel tends to be pronounced like the schwa vowel /ə/. The same stress pattern and relative change in vowel quality occurs in pairs like the noun and verb 'content,' where the first syllable in the noun retains the /ɑ/ vowel quality but changes to /ə/ in the verb. Some noun-verb pairs do not alternate stress but use the [= ˈ =] stress pattern for both noun and verb forms, as in 'campaign' and 'mistake.'

Three-Syllable Word Stress Patterns

Table 11–5 presents comparisons of common stress patterns for three-syllable words. The first comparison is between the [ˈ = = ˌ =] and [ˌ = = ˈ =] stress patterns, as exemplified by the pronunciation of the nouns 'overcharge' and 'interchange,' with primary stress on the first syllable, and the pronunciation of the verbs 'overcharge' and 'interchange,' with primary stress on the last syllable. Many other words fit these patterns, such as 'valentine,' with primary stress on the first syllable, and 'entertain,' with primary stress on the third syllable. In addition, there are verbs like 'separate' and 'estimate' which fit the [ˈ = = ˌ =] pattern and contrast with the adjective 'separate' and the noun

Table 11–5
Examples of contrasts between common stress patterns in three-syllable words (n, noun; v, verb; adj, adjective; [ˈ], primary stress; [ˌ], secondary stress; [=], syllable).

Pattern A	Pattern B
[ˈ==ˌ=]	[ˌ==ˈ=]
overcharge (n), interchange (n), valentine, candy stand, separate (v), estimate (v)	overcharge (v), interchange (v), entertain, understand, cigarette[a]
[ˈ===][b]	[ˈ=ˌ==]
separate (adj) estimate (n), rubbery, motherly, following, elephant	blueberry, library, primary, long-standing, kidnapper
[ˌ=ˈ==]	[=ˈ==][c]
substandard, old-fashioned, northwestern, archbishop	substantial, compassion, employer, allowing, assistant, aroma, museum, republic

[a]This word is also commonly pronounced with a [ˈ==ˌ=] stress pattern.
[b]This pattern occurs commonly in words with two-syllable stems that are stressed on the first syllable, attached to unstressed suffixes, such as '-ing,' '-er,' '-est,' '-y,' and '-ly,' as in 'following,' 'caterer,' 'cleverest,' 'rubbery,' and 'elderly.'
[c]This pattern occurs commonly in words with stems that are stressed on the final syllable, attached to unstressed suffixes, such as '-ing,' '-er,' '-est,' and '-ly,' as in 'enjoying,' 'employer,' 'severest,' and 'sedately.'

'estimate,' which fit the [ˈ===] pattern. The verbs maintain the /e/ vowel quality in the final syllable, but the vowel in the final syllable of the nouns shifts to the schwa vowel /ə/, in keeping with their reduction to weak stress.

The second comparison in Table 11–5 is between the [ˈ=ˌ==] pattern, as in 'blueberry,' and the [ˈ===] pattern, as in 'rubbery.' Like a number of other three-syllable words, 'blueberry' is a compound of two free morphemes, 'blue' and 'berry.' The primary stress on the first syllable of 'berry' is converted to a secondary stress when the compound is formed. On the other hand, 'rubbery' is formed by adding the bound morpheme '-y' to the free morpheme 'rubber.' Many two-syllable words that have a [ˈ==] stress pattern can add bound morphemes, for example, 'mother' plus '-ly,' and 'follow' plus '-ing,' to form words with [ˈ===] stress patterns.

The last comparison in Table 11–5 is between the [ˌ=ˈ==] pattern, as in 'substandard,' and the [=ˈ==] pattern, as in 'substantial.' These words are similar, but 'substandard' is a compound of the bound morpheme 'sub-' and the free morpheme 'standard,' while 'substantial' does not include a free morpheme. Other three-syllable compound words that fit the [ˌ=ˈ==] pattern are 'old-fashioned,' 'northwestern,' and 'archbishop.' Many words that fit the [=ˈ==] pattern are compounds formed by adding unstressed bound morphemes to words with [=ˈ=] stress patterns, like '-er' to 'employ,' '-ing' to 'allow,' and '-ant' to 'assist.'

Rhythmic and Recessive Word Stress

Table 11–6 presents comparisons between common word stress patterns that are basically rhythmic or recessive in nature. **Rhythmic** means that there is an alternation

Table 11–6
Examples of contrasts between rhythmic and recessive stress patterns in polysyllabic words (v, verb; adj, adjective; [ˈ], primary stress; [ˌ], secondary stress; [=], syllable).

Rhythmic	Recessive
[ˈ==ˌ==]	[ˈ====]
dormitory, secretary, inventory, dictionary, television	accuracy, permanently, preferable
[=ˈ==ˌ=][a]	[=ˈ===][b]
elaborate (v), associate (v), deliberate (v), appreciate, accumulate	elaborate (adj),[c] associate (adj),[c] deliberate (adj),[c] considerate, affectionate
[ˌ==ˈ==]	
constitution, revolution, invitation, manufacture	

[a]The '-ate' ending is pronounced with an /e/ vowel in the verb form.
[b]The '-ate' ending is pronounced with a schwa vowel /ə/ in the adjective form.
[c]These words are often pronounced with the third syllable omitted.

of stress on a sequence of syllables, as in the pronunciations of words like 'dormitory' [ˈ==ˌ==], 'constitution' [ˌ==ˈ==], and the verb 'elaborate' [=ˈ==ˌ=]. The **recessive** patterns are characterized by primary stress on the first or second syllable and weak stress on the remaining syllables, as in the [ˈ====] and [=ˈ===] patterns in Table 11–6. Words like 'dormitory' and 'accuracy' both have primary stress on the first syllable, but 'dormitory' has secondary stress on the third syllable and weak stress on the other syllables, while 'accuracy' has weak stress on all other syllables.

For some words, the contrast between the rhythmic [=ˈ==ˌ=] and recessive [=ˈ===] stress patterns is distinctive. Note that the verb 'elaborate' has the rhythmic pattern, while the adjective 'elaborate' has the recessive pattern. In addition, the /e/ vowel in the verb form changes to a schwa vowel /ə/ in the adjective form. There are many other words that fit these patterns which do not have this alternation, such as 'appreciate,' 'accumulate,' and 'homogenize' for the [=ˈ==ˌ=] pattern, and 'considerate,' 'affectionate,' and 'priority' for the [=ˈ===] pattern.

The final example of a rhythmic pattern is the [ˌ==ˈ==] one, exemplified by the pronunciation of words like 'constitution' and 'manufacture.' As in the [ˈ==ˌ==] pattern, stress alternates between the first and third syllables in 'constitution,' but primary stress falls on the third syllable instead of the first.

Stress in Intonation Contours

According to Crystal (1982), the stress in a sentence in adult language is on the last lexical item in 90% of cases. For example, in the sentence 'I am walking to the store,' greatest stress usually falls on 'store.' The sentence stress can be brought forward by changing the emphasis in the following ways: (1) Stress could be placed on 'walking' as a clarification for someone who thought that you were driving, (2) on 'am' as an emphatic rebuttal to someone who questioned whether you really were walking, and (3) on 'I' in order to contrast your intention with someone else's. In each case, the location of the tonic accent would be indicated by the primary change in the intonation that characterizes the sentence, an emphasis that is undoubtedly signaled by greater duration and loudness on the stressed word as well as a shift in pitch level.

Within intonation contours, or tone-units, certain words are usually stressed—nouns, main verbs, adjectives, and adverbs. Usually unstressed words include personal pronouns, auxiliary verbs, prepositions, conjunctions, and articles. In addition to being unstressed, these words often have reduced vowels, that is, vowels that have lost their original quality and are pronounced like schwa vowels. These changes are often referred to as vowel reduction or reduction of vowels. Of course, words that are usually unstressed may be stressed when the intended meaning requires it, as in the examples of shifting accent given above. In the final analysis, the tonic accent must be determined by where you perceive it to occur. The syllable that contains the tonic accent is marked by a primary stress symbol. All other syllables are marked as having secondary stress or no stress, depending on their word stress pattern. In the usual pronunciation of 'I am walking to the store,' primary stress occurs on 'store,' secondary stress on 'I' and the first syllable of 'walking,' and no stress on 'am,' the second syllable of 'walking,' 'to,' and 'the.'

RHYTHM

Rhythm is the pattern of stress location in speech and the duration of the intervals between stresses. In a sentence like 'I am walking to the store,' some syllables have primary or secondary stress and others have no stress. This is the usual stress pattern for English: Periodic stressed syllables alternate with one or more unstressed syllables. As noted previously, the vowels in the unstressed syllables often are reduced in quality to schwa vowels. Because of this pattern of stressing, phoneticians describe English as a **stressed-timed** language. Other languages, for example, French, are described as **syllable-timed** because each syllable is approximately equal in duration and vowels are not generally reduced.

The implication of the term *stressed-timed* is that speech rhythm involves the control of the location of stresses and the timing of the intervals between them. English is often described as having an isochronous rhythm pattern, that is, it is a language with approximately equal intervals between stressed syllables. For example, in the sentence, 'The elephant and man rule the jungle,' the interval that includes 'elephant and' is about equal in duration to the interval that includes 'rule the' even though they include four and two syllables, respectively. This means that 'elephant and' is spoken more rapidly than 'rule the,' so that the durations of each interval are close but not necessarily equal (Cruttenden, 1986). The alternate compression and expansion of syllables apparently give English its characteristic rhythm.

PROSODY DISORDERS

Tempo

Tempo disorders may involve speaking rates that are too slow or too fast (see Table 11–2). Excessively slow speech may be due to prolonged articulation or prolonged intersyllabic intervals. With prolonged articulation, syllables are lengthened, sometimes involving even unstressed vowels like the schwa /ə/ in 'the' and all consonants, even the VOT of voiced stops. In addition, the transitions between vowels and consonants may be prolonged. This type of tempo disorder is characteristic of some apractic speakers, as indicated by the spectrograms shown in Figure 11–11 (Kent & Rosenbek, 1982).

Excessively slow speaking rates may involve the prolongation of the usual pauses between syllables. In addition, they may involve the interjection of inappropriate pauses between syllables, as between the article 'the' and a following noun, or even between syllables in the same word. This pattern of slow speaking has been described as "syllable segregation" and is characteristic of some apractic speakers, as indicated by the syllable profiles in Figure 11–12 (Kent & Rosenbek, 1982).

With very fast speaking rates, consonant articulation cannot be fully achieved, so that the syllable boundaries usually formed by consonants are weak and indistinct. Since all syllables are shortened, there is very little or no distinction between the length of stressed and unstressed syllables. This pattern of syllable fusion is characteristic of speakers with parkinsonian dysarthria, as indicated in Figure 11–13 (Kent & Rosenbek, 1982).

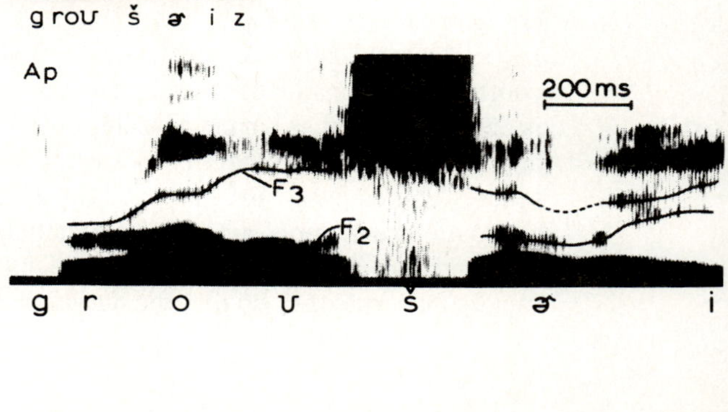

Figure 11–11
Spectrograms of 'groceries' produced in sentence context by a normal (N) and an apractic (Ap) speaker. The second and third formants (F_2 and F_3) are highlighted. Note the long segment durations and steplike formant shifts in the apractic pattern. This pattern of lengthened steady states and transitions is called *articulatory prolongation*.

Source: "Prosodic Disturbance and Neurologic Lesion," by R. D. Kent and J. C. Rosenbek, 1982, *Brain and Language, 15,* p. 265. Copyright 1982 by Academic Press, Inc. Reprinted with permission.

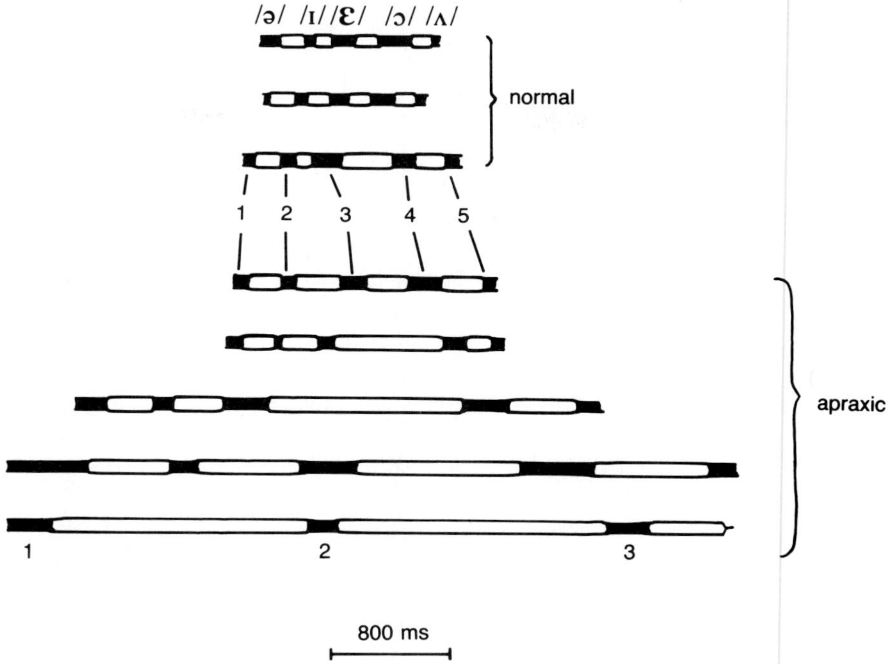

Figure 11–12
Profiles of syllable-nucleus time pattern for three normal speakers and five apractic speakers. The black portion in each pattern represents the durations of the voiced syllable nuclei associated with the vowels in the words 'The ship wreck washed up . . .' The appearance of widely spaced syllables in the apractic utterances is termed *syllabic segregation.*

Source: "Prosodic Disturbance and Neurologic Lesion," by R. D. Kent and J. C. Rosenbek, 1982, *Brain and Language, 15,* p. 267. Copyright 1982 by Academic Press, Inc. Reprinted with permission.

Figure 11–13
A wide band spectrogram of a speaker with parkinsonian dysarthria saying the words 'for something beyond his reach.' In this *fused* prosodic pattern, a seven-syllable utterance is attempted within an interval of 740 msec.

Source: "Prosodic Disturbance and Neurologic Lesion," by R. D. Kent and J. C. Rosenbek, 1982, *Brain and Language, 15,* p. 283. Copyright 1982 by Academic Press, Inc. Reprinted with permission.

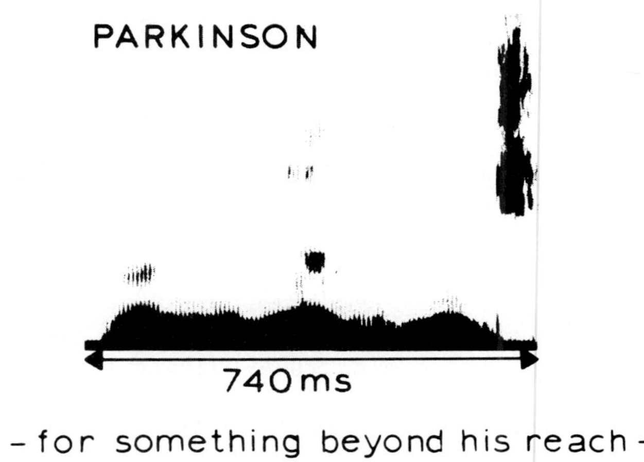

Intonation

There are two major types of intonation disorder, one which affects the number of intonation contours or tone-units used in the flow of speech, and the other which affects the degree of pitch fluctuation and continuity within them. The speech of some individuals is characterized by too few tone-units, while the speech of others is characterized by too many. The use of too few tone-units may occur in the rapid speech of some receptive aphasics or in the slow speech of individuals with mental retardation or expressive aphasia (Crystal, 1982). The first type is exemplified by the following example from the speech of a child: 'yes it was very hard to do very hard / but I did it anyway I did it / no sir I did not like to do it no way / ' Capital letters and punctuation marks were not used in the example so that you would not be biased to expect tone-unit boundaries. The [/] symbol is used by Crystal (1982) to mark boundaries determined from the intonation contours and pauses. In this example, the mean length of the tone-units is nine words, which is much greater than the mean of five words reported for adult language (Crystal, 1982). There should have been at least five additional boundaries, between 'yes' and 'it,' between 'do' and 'very,' between 'anyway' and 'I,' between 'sir' and 'I,' and between 'it' and 'no.' This speech pattern gives the impression of talking without paying attention to punctuation and the pitch fluctuations that accompany it.

The second type of intonation pattern, with too few tone-units but slow speech, is exemplified by the following example from the speech of a child: 'daddy + go + up + now + come + back + later / put + toys + away + be + quiet + go + sleep / '. Although the speech in the example above is broken up into one-word units by an excessive use of pauses, as indicated by plus signs in Crystal (1982), the intonation did not reflect more than two tone-units, one ending after 'later' and the other after 'sleep.' With this type of speech pattern, pitch is level almost throughout the entire utterance, and stress is about equal on every word. The mean length in words of the tone-units is seven. Assuming that the child is primarily using two-word phrases, the mean length should be about two.

Evidence suggests that spectrographic analysis may be needed to determine if a child is producing successive two-word utterances (car coming / house touch) rather than a series of separate single-word utterances (car / coming / house / touch). Contrary to most implications from the literature, it has been found that the successive single-word utterances of children between 1 1/2 and 2 years of age share some suprasegmental characteristics of multiple-word utterances—terminal juncture on the final words and shorter duration of the nonfinal one (Galligan, 1987).

Excessive use of tone-units may occur in the speech of language-delayed children, particularly when they are reading aloud (Crystal, 1982). In such cases, each word is pronounced as though it constitutes a separate tone-unit with falling or rising pitch, as in 'the / car / is / coming.' Overuse of tone-units may involve word groups in which the boundaries do and do not follow grammatical structure, patterns which might be observed in the speech of expressive aphasics, also referred to as Broca's or nonfluent aphasics (Crystal, 1982). The first type is exemplified by the following example: 'stale bread / is better / for toast /.' There are three boundaries rather than one, as would be expected, but they break up the sentence into grammatical units: noun phrase, verb phrase, and prepositional phrase. The second type is exemplified by the following example: 'stale bread is / better for / toast /.' In this case, the utterance is again broken up into three tone-units instead of one, but the boundaries occur at grammatically inappropriate intervals.

Intonation disorders may involve greater than normal or less than normal fluctuation of pitch within tone-units, as indicated in Figure 11–14. Shown in this figure are the intonation contours for a normal speaker and for speakers with dysarthria and apraxia (Kent & Rosenbek, 1982). Note that the intonation contours labeled "fused" and "dissociated" change very little in fundamental frequency as compared with the normal, but the contours labeled "segregated" and especially "sweeping" change considerably. Changes in the sweeping pattern, which are characteristic of speakers with ataxic dysarthria, within one syllable may be as great as or greater than the change across the entire contour for the normal speaker. Intrasyllabic changes for the segregated pattern, which is characteristic of speakers with ataxic dysarthria and apraxia, are also exaggerated, but the overall contour resembles the normal one.

The fused pattern, which is characteristic of speakers with parkinsonian and right-hemisphere dysarthria, shows almost no fundamental frequency change across syllables. Lack of fundamental frequency variation is evident in the dissociated pattern, which is characteristic of speakers with ataxic dysarthria and some with apraxia. In the dissociated pattern, however, there is no continuity in frequency from syllable to syllable, as there is in the fused pattern.

Stress and Rhythm

Two types of problems relate to the use of normal stress and rhythm: (1) incorrect location of the tonic accent in intonation contours, and (2) lack of differentiation between stressed and unstressed syllables. Incorrect location may be considered a problem of sentence stress, and lack of differentiation may be considered a problem of rhythm. Incorrect location of stress may vary in its nature, as in the following examples of shifting stress in the utterance 'I am going to play house': (1) The tonic accent may be moved forward from 'house' to 'play' when there is no contextual reason for doing so; (2) the tonic accent may remain on 'house' even when the question 'Who is playing?' should elicit a tonic accent on 'I,' and (3) the tonic accent may fall on 'to,' which is normally never stressed. These types of stress patterns appear in the speech of children with language disorders (Crystal, 1982).

Loss of differentiation between stressed and unstressed syllables is characteristic of individuals with ataxic dysarthria (Kent & Rosenbek, 1982). Not only are normal differences between the intensity and duration of contiguous syllables greatly reduced, but intersyllabic intervals are increased. This pattern alters the usual stress-timing of English speech.

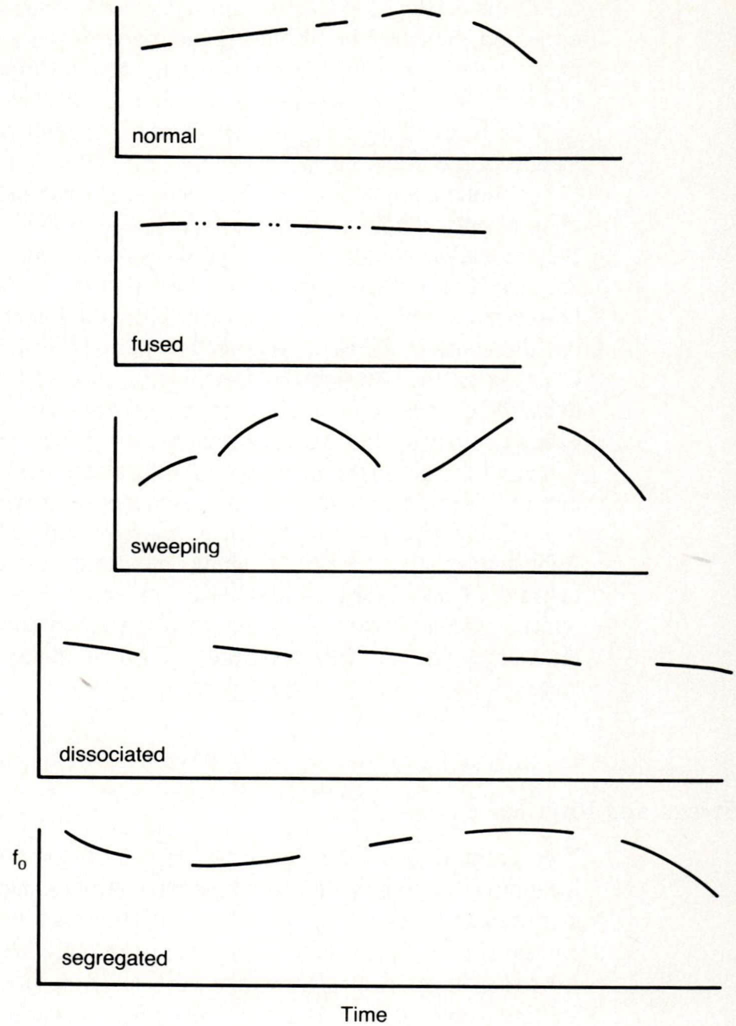

Figure 11–14
A schematic representation of the basic normal and disturbed prosodic patterns reviewed in this chapter. Each graph shows an intonation contour (f_0 as a function of time) for a five-syllable utterance. The properties of primary interest are the variations of f_0 within and across syllables and the duration of the voiced portion of individual syllables.

Source: "Prosodic Disturbance and Neurologic Lesion," by R. D. Kent and J. C. Rosenbek, 1982, *Brain and Language, 15,* p. 282. Copyright 1982 by Academic Press, Inc. Reprinted with permission.

Interaction between Prosodic and Phonetic Factors

There is increasing evidence to suggest that prosodic disorders may be influenced by articulation problems and that phonological problems may be influenced by prosodic problems (Klein, 1984). For example, it has been found (1) that a child who substituted /u/ for syllabic /l/ in the second syllable of words like 'table' and 'puzzle' tended incorrectly to put the greatest stress on the second syllable of such words, and (2) that a child who substituted a neutral vowel for /ɚ/ in the second syllable of words like 'paper,' 'corner,' 'hammer,' 'scissor,' and 'zipper' incorrectly put stress on the second syllable of such words that was equal to or greater than that placed on the first syllable.

It has also been found that the use of phonological processes is influenced by prosodic structure, phonotactic structure, and syllabification (Chiat, 1989). Stopping of /f, v, s, z/ occurred in a child from 4–7 to 4–10 years of age on fricatives: (1) between unstressed syllables, as on the /f/ of 'beautiful' and the second /s/ of 'exercise,' (2) in word-initial position, as in 'sun' and 'fat,' (3) between unstressed and stressed syllables, as on /s/ in 'decide' and on /f/ in 'before,' and (4) between stressed and unstressed syllables with a consonant plus fricative cluster that did not occur as a word-final cluster, as on /v/ after /n/ in 'anvil,' on /f/ after /m/ in 'comfort,' and on /f/ after /t/ in 'spiteful.' Stopping did not occur in word-final position, as in 'miss' and 'laugh,' or between stressed and unstressed syllables, as in 'person' and 'over.'

GLOSSARY

Close internal juncture. The articulatory transition between syllables within a word.

Falling contour. An intonation contour that involves a decrease in pitch from the tonic syllable. It is low falling if the decrease is from level 3, and high falling if the decrease is from level 4.

Fall-rise contour. An intonation contour that involves a decrease in pitch from level 3 to level 2 after onset and then an increase to level 3.

Heavy (strong) syllable. A syllable which (1) includes long (tense) vowels or diphthongs, as in the first syllable of 'tuba,' 'broken,' and 'baby' or in the second syllable of 'away,' 'believe,' and 'suppose'; or (2) includes short (lax) vowels terminated by a consonant, as in the first syllable of 'bunny,' 'penny,' and 'zipper,' or the second syllable of 'elect,' 'attack,' and 'arrest.'

Internal juncture. The articulatory transition between syllables within a word or between adjacent words.

Intonation. The systematic variation in the pitch of the voice that produces meaningful differences in units of speech comparable to phrases, clauses, and sentences.

Intonation contour. A unit of speech that includes a syllable or syllables with a tonic accent and an associated group of unaccented syllables across which meaningful patterns of pitch change occur.

Level contour. An intonation contour that involves no fall in pitch at the end.

Light (weak) syllable. A syllable which includes short (lax) vowels not terminated by a consonant, as in the first syllable of 'away,' 'believe,' and 'suppose,' or in the second syllable of 'tuba,' 'broken,' and 'baby.'

Open internal juncture. The articulatory transition between syllables across word boundaries.

Pitch. The perception of frequency; as related to intonation, it is the perception of the fundamental frequency—the frequency of vocal fold vibration.

Pitch contour. Intonation contour.

Recessive word stress. A stress pattern in which primary stress occurs on the first or second syllable in a word, and weak stress occurs on the other syllables.

Rhythm. The pattern of stress location in speech and the duration of the intervals between stresses.

Rhythmic word stress. A stress pattern in which alternate syllables in a word receive stress.

Rise-fall contour. An intonation contour that involves an increase in pitch to level 3 or 4 after onset and then a decrease to level 1.

Rising contour. An intonation contour that involves an increase in pitch from the tonic syllable. It is low rising if the increase is to level 3 and high rising if the increase is to level 4.

Segmental. Concerned with the sounds or phonemes of language; contrast with suprasegmental.

Stress. The relative prominence or emphasis with which syllables are produced in words or in larger units of speech.

Stress-timed. A pattern in which periodic stressed syllables alternate with one or more unstressed syllables that often include reduced vowels.

Suprasegmental. Concerned with the intonation, tempo, stress, juncture, and the rhythm of language; also called prosody.

Syllable segregation. The use of relatively long silent intervals between syllables.

Syllable-timed. A pattern in which each syllable receives approximately equal stress and vowels are not reduced in quality.

Tempo. The perception of the rate of speech production.

Terminal or external juncture. Pauses marking the termination of intonation contours; characterized by falling pitch (falling terminal juncture), rising pitch (rising terminal juncture), or level pitch (level terminal juncture).

Tone-unit. Intonation contour.

Tonic accent. The greatest emphasis placed on a syllable within an intonation contour.

Tonicity. The function of tonic accent placement.

REVIEW QUESTIONS

A. Indicate the likely implications of the following intonation patterns by matching them with the descriptive terms.

1. Low falling ________	a. matter-of-fact statement
2. Rising ________	b. emotional statement
3. Low level ________	c. enthusiastic incomplete statement
4. Fall-rise ________	d. cautionary statement
5. High fall ________	e. yes-or-no question

6. High level ________	f. bored incomplete statement
7. Rise-fall ________	g. definite statement
	h. wh- question

****

Key: 1. a; 2. e; 3. f; 4. d; 5. b; 6. c; 7. g

B. Indicate the usual stress pattern for the following by checking YES if you agree with the one presented or by checking the appropriate one if you do not.

	YES	a. ['==]	b. ['=,=]	c. [='=]	d. ['='=]
1. 'hap,py	________	________	________	________	________
2. 'base,ball	________	________	________	________	________
3. be'gin	________	________	________	________	________
4. ,sur'prise	________	________	________	________	________
5. 'flower	________	________	________	________	________
6. 'mailman	________	________	________	________	________
7. 'hu,man	________	________	________	________	________
8. ,ice'cold	________	________	________	________	________

****

Key: 1. a; 2. YES; 3. YES; 4. c; 5. YES; 6. b; 7. a; 8. YES

C. Indicate the usual stress pattern for the following by checking YES if you agree with the one presented or by checking the appropriate column if you do not.

	YES	a. ['===]	b. ['==,=]	c. [='==]
1. 'cere,al	________	________	________	________
2. 'cele,brate	________	________	________	________
3. ,valen'tine	________	________	________	________
4. po'liceman	________	________	________	________
5. 'different	________	________	________	________
6. 'e'lection	________	________	________	________
7. 'li,brary	________	________	________	________
8. 'sepa,rate (v)	________	________	________	________

****

Key: 1. a; 2. YES; 3. b; 4. YES; 5. YES; 6. c; 7. YES; 8. YES

LABORATORY ASSIGNMENT

Tape IV, Side A
IVA4: Suprasegmental Variations (Tape running time: 5:21; Elapsed time: 15:35–20:56)

The purpose of this section is to provide students with transcription practice on suprasegmental variations that occur in the speech of adults and children.

a. Stress Patterns in Two-Syllable Words

Listen to the words as they are pronounced by an adult and a child and indicate the stress for each syllable. In this section and subsequent ones, stop the tape if necessary, rewind, and listen again.

1. [= =]   2. [= =]   3. [= =]   4. [= =]   5. [= =]   6. [= =]

7. [= =]   8. [= =]   9. [= =]   10. [= =]

****

Consensus: 1. [ˈ=ˌ=] 2. [ˌ=ˈ=] 3. [ˈ=ˌ=] 4. [ˌ=ˈ=] 5. [ˈ=ˌ =]
6. [ˌ=ˈ=] 7. [ˌ=ˈ=] 8. [ˌ=ˈ=] 9. [ˈ=ˌ=] 10. [ˈ=ˌ=]

Variants: None.

b. Stress Patterns in Polysyllabic Words

Listen to the words as they are pronounced by an adult and a child and indicate the stress for each syllable.

1. [= = =] 2. [= = =] 3. [= = =] 4. [= = =]

5. [= = =] 6. [= = =] 7. [= = =] 8. [= = = =]

9. [= = = =] 10. [= = = =] 11. [= = = =] 12. [= = = =]

13. [= = = =] 14. [= = = =]

****

Consensus: 1. ['==ˌ=] 2. ['===] 3. [='==] 4. ['= ==] 5. [ˌ=='=] 6. ['==ˌ=] 7. ['==ˌ=] 8. ['==ˌ==] 9. [ˌ=='==] 10. ['== ==] 11. [='===] 12. [='==ˌ=] 13. ['==ˌ==] 14. ['==ˌ==]

Variants: 7. ['===] 10. ['===] 11. [='==ˌ=]

c. Internal Open Juncture

Listen to the words as they are pronounced by an adult and a child and indicate where the open juncture occurs (a or b).

1. ________ a. [kip+stɪkɪŋ] ________ b. [kips+tɪkɪŋ]
2. ________ a. [sim+ebəl] ________ b. [si+mebəl]
3. ________ a. [ɪts+prez] ________ b. [ɪt+sprez]
4. ________ a. [gre+de] ________ b. [gred+e]
5. ________ a. [ðæts+tʌf] ________ b. [ðæt+stʌf]
6. ________ a. [kip+stɪkɪŋ] ________ b. [kips+tɪkɪŋ]
7. ________ a. [sim+ebəl] ________ b. [si+mebəl]
8. ________ a. [ɪts+prez] ________ b. [ɪt+sprez]
9. ________ a. [gre+de] ________ b. [gred+e]
10. ________ a. [ðæts+tʌf] ________ b. [ðæt+stʌf]

****

Consensus: 1. b 2. b 3. a 4. a 5. a 6. a 7. a 8. b 9. b 10. b

Variants: None.

d. Intonation

Listen to the utterances as they are pronounced by an adult and a child. Indicate the intonation contours and write the word where the tonic accent occurs. Select from the following contours: (a) [231#] /\, (b) [241#] /\, (c) [23||] /, (d) [323 |] \/, and (e) [232 |] /\. If necessary, stop the tape at any time, rewind, and listen again.

1. ______________ 2. ______________ 3. ______________ 4. ______________

5. ______________ 6. ______________ 7. ______________ 8. ______________

9. ______________ 10. ______________ 11. ______________

****

Consensus: 1. a; store 2. c; store 3. e; store 4. b; am 5. b; am 6. a; careful 7. d; careful 8. a; name 9. c; name 10. c; store 11. a; store

Variants: 1. a; going 3. d; going store 4. a; am 5. d; I'm 6. e; better 11. d; going store

CHAPTER 12

Articulatory Assessment

In the preceding chapters, properties associated with physiologic, acoustic, and perceptual phonetics were reviewed and evaluated. The focus of this chapter is on articulatory assessment, particularly as it relates to the clinical functions of diagnosis and rehabilitation. Complementary to this chapter are appendixes D and E, which cover procedures for achieving accuracy, validity, and reliability in phonetic transcription.

In the clinical assessment of articulation, speech and language pathologists rely much more on perceptual phonetics than physiologic or acoustic phonetics. Although the quantitative approach offered by physiologic and acoustic phonetics is very desirable, there is too little information about the physiologic and acoustic correlates of misarticulated speech. Until there is a better understanding of these correlates and a practical way to translate this understanding into clinical practice, perceptual phonetics will remain the primary clinical basis of phonetic analysis. Perceptual phonetics also provides the additional advantage of expediency and direct analysis, which are not possible with either physiologic or acoustic phonetics.

In the discussion of perceptual phonetics in Chapter 1, reference was made to problems that might influence the accurate identification of speech sounds. If listeners are asked to identify the initial sound in a continuum of consonant-vowel (CV) stimuli that systematically vary in acoustic correlates differentiating /r/ and /w/, they will probably place the majority of these sounds, even ones that are acoustically ambiguous, into one category or another (see Figure 1–11). This tendency to categorize speech sounds is consistent with a basic pattern of categorization of other physical events occurring in the world (Repp, 1984). For example, in the process of categorizing speech, listeners presumably attend to certain acoustic correlates of speech and ignore others. Although it would be ideal if all listeners would attend to the same properties and perceive sounds identically, experience shows that this is not the case for either the perception of normal speech or synthetic analogs of misarticulated speech (Fitch, Halwes, Erickson, & Liberman, 1980; Sharf, Ohde, & Lehman, 1988).

If perception of normal and misarticulated speech is influenced by certain variables, it is important to evaluate potential parameters which may confound our analysis of errors in articulation. In this chapter the following are examined: (1) articulation testing, (2) analyses of articulation, (3) factors that influence the perception of sounds, (4) methods of calibration to minimize variation in perception of speech, and (5) the role of phonetic modification in articulation therapy.

ARTICULATION TESTING: GOALS, TYPES, AND ANALYSES

Goals

In assessing the articulation behavior of an individual, typically some type of **articulation test** is used which evaluates articulatory status. When administering these tests, one should be aware of the goals of articulatory assessment and of the inherent limitations of tests.

In general, the goals of articulation assessment can be divided into determining the nature of the articulation errors and deciding the implications of these errors for articulation therapy. The first goal is to discern whether any articulation errors are produced. Once it has been determined that a sound is produced incorrectly, age norms are consulted to determine if the error falls within normal limits. As shown in Figure 12–1, **articulation norms** typically consist of age levels by which most children produce sounds correctly (Sander, 1972). Recent research on one to three-year-old children has provided thorough analyses of sound acquisition during this period and indicates that the phonological processes occurring between one and four years are based on the phonetic tendencies of the prelinguistic period (Stoel-Gammon, 1985; Dyson, 1986, 1988; Vihman, Ferguson, & Elbert, 1986). If an articulation error is judged abnormal, then the nature of this error and its influence on intelligibility must be determined. Particular interest focuses on how frequently the error sound is used and how much its use produces confusions among words by increasing homonymity (Ingram, 1976; Vihman, 1981; Leonard, Schwartz, Allen, Swanson, & Frome-Loeb, 1989). **Homonymity** describes loss of distinction between words as a result of the use of phonological processes, as occurs between 'pick' and 'pig' when the final consonant of 'pig' is devoiced.

The ultimate goals of articulatory assessment involve the examination of articulatory errors as they relate to therapeutic intervention. Speech and language pathologists are particularly interested in determining the likelihood that the error sounds will self-correct or have a favorable prognosis for therapy. The frequency of error sound production and the potential for producing the sound correctly when provided an auditory model are important factors in determining the prognosis for self-correction and therapy. The final aim in this process is to synthesize the information on assessment so as to determine a plan for therapy.

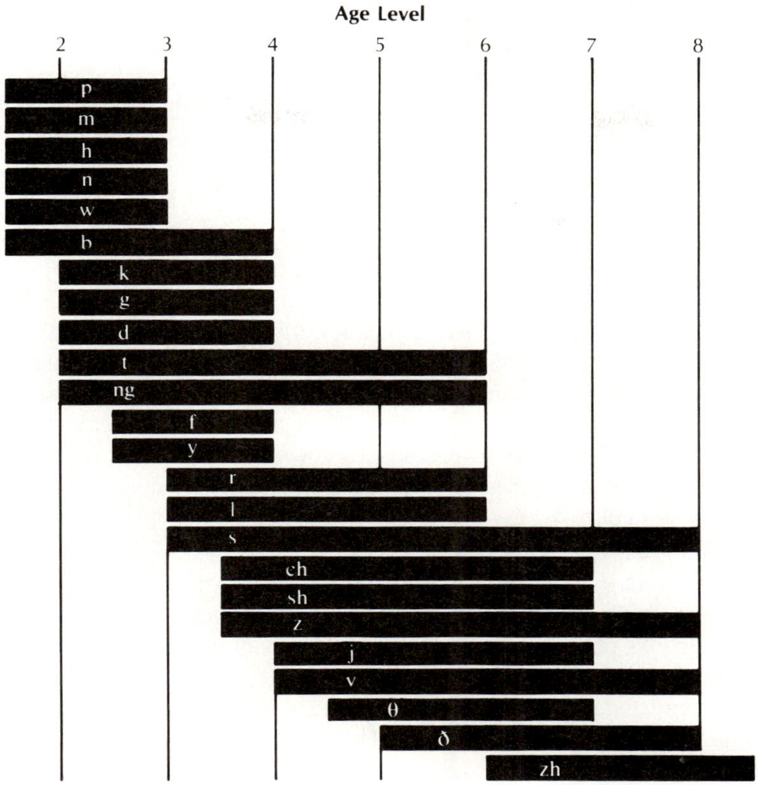

Figure 12–1
Average age estimate and upper age limits of sound acquisition. The solid bar corresponding to each sound starts at the median age of acquisition and stops at the age level when 90% of all children produce the sound correctly (ng = /ŋ/; y = /j/; ch = /tʃ/; sh = /ʃ/; j = /ʤ/; zh = /ʒ/).

Source: "When Are Speech Sounds Learned?" by E. K. Sander, 1972, *Journal of Speech and Hearing Disorders, 37,* p. 62. Copyright 1972 by the American Speech-Language-Hearing Association. Reprinted with permission.

Types

There are several general classes of articulation tests, ranging from screening procedures to more comprehensive phonemic inventory and phonological assessments. Although there are clear differences among tests, the rationales for tests of a particular type share certain characteristics.

Screening Tests

The purpose of **screening articulation tests** is to determine in an expedient manner if sounds are misarticulated. Screening tests can be as informal as asking the subject to count from one to ten or to name the days of the week. In addition to informal tests, several formal screening examinations are available. These tests usually consist of a limited number of items from a larger test battery such as the Templin-Darley screening test (Templin & Darley, 1969). They are most commonly used as an index of need for further, in-depth diagnostic tests. Results may vary among screening tests. One study reported that only one of eleven children failing at least one of three such tests failed all three of them (Ritterman, Zook-Herman, Carlson, & Kinde, 1982).

Articulation Tests

Perhaps the most common assessment tool is the articulation test. The general purpose of these tests is the systematic evaluation of the phoneme production of a speaker, usually through a set of pictures that represent words with sounds and consonant clusters in various positions. The subject's task is to name these pictures so that production of consonants can be assessed in prevocalic, intervocalic, and postvocalic position. Some of these tests also assess vowel and diphthong production, and several have sentence reading versions appropriate for older children and adults as well.

Phonological Process Tests

Because phonological processes represent certain patterns of language usage, a critical component of **phonological process tests** is to evaluate phonological patterns as comprehensively as possible. There are two schools of thought as to how to approach this problem. One school favors eliciting specific words through objects, pictures, or single-word delayed imitation tasks (Weiner, 1979; Hodson, 1986). This is akin to the phonemic inventory approach discussed above. The other school bases word analysis on samples of continuous speech (Shriberg & Kwiatkowski, 1980). Other proponents of phonological process assessment leave the method of elicitation to the individual clinician (Ingram, 1981; Grunwell, 1985). The common thread linking all phonological process tests is that patterns of sound production are evaluated through whole-word responses.

Generative Phonological Tests

The generative phonological assessment approach can best be described as a gestalt approach which attempts to evaluate a child's phonological development as an entity independent of the correct underlying adult forms (Maxwell & Rockman, 1984). But some practitioners of the generative approach compare data to adult models (Elbert & Gierut, 1986). There is no single **generative phonological test** which assesses phonological development from the generative perspective. Instead, several procedures are used in assessment. These procedures include both tests of phonemic inventories and conversational analyses. Generative phonological and phonological process tests include similar examinations, but only the generative approach consistently uses the conversational procedure.

Analysis of Results

It is possible to evaluate the results for a particular type of test according to different theoretical frameworks. For example, the results of a phonemic inventory test could easily be examined from the perspective of speech segments, place of articulation, distinctive features, or phonological processes. Procedures to assess phonological processes have been developed using either the Goldman-Fristoe or the Templin-Darley phonemic inventory tests of articulation (Lowe, 1986). Moreover, results from articulation tests form part of the data base of the generative phonological assessment. The restrictive data set of a phonemic inventory test does limit interpretations of analyses other than segmental. From a historical perspective, the major approaches to the evaluation of phonological data are segmental, distinctive feature, phonological process, and generative phonological analyses. The latter three share an approach that views the articulatory system according to certain patterns of sound production.

Segmental Analysis

The earliest and most basic approach to sound assessment was the **segmental analysis** of speech (Van Riper, 1978). The data for this analysis generally are derived from an articulation test. Each sound in error is evaluated as a single entity requiring intervention. The relationship among sounds, as well as changes in sound patterns and phonological rules, is not evaluated in this approach. The clinician determines the number and word position of sound errors, and therapy proceeds with training for each misarticulation. Segmental analysis is most appropriate for individuals with relatively few articulation errors.

One of the earliest attempts to determine the relationships among articulation errors was an outgrowth of applying the segmental approach to children with multiple articulation errors (Elbert & Gierut, 1986). Proponents of the segmental approach found a certain elegance in examining children with multiple articulation errors according to place, voicing, and manner of articulation. For example, the results of a segmental analysis of child A might reveal substitutions of voiceless cognates for final voiced stops. Because these misarticulations represent a rather limited set, the general pattern of voicing changes may not be striking. On the other hand, child B might substitute voiceless cognates for all final voiced obstruents and homorganic voiceless stops for final nasals, e.g., /p/ for /m/. Although the incorrect use of the voicing feature characterizes the speech of both children, the pervasive nature of child B's problem as compared with child A's problem becomes clear only after analysis of patterns of misarticulation.

Distinctive Feature Analysis

Distinctive feature analysis views articulation errors as comprising **distinctive features.** It is used to analyze misarticulations according to certain patterns. For years, linguists had been interested in various patterns of sounds which could be differentiated on the basis of discrete features (Jakobson, Fant, & Halle, 1951). Table 12–1 includes descriptions of selected features from a system that was devised to provide a set of distinguishing characteristics of phonemes by using a relatively small number of binary descriptive terms. In the case of voicing, the binary distinction is between voiced and voiceless sounds. Since the system was introduced, it has undergone extensive modifications (Jakobson et al., 1951; Jakobson & Halle, 1956; Chomsky & Halle, 1968). The features shown in Table 12–1 are those that are most useful in describing the phonemes of English. Some features, like nasal, round, and voiced, are very similar to the phonetic terminology already covered. Other features, like strident and coronal, are similar to phonetic terms like sibilant and apico-alveolar, but differ enough so that they sort out the sounds of English in slightly different ways. For example, the category strident includes all the sounds identified as sibilants, but it also includes /f/ and /v/, which are not classified as sibilants.

Although the system was devised primarily for the use of linguists in describing the structure of different languages with one feature system, it has been used to analyze

Table 12–1
Distinctive features used in characterizing phonemes of English.

Term	Description	Sounds Included
Manner Features		
Consonantal	Restriction that: (1) stops air flow completely or centrally or (2) produces frication	All consonants except /w, j, h/
Vocalic	Narrowing no smaller than for highest vowels /i, u/	All vowels plus liquids /r, l/
Continuant	Free passage through vocal tract for airflow	All vowels and consonants except nasals and stops
Nasal	Airflow emitted through nasal cavity	Nasal consonants
Lateral	Lingua-alveolar contact with tongue margins lowered	Lateral consonants; only /l/ in English
Strident	Relatively great noise	Sibilants and /f, v/
Delayed Release	Relatively slow release of stop closure	Affricates
Sonorant	Relatively open oral tract that allows for spontaneous voicing	Vowels, glides, liquids, and nasals
Place or Cavity Configuration Features		
Coronal	Closure/restriction involves front portion (corona) of tongue	All tongue tip and blade consonants; /r/
Anterior	Closure/restriction at or anterior to alveolar ridge	All labial and alveolar consonants
Round	Narrowing of lip opening	Rounded vowels
High	Tongue body raised above neutral vowel position	All vowels above /e, o/; /w, j/
Low	Tongue body lowered below neutral vowel position	All vowels below /ɛ, ɔ/
Back	Tongue body retracted from neutral vowel position	All back vowels and velar consonants; /w/
Source Features		
Voiced	Vocal folds are in position to vibrate	All voiced sounds

speech problems and speech sound development. This form of analysis has been used by some speech and language pathologists in the study of misarticulations (McReynolds & Engmann, 1975). Most important, distinctive feature analysis provides a basis for using minimal or maximal pair contrast treatment as new approaches to articulation therapy (McReynolds & Bennett, 1972; Costello & Onstine, 1976; Blache, Parsons, & Humphreys, 1981; Gierut, 1989). For example, McReynolds and Bennett (1972) taught a child the contrast between /ʃ/ and /tʃ/, which differ in that the former is plus continuant and the latter is minus continuant. Following treatment, other continuant sounds, /f, v, s, z/, were produced correctly. Thus, focusing attention on a single feature not only resulted in learning this distinction for the particular phoneme treated but also led to generalizing the distinction to include other phonemes.

Table 12–2 includes descriptions of the feature differences between target and replacement sounds for a number of common misarticulations. Using the conventional notation for distinctive features, the presence and absence of a feature in a sound are indicated as plus and minus, respectively. For some misarticulations there is a minimal feature difference between target and replacement. For example, /θ/ and /f/ differ only in that the former is − strident and + coronal and the latter is + strident and − coronal. For other misarticulations, there are multiple feature differences, as in the case of target

Table 12–2
Distinctive feature differences between target and substituted sounds associated with common misarticulations (Cons = consonantal; Voc = vocalic; Cont = continuant; Cor = coronal; Ant = anterior; Strid = strident).

Error[a]	Cons	Voc	Cont	Cor	Ant	High	Back	Strid
r/w	+/−	+/−	+/+	+/−	−/−	−/+	−/+	−/−
l/j	+/−	+/−	+/+	+/−	+/−	−/+	−/−	−/−
l/w	+/−	+/−	+/+	+/−	+/−	−/+	−/+	−/−
s/t	+/+	−/−	+/−	+/+	+/+	−/−	−/−	+/−
s/θ	+/+	−/−	+/+	+/+	+/+	−/−	−/−	+/−
z/d	+/+	−/−	+/−	+/+	+/+	−/−	−/−	+/−
z/ð	+/+	−/−	+/+	+/+	+/+	−/−	−/−	+/−
θ/t	+/+	−/−	+/−	+/+	+/+	−/−	−/−	−/−
θ/f	+/+	−/−	+/+	+/−	+/+	−/−	−/−	−/+
ð/d	+/+	−/−	+/−	+/+	+/+	−/−	−/−	−/−
ð/v	+/+	−/−	+/+	+/−	+/+	−/−	−/−	−/+
k/t	+/+	−/−	−/−	−/+	−/+	−/−	+/−	−/−
g/d	+/+	−/−	−/−	−/+	−/+	−/−	+/−	−/−
f/p	+/+	−/−	+/−	−/−	+/+	−/−	−/−	+/−
v/b	+/+	−/−	+/−	−/−	+/+	−/−	−/−	+/−

[a]First sound is target, second sound is replacement; first + or − indicates feature of target, second + or − indicates feature of replacement.

/r/ and replacement /w/, which differ in consonantal, vocalic, coronal, high, and back features. What is most important is that a number of pairs differ on the basis of the same feature. Each of the pairs /s, t/, /s, θ/, /z, d/, /z, ð/, /θ, f/, /ð, v/, /f, p/, and /v, b/ differ with regard to stridency. The therapeutic implication of such feature commonality is that the cognition achieved by teaching a child the contrast between + and − stridency in one pair will generalize to all the others.

Although distinctive features appear to offer a basis for effective planning of speech therapy, some have raised serious questions about their clinical application (Leonard, 1973; Walsh, 1974; Parker, 1976). In particular, it has been pointed out that distinctive features were designed to differentiate phonemes, not to provide complete descriptions of productive variations in sounds. The binary system used for distinctive feature analysis is convenient for linguistic analysis of meaningful distinctions within a language but may oversimplify the differences between a misarticulated target sound and its substitute. Since distinctive features relate to the normal use of phonemic distinctions, they are not useful for the analysis of distortions of sounds like /r/, /l/, and /s/.

Phonological Process Analysis

Phonological process analysis overcomes some of the limitations of distinctive features in analyzing speech production by describing speech errors according to certain characteristics of phonology. These characteristics of phonology, or phonological patterns, have been described as simplifications of the adult sound target (Ingram, 1976; Grunwell, 1988). According to phonological process analysis, children who substitute voiceless cognates for final voiced obstruents are using final consonant devoicing. Through this process of simplification, these children have eliminated the voicing contrast so that 'bad' and 'bat' are both /bæ t/. Although a number of different analysis procedures employ phonological processes, they all are based on a theory of Natural Phonology (Stampe, 1972) which attempts to characterize sound variations according to patterns of production. The results obtained with different procedures appear to be comparable (Benjamin & Greenwood, 1983; Paden & Moss, 1985; Dyson & Robinson, 1987).

Two theoretical assumptions underlie phonological process analysis. First, phonological processes are assumed to be simplifications of adult phonology, a concept shared with distinctive feature analysis. Children replace difficult adult targets with simplified versions or versions that are easier to produce.

The second assumption of phonological process analysis is that the child, while knowing the adult target form, still produces a different sound. It is assumed that there is a one-to-one correspondence between the simplified production and the adult target form.

Generative Phonological Analysis

Generative phonologists believe that claiming a child's productions are based on the adult target form is a conceptual flaw (Maxwell & Rockman, 1984; Elbert & Gierut, 1986). The foundation of **generative phonological analysis** is determining the phonological knowledge of the child using a linguistic methodology and an analysis procedure which evaluate the child as an independent system. Care is taken not to use substitution and error analysis based on the adult model.

Generative phonological analysis is based on two types of data, a spontaneous speech sample and some form of elicited speech sample. No a priori assumptions are made about the phonological knowledge of the child, and all analyses are based on empirical data. Some proponents of the generative phonological approach have left the organization of data largely up to the individual clinician (Maxwell & Rockman, 1984); others have provided a general analytical framework based on various types of phonological knowledge (Elbert & Gierut, 1986).

The framework proposed by Elbert and Gierut (1986) consists of three main components of phonological knowledge: (1) the breadth of the distribution of sounds, (2) phonological rules, and (3) the nature of the child's lexical representations. Analysis of the breadth of the distribution of sounds includes complete inventories of the sounds that are phonemically contrastive. For example, /m/, /n/, /d/, and /æ/ are part of the phonetic inventory of a child who produces 'man' and 'mad' correctly, and /n/ and /d/ are part of the phonemic inventory. The child's phonemic inventory is further analyzed according to the distribution of these contrasts in word positions and morphemes. In the above example, /n/ and /d/ are used contrastively in word-final position.

The sounds in the child's phonetic and phonemic inventories should be constrained by the phonological rule component of linguistic knowledge. Two types of rules can influence sound production, static and dynamic. **Static rules** are phonotactic constraints which can either restrict the production of sounds in certain word positions or sequences, or entirely exclude the production of other sounds. A child may, for example, produce /s/ and /p/ word-initially in the context of /ɑɪ/, but may fail to combine /s/ and /p/ in the consonant cluster production /spɑɪ/, instead producing /pɑɪ/. The child's production of 'spry' could also be /pɑɪ/ because of the omission of /r/ in all sound positions.

Dynamic rules serve to alter the production of sounds in various contexts due to **allophonic rules** and neutralization rules. For example, the production of /p/ in 'pie' is aspirated, but the production of /p/ in 'spy' is unaspirated, which is an allophonic variation in English. Neutralization rules collapse a phonemic distinction in a particular context. For example, a child may produce /k/ and /g/ correctly in initial position, but only /k/ in final position. Such a child says /pɪk/ for 'pig,' neutralizing the difference between /k/ and /g/. Further evidence for such a neutralization rule is obtained if the child says /g/ in 'piggy.' The pair /pɪk/ 'pig' and /pɪgi/ 'piggy' represents a morphophonemic alternation of velar production.

The last component of phonological knowledge examines the nature of a child's "lexical representations," or the words he/she uses to indicate meanings, which reflect the relationship between sound production and meaning. The goal of this analysis is to determine if the child's morphemes are similar to the adult target productions. This is particularly important because the nature of a child's lexical representations is controversial. Some view them as identical to the adult target (N. V. Smith, 1973; Ingram, 1976; Menn, 1978; Donegan & Stampe, 1979), and others view them as unique (Kornfeld & Goehl, 1974; Macken, 1980; Maxwell, 1981b; Weismer, Dinnsen, & Elbert, 1981; Dinnsen, 1984).

DIAGNOSTIC FACTORS: ACCURACY, VALIDITY, AND RELIABILITY

Accuracy

The choice of which of the wide range of articulation tests and analyses to use should be made by the examiner with the intent of obtaining the most accurate impression of an individual's speech. With this goal, the examiner should be aware of factors that can affect the accuracy of any test. These range from such basic issues as recording procedures to more complicated problems such as the recording skill of the transcriber. (See Appendix D for procedures to achieve accuracy.)

Audio Recording

When examining articulation, individuals are frequently tape-recorded so that an in-depth analysis and transcription can be completed after the test session. If a conversation is included in the testing protocol, then a recording is imperative because of the difficulty involved in trying to transcribe such a sample. The need to obtain a high-quality audio recording should not be overlooked; a poor recording can be so noisy that it precludes accurate transcription by even the most skilled clinician. Recordings should be made in environments that are reasonably quiet and with equipment that can provide an accurate representation of speech.

The principal aspects of recording include noise reduction, recording mode, and equipment (Allen, 1984). Background noise can be reduced by having the child play with toys that minimize noise, by not talking while the subject is speaking, and by recording in a closed room to reduce extraneous environmental sounds. Recording in stereo results in a wider dynamic range of the recorded voice signal and enables the transcriber to utilize binaural auditory acuity in later transcriptions. A moderately priced stereo cassette recorder with output level controls, a review button, and lavaliere microphone are usually sufficient for audiotape recordings. (See Appendix D for information on standards used in recording the transcription tapes for this book.)

Method of Recording

Although it is not uncommon to transcribe audiotape recordings in the assessment of articulation skills, the method most frequently used is the live articulation test. Other techniques used in the assessment of articulation include audio recordings and videotape recordings. At least two basic questions relate to the method of recording. First, is one technique better than another? There is little information on this topic, but research indicates that transcription of /s/ from live articulation is more accurate than that from audiotapes (Shriberg, 1972; Stephens & Daniloff, 1977). Second, is accuracy compromised if comparisons are made between two different methods of recording? Wright (1954) found that examiner agreement was higher as determined from a tape recording of an articulation test played on two different occasions than as determined from the live articulation test and the tape recording of it. The findings of Hoffman and Schuckers (1978) contradicted those of Wright (1954) in finding that interjudge reliability was unaffected by mode of stimulus presentation. Judges tended, however, to identify unstressed vocalic /r/ more often as incorrect in the recorded mode compared to live analyses.

As for videotape recordings, their disadvantages appear to outnumber their advantages (Shriberg & Kent, 1982). Among the disadvantages (as compared with medium-priced audiotape recorders) are the following: (1) higher cost, (2) more time to set up, and (3) poorer audio signal. But videotape recordings have at least two distinct advantages. They may capture both important visual gestures of production and the context of the recording, which can be reviewed later for a better understanding of a subject's articulation behavior.

Notational System

The choice of notational system appears very often to relate to convenience, skill, and the clinician's purpose. Common notational systems range from the simple right-wrong system to the detailed allophonic, or narrow phonetic, system. If a quick assessment of articulation behavior is desired, then a right-wrong system may be used. This analysis indicates only whether a subject's articulation is the same or different from the phonology of a language. If the test reveals that the subject's articulation is different, the notation provides no information about the variations in production and the possible physiological processes involved. The traditional notational system is only slightly better in describing the articulatory behavior of an individual. This system classifies errors as omissions, additions, substitutions, or distortions. An omission is the deletion of a phoneme from a word, an **addition** the insertion of an additional phoneme in a word, a substitution the replacement of one phoneme by another in a word, and a **distortion** a variation of a target sound that is not allophonic but does not fall into another phoneme category.

Except for the transcription of substitutions, the notational systems covered so far provide only a limited analysis of a subject's speech production. These systems give little information for both the diagnosis of articulatory skills and the design of treatment strategies. The most detailed and comprehensive notational system utilizes the International Phonetic Alphabet (IPA), which has two components. One component is a set of symbols representing the phonemes of a language, and the other component is a set of symbols representing allophonic variations of these phonemes.

Although broad transcription may be sufficient for some purposes, a more thorough notational system provides a better indication of an individual's articulation. There are clear cases of productions that demand narrow transcription for correct and accurate assessment. Some of these cases are critical because of the implications for remediation. For example, in the transcription of a production of /wed/ 'wade' by a child who deleted the final consonant but lengthened the vowel, clinician A broadly transcribed the production as /we/, whereas clinician B narrowly transcribed the production as [weː] based on minimal pair contrasts ('wait'/'wade'). Clinician B's transcription reflects the child's phonological cognition of postvocalic voicing much better than clinician A's. According to clinician B's transcription, the child is producing durational differences that occur normally before final voiced and voiceless consonants. The two different transcriptions could very easily lead to different conclusions about the child's phonological maturity and need for therapy.

In another example, the production of 'rip' by a child who did not release the final /p/ was transcribed by clinician A as /rɪ/, while clinician B transcribed the same production as [rɪp˺]. The release of stops in postvocalic position in English is in free variation, and it is important to differentiate between stops that are unreleased and those that are omitted. Again, the child's level of phonological cognition is substantially better according to clinician B's transcription than it is in clinician A's transcription. (See Appendix D for further details about variants which should be transcribed in children's speech.)

Background of Transcriber

Differences in transcriptions like those in the examples presented above may be due to the background of the transcribers, that is, their natural skill and training. Although there may not be an unequivocal reason for these differences, the skill and the training of these individuals may be quite different. A speech and language pathologist without training in narrow transcription is unlikely to transcribe as accurately as one who has such a background. If both individuals received identical training, one probably has more natural ability than the other. The existence of such differences in background is supported by preliminary data (Sharf, Ohde, & Lehman, 1988).

Validity

Validity refers to the extent to which a test adequately measures speech behavior. In particular, we are interested in construct validity, which most likely influences perceptual judgment of speech sounds. Construct validity requires evidence that a test provides a representative sample of the subject's speech behavior. The four critical components of construct validity are type of sample, size of sample, frequency of sample, and context of sample.

Type of Sample

The major types of speech samples used in articulation tests are imitation, picture naming, reading, and conversation. Although the conversational sample presumably best reflects normal speech, it is the basic test of only the generative phonological assessment. A conversational sample is used in other assessment procedures, but not consistently, even though some clinicians believe that it should be.

For practical reasons it may be important to include a picture naming test in evaluating speech production. This procedure provides the certainty of obtaining systematic responses to all consonants in several word positions, which cannot be assured in a conversational sample. Another reason for selecting a picture naming sample is that it may provide information on articulatory potential that is not observed in a conversational sample, particularly for an unintelligible child.

If the picture naming sample reveals extensive articulation errors, then an imitation test may provide more information on articulatory potential. In general, children produce target sounds correctly more often when asked to imitate them than when asked to pronounce them spontaneously (Snow & Milisen, 1954; Carter & Buck, 1958; Siegel, Winitz, & Conkey, 1963; Smith & Ainsworth, 1967). Although the reason for the difference is unclear, demands on memory and lexical access appear to be minimized in the imitation task (Best & Wilkenfeld, 1988). Other advantages of the imitation sample compared to picture naming include the potential for using nonsense target words, direct knowledge of the child's intended target, and the opportunity directly to compare phonetic and acoustic properties of child and adult utterances.

If subjects can read, speech samples may be obtained by having them read. But this approach may not yield a valid assessment of articulation skills because subjects may employ a different speech pattern when reading. Fewer errors tend to occur in reading than in conversational speech (Wright, Shelton, & Arndt, 1969).

The type of sample used may influence the outcome of an articulation test. Of those reviewed, the conversational sample is the one most analogous to natural speech. One should be aware, however, that a conversational sample may not get a cross section of all English sounds because of the low frequency of occurrence of some sounds and/or selective avoidance of problem sounds by an individual. Tables 12–3 and 12–4 show the frequency of occurrence of common error sounds observed in the speech of children. Although it is clear that some sounds commonly misarticulated by children, such as /r/, /l/, and /s/, occur frequently, others, such as /f/, /ʃ/, and /tʃ/, occur much less frequently. Table 12–3 reveals that the frequency of occurrence of these sounds is quite consistent across grade levels, while Table 12–4 shows that the proportion of these sounds across word positions is rather inconsistent. For example, voiceless fricatives occur more frequently in prevocalic position, while voiced fricatives generally occur more frequently in postvocalic position.

Table 12–3
Frequency of occurrence (% of all consonants spoken) of common error sounds of first-grade, third-grade, and fifth-grade children's speech (Carterette and Jones, 1974). Values in parentheses are rankings of error sounds from highest (1) to lowest (14).

Error Sounds	1st Grade	3rd Grade	5th Grade
/r/	8.2 (1)	8.7 (1)	9.0 (1)
/l/	4.9 (3.5)	5.0 (3)	5.2 (3)
/s/	6.9 (2)	7.4 (2)	7.3 (2)
/z/	4.5 (5)	4.2 (6)	4.6 (5)
/k/	4.9 (3.5)	4.7 (4)	4.8 (4)
/g/	2.9 (7)	2.5 (7)	2.5 (7)
/θ/	1.0 (10)	0.9 (10)	1.0 (11)
/ð/	4.4 (6)	4.5 (5)	4.5 (6)
/f/	2.2 (8)	2.1 (8)	2.3 (8)
/v/	1.6 (9)	1.5 (9)	2.1 (9)
/ʃ/	0.8 (11)	0.9 (11)	1.3 (10)
/ʒ/	0.0 (14)	0.0 (14)	0.0 (14)
/tʃ/	0.5 (13)	0.5 (12)	0.7 (12)
/dʒ/	0.5 (12)	0.5 (13)	0.6 (13)

Table 12–4
Frequency of occurrence (of 100 consonants spoken) of common error sounds of first- through third-grade children's speech according to a study by Mader (1954). Values in parentheses are rankings of error sounds from highest (1) to lowest (14). Proportions according to word position are given for each sound.

		Position		
Error Sounds	**1st–3rd grade**	**Prevocalic**	**Intervocalic**	**Postvocalic**
/r/	7.8 (1)	14	46	40
/l/	5.5 (4)	23	41	36
/s/	6.5 (2)	50	20	30
/z/	3.7 (6)	0	6	94
/k/	4.2 (5)	41	29	30
/g/	2.3 (7)	77	13	10
/θ/	0.9 (10)	45	22	33
/ð/	6.4 (3)	93	7	0
/f/	1.8 (9)	64	17	19
/v/	1.9 (8)	4	36	60
/ʃ/	0.8 (11)	76	17	7
/ʒ/	0.0 (14)	0	0	0
/tʃ/	0.5 (13)	31	24	45
/dʒ/	0.6 (12)	78	12	10

Number and Frequency of Sounds in Sample

In addition to the type of sample selected, it is important to be aware of how many different sounds are tested and how frequently they occur in the sample. With the exception of a conversation, which cannot be easily controlled, samples should include all vowel and consonant phonemes and a representative sampling of consonant clusters. The consonants should be evaluated in all phonologically permissible word positions. Sounds should be repeated more than once during testing. Sound acquisition is a gradual process, and sound production may be variable, particularly in children (Kent, 1976; Ohde, 1985). Only one presentation of a target sound, resulting in 100% or 0% correct is rather meaningless.

There is no research basis for how often sounds should be tested to obtain a valid sample. In the case of distinctive feature analysis, McReynolds and Engmann (1975) recommend ten samples for each sound. Studies examining speech production characteristics of both children and adults typically have collected three to five samples for each sound (Kent & Forner, 1980; Ohde, 1984, 1985). There is no absolute rule for sample size, but five to ten tokens per sound seem desirable (Weismer, 1984).

Context of Sounds in Sample

The importance of sound context in effecting changes in the articulatory gestures of speech has been viewed from both diagnostic (McDonald, 1964a) and therapeutic perspectives (Winitz, 1975; Prather & Whaley, 1984). It should be very clear from previous discussions of phonological processes that sound context forms the basis of assimilatory processes. In assessing speech sound production, we are interested in variations that result as a function of changes in sound position, sound context, and the complexity of the linguistic material. Sounds can be assessed in simple linguistic contexts like monosyllables or in more complex utterances like polysyllables, phrases, and sentences, which may produce variations in production due to coarticulatory and assimilatory processes as well as changes in prosody.

The traditional phonemic inventory test was designed with the knowledge that any sound may be produced differently, depending on its position in a word. But the results of research into which position most facilitates correct sound production are equivocal. In one study, sounds were generally produced more correctly in initial position than in medial position, and more correctly in medial position than in final position (Scott & Milisen, 1954). In another study, however, errors on a picture articulation test for any one sound were similar across word position (Snow, 1963).

Sound context influences speech production for both normal speakers and those with articulatory disorders (Sharf & Ohde, 1981). In the discussion of phonological disorders it was pointed out that both contiguous and noncontiguous assimilatory processes exist. For example, the production /fwɪnz/ for /twɪnz/ is a contiguous labial assimilation, and the production /maɪp/ for /naɪf/ is a noncontiguous labial assimilation. In both examples the labial feature of one sound seems to influence the production of either an adjacent or a nonadjacent sound.

Sound context has typically been examined according to the effects of features, transitions, and direction of sound influences. The goal of evaluating the effects of these properties on sound production is to determine potential facilitating effects on correct sound production (Kent, 1982). For example, /t/ might facilitate correct /s/ production in 'stay' because both are alveolar sounds. The influence of place of articulation on correct sound production has been observed to be either limited (Siegel et al., 1963; Zehel, Shelton, Arndt, Wright, & Elbert, 1972) or contradictory, at least in the cases of /t/ versus /p/ influence on /s/ production (Gallagher & Shriner, 1975a; Mazza, Schuckers, & Daniloff, 1979), /p/ versus /t/ and /k/ influence on /r/ production (Curtis & Hardy, 1959; Hoffman, Schuckers, & Ratusnik, 1977), and stop versus fricative influence on /s/ and /r/ production (Curtis & Hardy, 1959; Gallagher & Shriner, 1975a; Kenney, Prather, Mooney, & Jeruzal, 1984).

Contradictory evidence has also been compiled about the direction of contextual influence on correct sound production. This is true in the case of the effect of the preceding versus the following consonant on achieving correct /s/ production (Zehel et al., 1972; Mazza et al., 1979); in the case of the effect of the manner feature of preceding versus following consonants on achieving correct /s/ and /z/ production (Gallagher & Shriner, 1975a), and in the case of the effect of the preceding versus the following consonant on achieving correct /ɝ/ production (Hoffman et al., 1977).

Our discussion of contextual effects has generally been restricted to influences at the word level, particularly in monosyllabic words. But the influence of context extends beyond monosyllabic words (Sharf & Ohde, 1981). Even when discussing relatively simple effects like the influence of word position, one must be mindful of potential confusion between word position and prosodic components of language. Some believe that in speech production consonants do not occur in initial, medial, and final positions, but rather serve either to release (prevocalic consonant) or arrest (postvocalic consonant) a syllable (McDonald, 1964b). These releasing and arresting gestures encompass word boundaries and juncture influences, clearly increasing the linguistic complexity of context. No differences in correct /s/ and /z/ production occurred between contexts preceding and following word boundaries for normal children (Gallagher & Shriner, 1975b), but they did occur for children who misarticulated /s/ (Mazza et al., 1979). Although /s/ was produced correctly more often in a cluster within word boundaries, as in 'stop,' than across word boundaries, as in 'this time' (Gallagher, 1975), /r/ was produced correctly more often in a cluster across word boundaries, as in 'jeep ride,' than within word boundaries, as in 'pried' (Hoffman et al., 1977).

Our understanding of the influences of other aspects of context and prosody on correct sound production is quite limited. There is evidence that as one increases the length and/or complexity of an utterance, correct sound production decreases, as in sounds in isolation compared to nonsense syllables and words (Scott & Milisen, 1954), sounds in monosyllabic and polysyllabic words (Ingram, 1978), and sounds in isolation and conversation (Faircloth & Faircloth, 1970). As pointed out in Chapter 11, the use of stopping is influenced by prosodic structure, phonotactic structure, and syllabification (Chiat, 1989).

Increases in the length of production involve concomitant prosodic effects like juncture. In contrast to sound segments, no developmental norms exist for the acquisition of prosody. Nor is it known whether abnormal prosodic development plays any role in abnormal sound development. The imitative productive abilities of normal children and children with misarticulations enrolled in therapy were found to be similar on tests of rhythm, tempo, and intonation (Shadden, Asp, Tonkovich, & Mason, 1980), but lack of controls for therapy in the study makes interpretation of the data difficult.

Reliability

Reliability refers to the extent to which a test provides a measure of speech behavior which is relatively invariable. In a sense, reliability measures serve to calibrate an examiner's responses. Several sources can undermine reliability by contributing to variability in testing. These include subject variability, examiner variability, and subject-examiner variability.

Subject Variability

At least two factors may produce variability in an individual's articulation. One of these is the status of the individual due to such temporary conditions as fatigue and emotional state. Changes in these conditions from test to test could produce different results in articulation measures. A critical variability factor for children is the time span of speech sound development. If tests are repeated across a relatively long period of time, improvements in articulation measures may occur simply because of development. Articulation tests given within a short time span should not be influenced by development, as indicated by the findings on group articulation scores obtained within seven or eight days (Templin, 1947a; Siegel, 1962; Winitz, 1963). But fatigue and emotional state could change within a week and influence articulation, which may explain the intrasubject variability found for kindergarten children on specific sounds (Winitz, 1963).

Examiner Variability

In order to determine whether an examiner's perceptual judgments are accurate, there must be calibration both within and between judges. Such measures are referred to as intrajudge reliability and interjudge reliability. Both sources of variance are susceptible to the examiner's biases, which may include the age and sex of the subject, the etiology of the problem, and an examiner's knowledge of acoustic and perceptual phonetics. For example, the knowledge that boys make significantly more articulation errors than girls could influence an examiner toward the identification of more sound errors in boys than in girls (Kenney et al., 1984). Similarly, if a child has a cleft palate, the examiner may perceive hypernasality whether or not it is present. And transcriptions may differ when the intended word is known or unknown (Oller & Eilers, 1975).

Several factors in addition to examiner bias can influence scores. The method of performing judgments should be kept constant from one session to the next. Although Henderson (1938) found intrajudge reliability to be 90–98% for judgments made from audiotapes, others have found agreement to be lower for judgments made first from a live transcription and then from an audio recording (Wright, 1954). Subjects' responses may be different if they are first given a spontaneous naming test and then an imitation test (Snow & Milisen, 1954).

The system of notation employed in intrajudge reliability measures can affect scores substantially. When intrajudge scores were computed on correct or incorrect judgments, 90% to 100% self-agreement values were obtained, but these fell to 82% to 97% for the specification of articulation errors (Norris, Harden, & Bell, 1980).

Interjudge reliability is influenced by factors similar to those for intrajudge reliability. When judgments are based on the simple correct or incorrect notational system, agreement between examiners is generally above 80% (Henderson, 1938; Norris et al., 1980). The level of reliability is not as high for judgments of error responses only, and when the type of error is judged, reliability tends to drop even further. Mean reliability in one study for substitution of an English phoneme, substitution of a sound comprising features not characteristic of an English phoneme, and error type (weighted average of agreement for specification of types of features in error) was 76%, 63%, and 71%, respectively (Norris et al., 1980). Place and manner of articulation of the sounds being judged also influence the level of interjudge reliability in ways difficult to interpret but voicing has no influence.

One other parameter that can influence reliability is the method of scoring. The two methods of scoring are point-to-point agreement and overall comparison of judgments. To determine the percentage of point-to-point agreement, the number of items agreed on by both judges is divided by the total number of items judged. To determine overall agreement, the number of items judged correct and incorrect by both judges is divided by the total number of items judged. An example shows the difference between methods. In a ten-item articulation test, examiner A found 9 correct and 1 incorrect, while examiner B found 8 correct and 2 incorrect. But their correct and incorrect judgments were in agreement on only 7 of the items. Thus, the overall agreement is 90% (8 items correct plus 1 item incorrect), but the point-to-point agreement is 70%. Using an 85% criterion to assess the agreement between A and B (Bernthal & Bankson, 1988), reliability is sufficient according to the overall comparison, but insufficient according to the point-to-point comparison.

The importance of establishing intrajudge and interjudge reliability relates to both diagnostic and therapeutic issues. In the diagnostic identification of error features, it is necessary to establish whether they are consensus identifications both within and across listeners. From a clinical perspective, the stability of judgments about potentially changing or moving sound targets must be established both within and across listeners. Interjudge and intrajudge pretreatment reliability scores should be obtained, as well as interjudge post-treatment reliability scores. If a low interjudge reliability score is obtained, evaluate the criteria and standards used in making decisions with the other examiner and then redo the test. If agreement is still low, then bring in a third observer. Some suggest that less than 80% to 90% agreement is unacceptable, while others set the level at 70% agreement (Shriberg & Kent, 1982; Bernthal & Bankson, 1988). (See Appendix E for transcription tests to use in assessing reliability of normal and abnormal speech.)

Subject-Examiner Variability

In any situation that requires the interaction of two individuals, the interpersonal dynamics of the meeting can influence speech behavior, and this is true as well of the subject-examiner relationship (Winitz, 1969). There are few data on this factor because of the difficulty of quantifying its effects. Certain factors that influence rapport and test performance include physical anomalies and the severity of the subject's articulation disorder. Subjects with orofacial anomalies and severe articulation errors may receive negative or limited feedback, which could influence their speech behavior. Children's test performance can change if the examiner's overt and/or covert reactions influence the children's articulatory behavior (Siegel, 1962).

PROGNOSTIC FACTORS: CONSISTENCY AND STIMULABILITY

In the phonetic analysis of normal speech, production variations rarely alter the phonemic identity of a sound. Those who misarticulate speech, however, may produce variations in a target sound over time. Although the basis of diachronic changes in production may be unclear, they must be accurately identified and assessed, particularly during the therapeutic process. One view is that through sound consistency and stimulability testing, a measure of reliability can be obtained during the therapeutic process which helps differentiate diachronic variations in sound targets from changes due to therapy.

Consistency

Consistency refers to the frequency of occurrence of the same misarticulated sound. Although the term is generally defined in this way, it can also be used to describe how correctly a sound is produced when repeated in the same context. In the most extreme cases, the sound is never produced correctly and never approximates the target. Two assumptions form the theoretical basis of sound consistency. First, sounds produced incorrectly in all contexts are less amenable to remediation than those that are produced correctly in some contexts. Second, certain contexts are more conducive to correct sound production than others. Contexts in which a sound is produced correctly or the target is approximated are usually considered appropriate for the initiation of therapy.

Children who inconsistently misarticulate sounds may be more amenable to the improvement of error sounds than children who consistently misarticulate speech sounds (Brungard, 1961; Ryan, 1969). Error consistency, however, does not appear to be linearly related to improvement for children grouped according to high (22.7), average (11.0), and low (1.3) mean error levels for /v/ (Baer & Winitz, 1968). As shown in Figure 12–2, significantly less improvement as a function of training on /v/ was observed for the high and the average groups compared to the low group, but the high and the average groups did not differ.

The influence of context on production tends to support the notion that sound inconsistency can be explained on the basis that sounds are easier to produce in some contexts than in others (Sharf & Ohde, 1981). Two hypotheses imply a relationship between sound consistency and sound context. First, due to coarticulatory influences, error sounds are more likely to occur in the context of certain sounds than in the context of others. Second, due to coarticulatory influences, it is easier to achieve correction of an error sound in certain sound contexts than in others. There is general support for the first hypothesis, but to our knowledge no data are available to support or disprove the second hypothesis.

The implication of these hypotheses is that there is a need to test for error sound production due to context. Some changes in articulation may relate as much to contextual facilitation as to therapeutic intervention. Several kinds of tests have been used to examine the influence of context on the consistency of articulation errors. Conversational samples may be used, but for reasons cited earlier they may not adequately test the particular sounds and contexts. An early formal test designed to assess sound context systematically was the Deep Test of Articulation (McDonald, 1964a). The Deep Test examines the effects of adjacent sounds on consonant articulation through two-word utterances. For children who misarticulate /s/, for example, one might predict more accurate production of /s/ in 'hatsun' than in 'capsun' because of the compatible alveolar feature of /t/ and /s/.

The Sound Production Task is another procedure used to assess systematically the influence of context on consistency. Its design relies in part on the Deep

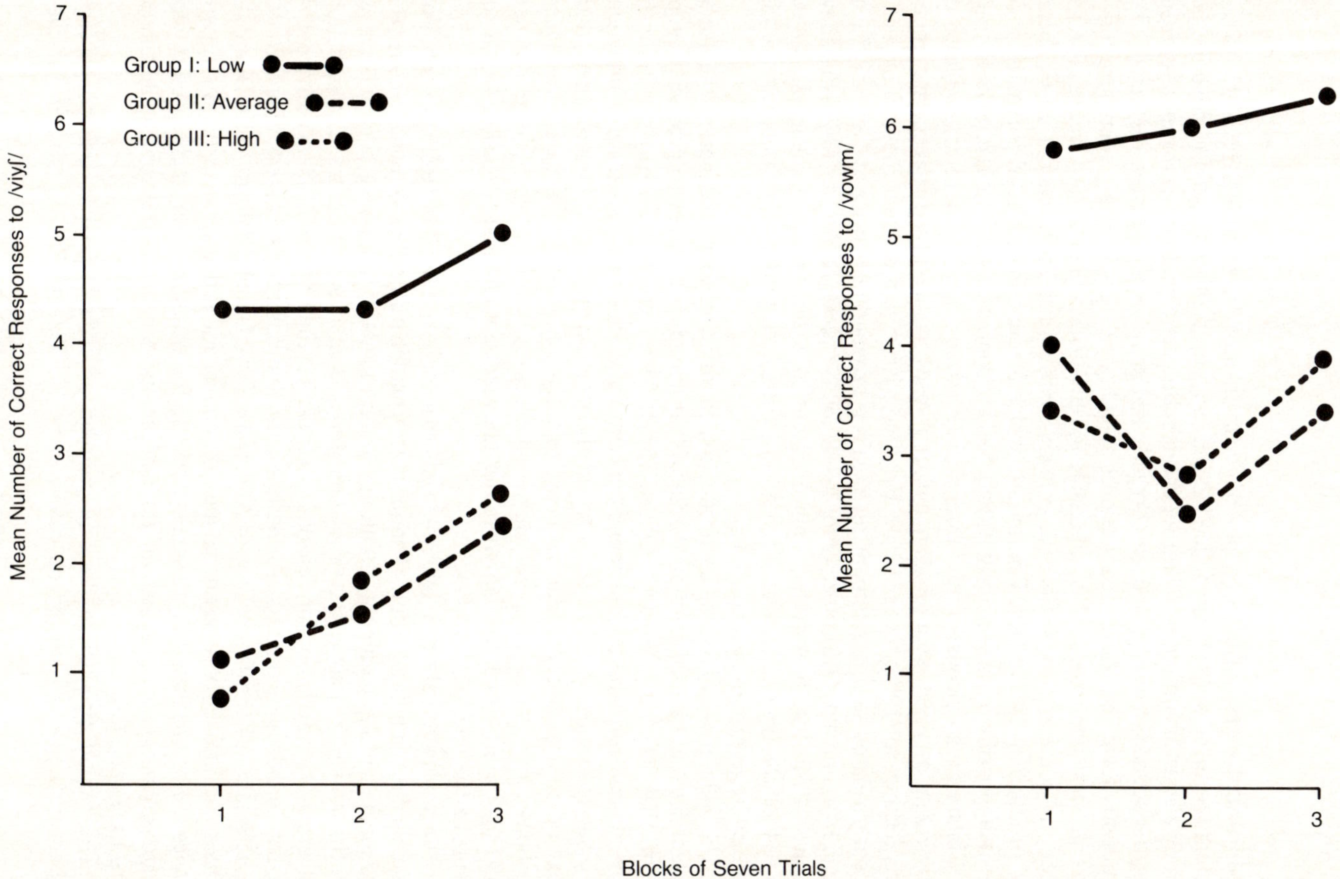

Figure 12–2
Mean acquisition curves for the test syllables /v i y ʃ/ (left panel) and /v o w m/ (right panel) for three groups of subjects divided according to their frequency of /v/ errors.

Source: "Acquisition of /v/ in 'Words' as a Function of the Consistency of /v/ Errors" by W. P. Baer and H. Winitz, 1968, *Journal of Speech and Hearing Research, 11,* p. 330. Copyright 1968 by the American Speech-Language-Hearing Association. Reprinted with permission.

Test (Elbert, Shelton, & Arndt, 1967). This test examines sound production in a number of different contexts ranging from the isolated sound to the sound in conversation. Table 12–5 shows how /s/ is examined alone and in syllables, words, and phrases.

Although the evidence is not unequivocal, there is reason to assume that inconsistency of error production indicates a greater potential for improvement of articulatory skills, and that certain contexts may produce greater improvement than others. These assumptions can be used as a basis for planning therapy. Remedial techniques based on these assumptions, however, may not work any better than other remedial techniques.

Table 12–5
An example of the Sound Production Task test for /s/ (Elbert et al., 1967). When /s/ appears in isolation or in nonsense syllables, phonetic transcriptions are provided. For words, phrases, or sentences, transcriptions of sounds preceding and following /s/ are provided to the right of the target utterance (# indicates an intervening word boundary).

Production Contexts for /s/	
Isolation/ Syllables	**Words/Phrases/ Sentences**
/us/	musty /ʌst/
/sæ/	household /aʊsh/
/s/	glasszoo /æsz/
/sɑ/	I'm on your side /r#sɑɪ/
/is/	placemat /esm/
	missing /ɪsɪ/
	The dog sits up /g#sɪ/
	houseknife /ɑʊsn/
	I will get some /t#sʌ/
	Bob sent me /b#sɛ/
	busboy /ʌsb/
	classday /sde/
	Please breathe softly /ð#sɔ/
	He has on a clean suit /n#su/
	pass that /s#ðæ/
	iceroom /sru/
	Will he be home soon /m#su/
	husky /ʌsk/
	Will you be up Sunday /p#sʌ/
	asleep /əsl/
	Who took his seat /z#si/
	I like soup /k#su/
	The dress is all silk /l#sɪ/
	icewater /ɑɪsw/
	I lost my red socks /d#sɑ/

Stimulability

Stimulability is the ability of an individual to imitate the correct production of a sound he/she misarticulates. Stimulability may result in subjects' superior performance on articulation tests involving imitation of auditory stimuli, as compared with those involving spontaneous naming of pictures or reading of words. Along with error consistency, stimulability testing has been viewed as an important parameter in the diagnosis, prognosis, and therapeutic intervention of articulation disorders (Diedrich, 1983). On the basis of imitation testing, about 74% correct predictions for improvement were obtained for first-grade children with articulation disorders (Carter & Buck, 1958).

There has been interest in the relationship between stimulability and error consistency. A particular concern is whether data from either of these parameters sufficiently characterizes the articulatory potential of a speaker. A significant correlation has been found between the Deep Test of Articulation (McDonald, 1964a) and the Carter and Buck (1958) test of stimulability for /s/ (Lapko & Bankson, 1975). These data suggest that high stimulability scores may eliminate the need for contextual testing. Others have come to similar conclusions with respect to therapy. For children who are highly stimulable, context may be relatively unimportant in the therapeutic process (Zehel et al., 1972; Moore, Burke, & Adams, 1976; Elbert & McReynolds, 1978).

Research findings on stimulability are controversial. Some studies have found that children with articulation disorders perform better on an imitative test than on either spontaneous picture or word tests (Snow & Milisen, 1954; Farquhar, 1961; Smith & Ainsworth, 1967; Sommers et al., 1967), while others have found no difference between imitative and spontaneous picture tests (Templin, 1947b; Paynter & Bumpas, 1977). The range of differences in methodology across studies, coupled with the diverse causes of articulation disorders, are most probably the primary contributors to variability in the results of stimulability studies.

Critical to the issue of stimulability testing are the basis of the change in sound production from spontaneous to imitative and the relationship of this change to articulatory improvement. A simple view of this change is that the child demonstrates the capability of performing the motor gestures associated with a particular sound. This interpretation suggests that the basis of the change in stimulability testing is phonetic, because of the ability of the child appropriately to modify the neuromotor gestures associated with an error sound and to produce the correct target features (Turton, 1973). According to this view, stimulability lends no insights into the integrity of the phonemic system. But another view sees stimulability functions as representing knowledge of the phonemic system. Stimulability measures may show either absence of phonemic competence (Pollack & Rees, 1972) or presence of phonemic competence (Dinnsen & Elbert, 1984; Best & Wilkenfeld, 1988). In this view, high stimulability occurs when the child has the correct underlying representations of the target sound features, and the child's productions demonstrate a relatively high level of phonological cognition.

If high stimulability scores represent both phonetic capability and phonemic competence, then a relatively rapid generalization of articulatory skills to spontaneous speech can be predicted during therapy. As shown in Figure 12–3, a study of the relationship between spontaneous speech (TALK) and stimulability (SPT) during therapy did not support this prediction for most children (Diedrich & Bangert, 1980). Generally, the children followed the patterns of little or inconsistent relationship or of very gradual but close relationship in the development of skills ("Immediate" in the figure). Some children supported the prediction by following the pattern of rapidly improving the production of their error sounds, but only several weeks after achieving high stimulability scores ("Delayed").

At a minimum, stimulability testing provides information on the phonetic capability of a speaker. The relationship between stimulability and change in articulatory behavior during therapy is less clear. Although it is logical to infer that good stimulability indicates a more advanced stage of sound development than poor stimulability, empirically there is only indirect support for this inference. The following clinical implications of stimulability testing have been proposed (Madison, 1979): (1) priority should be given to highly stimulable sounds in isolation; (2) self-correction may occur for children who are highly stimulable on syllables and words; and (3) for children highly stimulable on syllables and words, intervention is likely to be successful.

PHONETIC MODIFICATION USED IN ARTICULATION THERAPY

In planning sound modification intervention strategies, speech and language pathologists use their phonetic knowledge and skills to modify error sound production. Three procedures are commonly used: progressive approximation, phonetic facilitation, and phonetic placement. Progressive approximation is closely linked to the principles of facilitating contexts previously reviewed and is based on the approximation of a target sound from correctly produced sounds that share certain features. For example, the target for the error sound /s/ can be approximated from /t/, with which it shares voiceless and apico-alveolar features. Spectrograms of /z/ and sounds that share the alveolar feature with it /d, n/ are shown in figures 12–4 and 12–5 for a child and an adult. The voiced cognates of /t/ and /s/ were analyzed because the duration of the formant transitions is longer for them than for voiceless sounds. Note that the position and the trajectory of change in the F_2 transition, which is influenced most by changes in tongue position, are quite similar for the three sounds in a given vowel context. Thus, for children who misarticulate /s/ and /z/, it is not surprising that some intervention strategies begin with the /t/ or /d/ sounds which are produced correctly.

In a particular session a child may be asked to produce /t/ rapidly a number of times and then prolong the last production into /s/. Conceptually, this type of intervention is similar to the phonetic context approach utilized in the diagnosis of articulatory disorders (McDonald, 1964a). The difference is that progressive approximation begins with isolated sounds, whereas the diagnostic approach to phonetic context utilizes disyllabic utterances.

The second procedure based on phonetic knowledge is phonetic facilitation, or the use of a particular context to facilitate correct production of an error sound. For

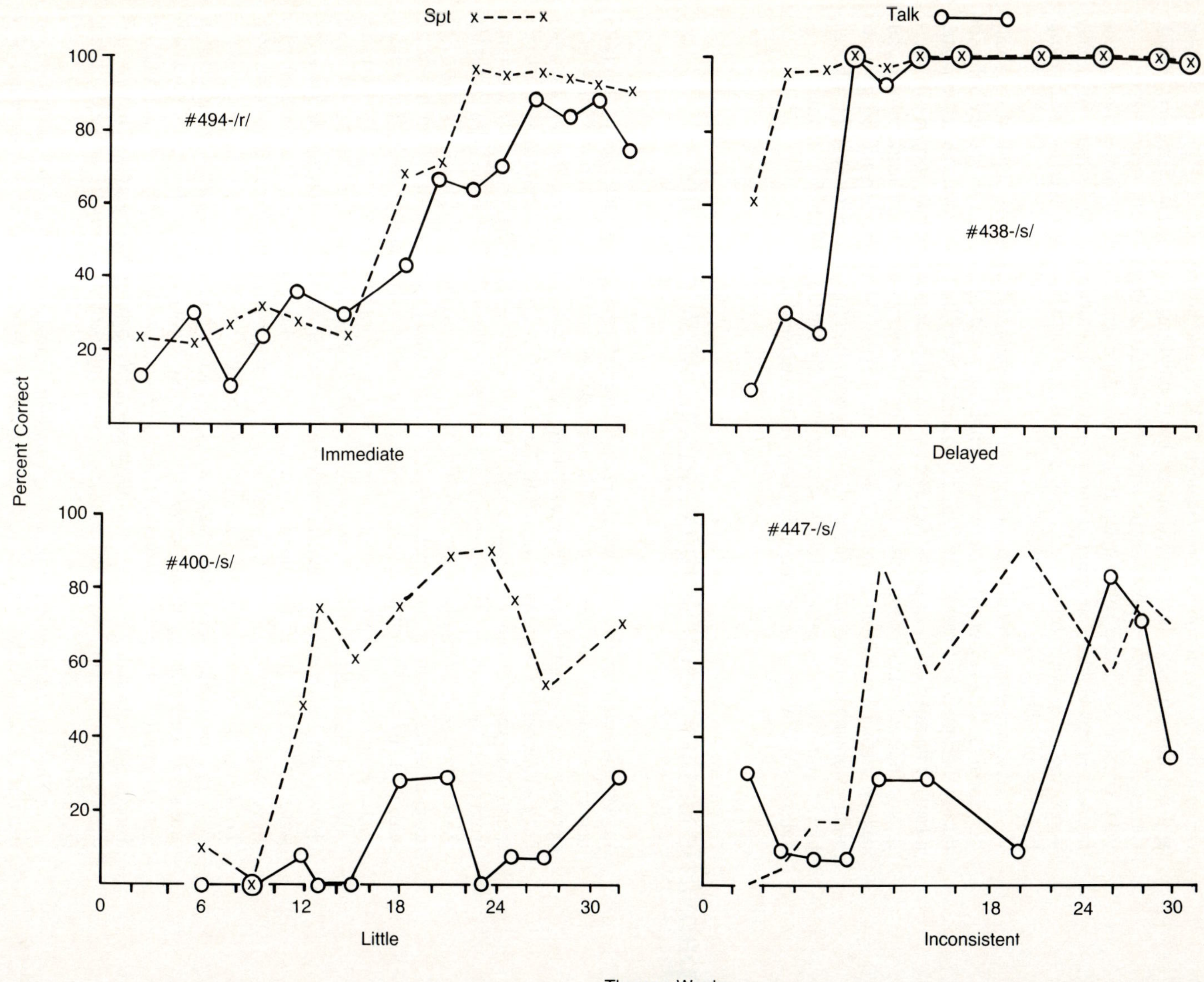
Spt x - - - - x
Talk o——o
Percent Correct
#494-/r/
Immediate
#438-/s/
Delayed
#400-/s/
Little
#447-/s/
Inconsistent
Therapy Weeks
100
80
60
40
20
0
6
12
18
24
30

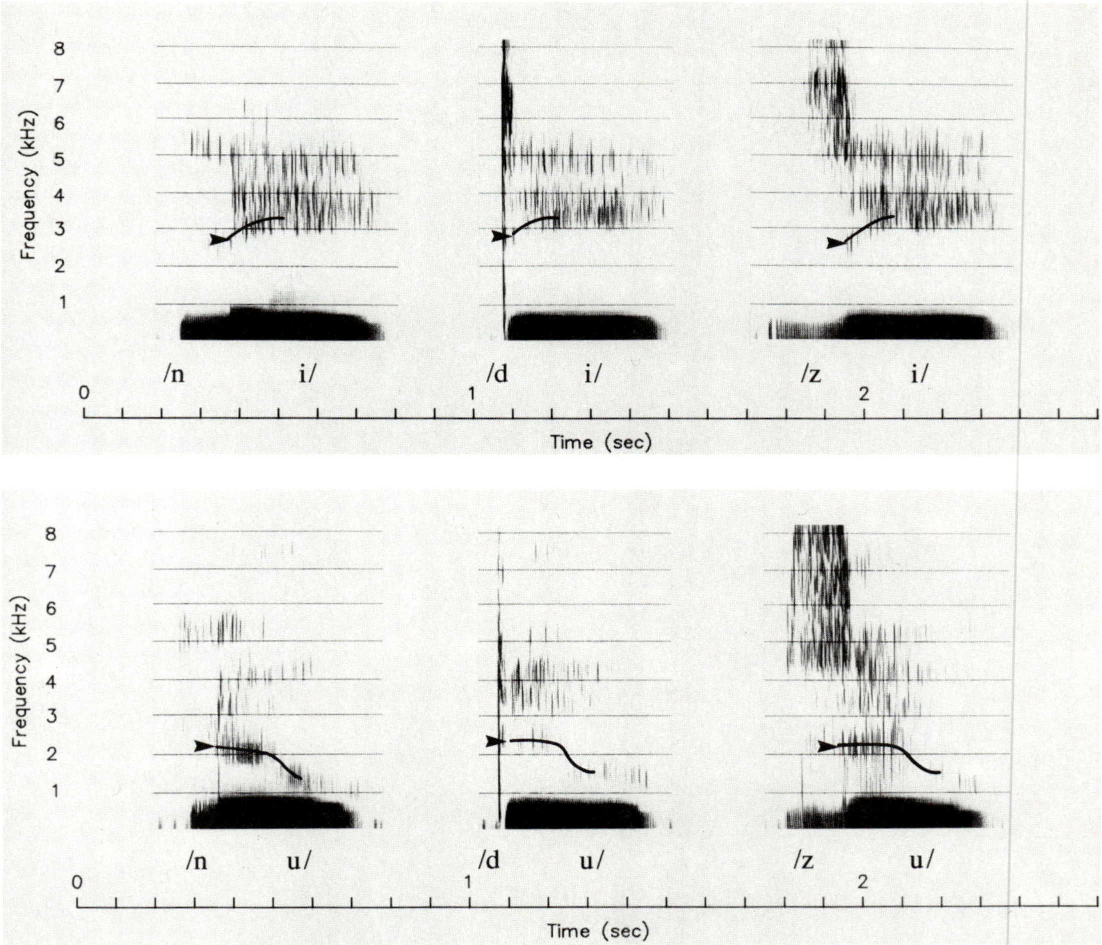

Figure 12–4
Spectrograms of /n i/, /d i/, and /z i/ (top panel), and /n u/, /d u/, and /z u/ (bottom panel) produced by a child. Arrows along the *y* axis (ordinate) indicate the onset frequency of the second formant (F_2), and lines along both *y* and *x* axes indicate the trajectory of change in F_2.

Figure 12–3
Four classes of error sound generalization to spontaneous speech (TALK) as a function of therapy. SPT (imitative or stimulability) and TALK probes were systematically sampled throughout therapy. Panels represent examples of subjects fitting the following four patterns: Immediate—correct sound production in imitative and spontaneous speech was nearly identical; delayed—correct sound production in spontaneous speech lagged several weeks behind imitative speech; little—improvement in correct sound production occurred in imitative speech but not in spontaneous speech; and inconsistent— improvement in correct sound production was particularly erratic in spontaneous speech.

Source: Articulation Learning (p. 212) by W. M. Diedrich and J. Bangert, 1980, San Diego: College-Hill Press. Copyright 1980 by College-Hill Press. Reprinted with permission.

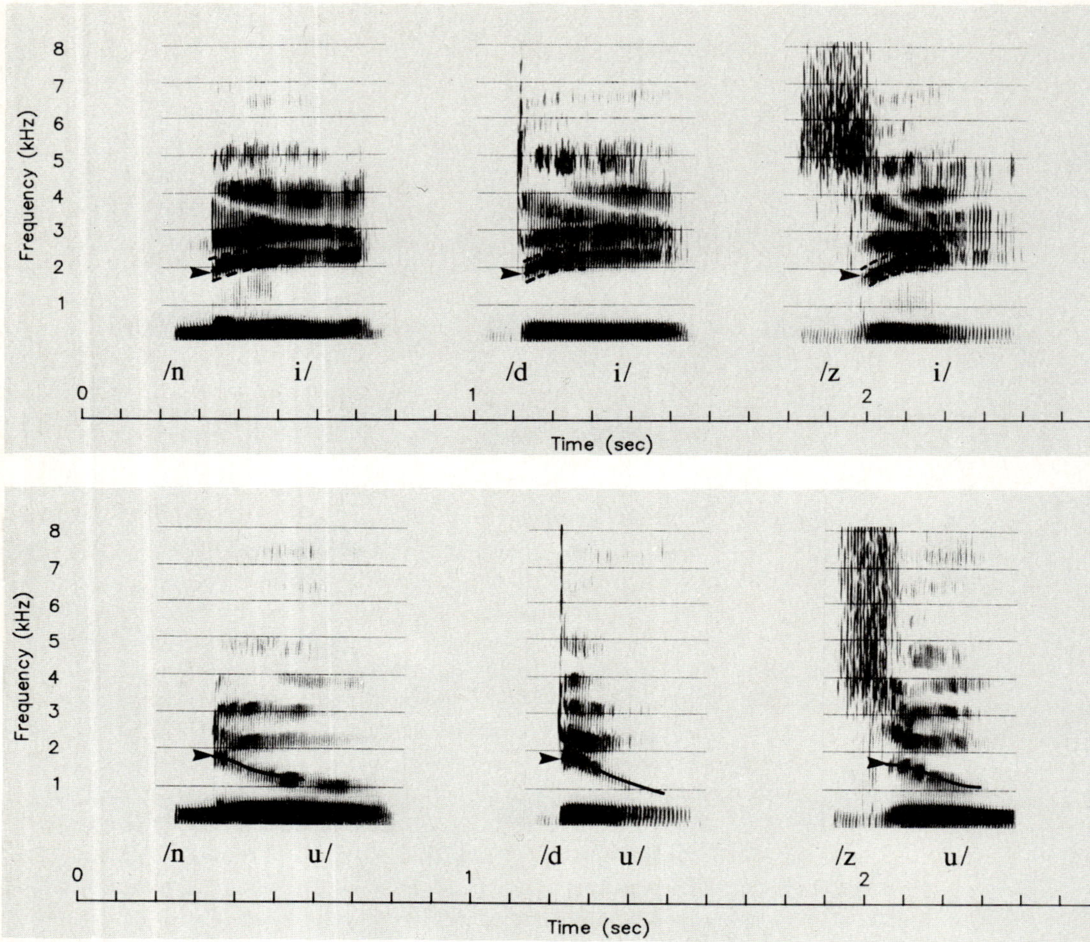

Figure 12–5
Spectrograms of /n i/, /d i/, and /z i/ (top panel), and /n u/, /d u/, and /z u/ (bottom panel) produced by an adult male. Arrows along the *y* axis indicate the onset frequency of the second formant (F_2), and lines along both *y* and *x* axes indicate the trajectory of change in F_2. For /i/, dashed lines along the border of F_2 are also included, because the relative intensity of this formant obscures the single line.

example, /s/ production is initiated in the /s/ plus /t/ context provided by the cluster in a word like 'stew' rather than in the /s/ plus vowel context provided by a word like 'sigh' (see Gallagher & Shriner, 1975a, 1975b). Although phonetic facilitation presumably works because of compatibility between features of a target sound and an adjacent one, not all research supports it. It has been found that /p/ facilitates correct production of /s/ and /r/ even though it shares no critical place of articulation feature with /s/ or /r/ (Curtis & Hardy, 1959; Swisher, 1973; Gallagher & Shriner, 1975a; Elbert & McReynolds, 1978; Mazza et al., 1979). Facilitation in such cases may occur because of minimal contextual interference with the place of articulation feature of the target sound (Kent, 1982).

One other caution relates to the multifactorial nature of articulatory disorders. For any misarticulated sound, a number of different articulatory disorders may be observed. Chapter 8 described three categories of lisps for /s/ and /z/—protruded, dentalized, and lateralized. The principle of sound feature compatibility does not differentiate among these disorder types, and correction for /s/ would in all probability start with /t/ for the entire lisp category. It is possible that different errors require an intervention approach as diversified as the disorder types observed for a particular sound.

The third procedure based on phonetic knowledge is phonetic placement. In using this procedure the therapist gives specific instructions for positioning articulators for a target sound and/or tactile and biofeedback cues to indicate sound target position. For example, a child who misarticulates /s/ is asked to raise his/her tongue so that the sides contact the upper back teeth, then is directed to position the tongue tip just behind the upper or lower front teeth, and finally is asked to direct the airstream toward the cutting edges of the front teeth. These instructions are based on our knowledge of the physiological events and the features that comprise apico-alveolar sounds.

The modification strategies reviewed here could be classified as static. Clinicians facilitate the correct production of error sounds in isolation or in positions of limited linguistic complexity. Variations in context and linguistic complexity will most probably produce changes in target sound positions, and the attainment of these target sound positions may be complicated by the type of articulation disorder for a particular sound. In facilitating correct productions with these modification strategies, one must be mindful of both speech context and the type of articulatory disorder giving rise to a particular sound.

GLOSSARY

Addition. Insertion of an additional phoneme in a word; a misarticulation.

Allophonic rules. Rules governing the occurrence of variants of a sound in different contexts.

Articulation norms. Age levels at which most children produce sounds correctly.

Articulation test. A systematic evaluation of the phoneme production of a speaker, usually through a set of pictures representing words with consonants and consonant clusters in various positions; vowels and diphthongs are also frequently evaluated.

Consistency. The extent to which an individual produces a misarticulated sound in different contexts, or, less frequently, how often a misarticulated sound is repeated in the same context.

Distinctive feature. A speech sound characteristic described according to a relatively small inventory of binary descriptive terms. Originally devised primarily for the use of linguists in describing the structure of different languages but also used as a basis for the analysis of misarticulations.

Distinctive feature analysis. A systematic evaluation of misarticulations in terms of binary features. Designed to find patterns of common error features.

Distortion. A nonallophonic variation of a target sound but not another phoneme; a misarticulation.

Dynamic rules. Rules which serve to alter the production of sounds in various contexts. May be allophonic rules or neutralization rules.

Generative phonological analysis. A procedure to determine the phonological knowledge of a child using a linguistic methodology which evaluates him/her as an independent system.

Generative phonological test. A systematic evaluation of a child's phonological development, sometimes including phonemic inventories but always including conversational analyses, in which the child's speech is usually considered an entity independent of the correct underlying adult forms.

Homonymity. The loss of distinction between two or more words. Results from the use of phonological processes, as when final consonant devoicing causes 'pick' and 'pig' to be pronounced alike.

Phonological process analysis. A procedure in which sound variations are characterized according to patterns of production. Its theoretical assumption is that phonological processes are simplifications of adult phonology, and that the child knows the adult target form but produces an easier sound or deletes one or more sounds.

Phonological process test. A systematic evaluation of the use of phonological processes by children through whole-word responses elicited by naming objects and/or pictures, by single-word delayed imitation tasks, or by sampling continuous speech.

Screening articulation test. A short test of the ability of an individual to produce speech sounds, usually those that are most frequently misarticulated.

Segmental analysis. The evaluation of individual error sounds or misarticulations as single entities requiring intervention. Often includes the analysis of multiple articulation errors according to place, voicing, and manner of articulation.

Static rules. Rules of phonotactic constraints which can either restrict the production of sounds in certain word positions or sequences or entirely exclude the production of other sounds.

Stimulability. An individual's ability to imitate the correct production of a sound he/she misarticulates.

REVIEW QUESTIONS

A. Indicate which descriptions most accurately characterize each of the following assessment procedures: a = segmental; b = distinctive feature; c = phonological process; d = generative phonological.

1. Binary distinctions ____________________
2. Morphophonemic alternations ____________________
3. Sound simplification ____________________

4. Traditional approach ____________

5. Limited utility for sound distortions ____________

6. Based on a theory of Natural Phonology ____________

7. Phonotactic constraints ____________

8. Phoneme production ____________

****

Key: 1. b; 2. d; 3. c; 4. a; 5. b; 6. c; 7. d; 8. a

B. Indicate if the statements below about diagnostic factors are true (T) or false (F).

1. ________ Transcription of live articulation tends to be more accurate than transcription of audiotapes.

2. ________ Narrow transcription is a more thorough notational system than broad transcription.

3. ________ The transcriptions /rɛ/ and [rɛ:] reflect the same level of phonological cognition of final consonant voicing.

4. ________ Validity requires evidence that a test provides a representative sample of speech.

5. ________ A conversational sample is generally not considered a critical part of a speech evaluation.

6. ________ It is generally not important to test a particular sound more than once.

7. ________ Certain sound contexts may interfere with the correct production of a misarticulated sound.

8. ________ A reliable articulation test provides a measure of speech behavior which is relatively invariable.

9. ________ Temporal variability has no effect on articulation scores.

10. ________ Reliability judgments are not influenced by type of notational system.

****

Key: 1. T; 2. T; 3. F; 4. T; 5. F; 6. F; 7. T; 8. T; 9. F; 10. F

C. Indicate if the statements below about prognosis and phonetic modification are true (T) or false (F).

1. ________ Children who inconsistently produce an error sound may show more improvement from therapy than children who consistently produce an error sound.

2. ________ There are no diagnostic tests which attempt to assess the effects of sound context on articulation.

3. ________ Only one procedure has been used in calculating stimulability scores across studies.

4. ________ High stimulability scores have been interpreted as support for phonetic knowledge only.

5. ________ High stimulability scores for sounds in syllables and words may indicate success in therapy.

6. ________ Not all sound contexts that facilitate correct production of error sounds are composed of the most compatible phonetic features.

7. ________ There is no need to be concerned about the type of articulatory disorder for a particular sound when applying the principles of sound compatibility in intervention strategies.

****

Key: 1. T; 2. F; 3. F; 4. F; 5. T; 6. T; 7. F

APPENDIX A

Terminology of Articulatory/Phonological Disorders

In this appendix, brief descriptions are given of articulatory and phonological disorders. Text locations for more thorough coverage of these terms are given in the Subject Index.

OMISSIONS

SYLLABLE REDUCTION

Syllable reduction is a syllable simplification process. It functions to reduce VCV and CVCV words to CV words and CVCVCV words to CVCV words by eliminating the initial syllable or the vowel in it. For example, 'away,' 'potato,' and 'believe' are pronounced as 'way,' 'tato,' and 'blieve.' The syllable reduction process may also influence VCV and CVCV words with weak stress on the second syllable, as in 'ted' for 'teddy,' and it occurs also in polysyllabic CVCVCV words like 'banana,' shortened to 'nana.' This process does not occur after four years of age in the speech of normally developing children (Ingram, 1976).

CLUSTER REDUCTION

Cluster reduction is a phonological process in which children simplify complex consonant combinations by deleting one or more of the consonants or by substituting another consonant for one of those in the cluster (Ingram, 1976). It has been proposed that children pass through the following four stages as they develop the ability to produce clusters (Greenlee, 1974): (1) the entire cluster is omitted, as in /ɑ p/ for 'stop'; (2) one of the consonants is eliminated, as in /t ɑ p/ for 'stop'; (3) the previously deleted consonant is replaced by another, as in /θ t ɑ p/ for 'stop'; (4) the correct cluster is produced. Although cluster reduction is characteristic of normal development, it is not clear that all children go through four stages. Cluster reduction frequently occurs in the speech of children with abnormal articulation (Khan, 1982). A large number of cluster reductions involve /s/ deletions, as in the following: /dip/ for 'sleep'; /pɑt/ for 'spot'; /mɔ/ for 'small'; /dɛk/ for 'desk.'

FINAL (POSTVOCALIC) CONSONANT DELETION

Final consonant deletion is a syllable simplification process by which VC and CVC syllables are reduced to V and CV syllables. For example, 'bed' becomes /bɛ/, and 'beat' becomes /bi/. Although many children omit final consonants, it is not always clear that the omissions constitute a phonological process. Clarification of the question requires evidence of cognition on the part of the child that a final consonant is present in a word. Such evidence could be one or both of the following: (1) the child deletes the /t/ in 'eat' but includes it in 'eating'; (2) the child differentiates words like 'beat' and 'bead' from which he/she omits the final consonants by making the vowel longer in 'bead' than in 'beat.' Evidence of vowel lengthening has been noted in acoustic analyses of children who delete final consonants. Deletion of final stops, for example, /bi/ for 'bead,' and deletion of final fricatives, for example, /lu/ for 'lose,' is a complex process since it involves the elimination of the contrast between the closed and open syllables 'bee'/'bead' and 'Lou'/'lose,' as well as the elimination of the voicing contrast, 'bead'/'beat' and 'lose'/'loose.' This process is commonly found in the speech of misarticulating children (Ingram, 1976). Acoustic studies have shown that some of these children use differential vowel duration to signal the voicing of final stops (Weismer, Dinnsen, & Elbert, 1981; Weismer, 1984). This evidence, plus the children's use of morphophonemic alternations, such as [pɪ:] for 'pig' and /pɪgi/ for 'piggy,' suggests that they have an underlying knowledge that 'pig' includes a final consonant (Weismer et al., 1981; Elbert & Gierut, 1986).

STRIDENCY DELETION

Stridency deletion covers a number of phonological processes that influence the strident sounds /f, v, s, z, ʃ, ʒ, tʃ, dʒ/, including initial consonant deletion, final consonant deletion, cluster reduction, deaffrication, and stopping. Stridency deletion is a common symptom of disordered phonology (Hodson & Paden, 1983). Omissions occur for stridents as a function of initial consonant deletion in /op/ for 'soap,' final consonant deletion in /haʊ/ for 'house,' and cluster reduction in /tɑp/ for 'stop.' Substitutions occur for stridents as a function of stopping in /pɔɚk/ for 'fork,' and deaffrication in /tɛɚ/ for 'chair' (Hodson & Paden, 1983).

PLACE SUBSTITUTIONS

FRONTAL LISP

The frontal lisp is one of the three major types of lisp; it is also called a protruded lisp in this book. In this misarticulation the tongue tip is in position for /θ/, so that /θ/ is substituted for /s/ and /ð/ is substituted for /z/. This type of lisp results in the loss of phonemic distinction in minimal pairs like 'some' and 'thumb' and 'close' (verb) and 'clothe.' The intensity of the high frequency noise characteristic of sibilants is lost.

GLIDING

The phonological process of gliding applies to /l/ and /r/. For /r/, gliding involves the substitution of /w/ for the /r/ onglide in words like 'round' and 'around.' For the /l/ onglide, the substitution may involve /w/ or /j/. Although the process is not completely predictable in all children, /w/ may more often replace /l/ when it precedes back vowels, as in 'low' and 'below,' and /j/ may more often replace /l/ when it precedes front vowels, as in 'leave,' 'lip,' and 'believe.' In earlier terminology these errors were always described as substitutions. Current terminology characterizes them as gliding errors.

PALATALIZATION

Palatalization, depalatalization, and fronting are related phonological processes. All involve changes in place of articulation for fricatives and affricates. Palatalization involves the substitution of the palatal for the alveolar fricative, as in /ʃop/ for 'soap.' This substitution results in the loss of distinction in minimal pairs like 'sew' and 'show.'

DEPALATALIZATION

Depalatalization is the reverse of palatalization in that 'watch' may be pronounced as /wɑts/ and 'shoes' as /suz/. The distinction in minimal pairs like 'cats'/'catch' and 'sue'/'shoe' is lost.

FRONTING

Fronting is a phonological process that results in the substitution of alveolar for velar stops, as in /do/ for 'go.' There is nothing in the context to explain the substitution. Fronting is relatively common among children with the most severe articulatory disorders (Hodson & Paden, 1983).

DENTALIZING

In words where apico-alveolar sounds abut /θ/ or /ð/, dentalizing occurs allophonically, as in 'health,' in which dentalized /l/ is an allophone of the /l/ phoneme. Some speakers dentalize apico-alveolar sounds no matter where they occur in context, an abnormal pattern. The difference between alveolar and dental sounds is not always easy to hear, but it is easy to see if the tongue tip protrudes between the teeth. If the tongue tip contacts the inner surface of the upper teeth, several repetitions of an utterance may be necessary to perceive the misarticulation. The dentalization of any one alveolar sound is easier to identify if it is part of a pattern that includes dentalization of all apico-alveolar consonants, /t, d, n, l, s, z/.

LABIALIZATION AND LABIAL ASSIMILATION

Labialization and labial assimilation are phonological processes that cause alveolar and interdental sounds to become bilabial or labiodental. Such changes are called labialization when they cannot be accounted for by context, as in /fɪŋ/ for 'thing.' Labial assimilation, however, involves the substitution of a bilabial for another consonant occurring in the context of a bilabial consonant. For example, in /bebu/ for 'table,' /b/ is substituted for /t/ because of the influence of the following /b/; in /pɪm/ for 'pin,' /n/ changes to /m/ under the contextual influence of the /p/ sound.

BACKING AND VELAR ASSIMILATION

Backing and velar assimilation are phonological processes that cause front sounds to become back ones. Such changes are called backing when they cannot be accounted for by contextual influences, as in /k u/ for 'two.' In velar assimilation, changes are accounted for by contextual influences, as in /k w ʌ k/ for 'truck,' in which /t/ changes to /k/ under the influence of final /k/.

NEUTRALIZATION

Neutralization is a phonological process that influences vowels. For the most part, correct production of vowels is not a problem for native speakers of English. During early speech development, however, children often neutralize vowels, substituting /ɑ/ and /ʌ/ for the target vowels, as in /bɑ t/ for 'boat,' /bʌ d/ for 'bed,' and /t ʌ f/ for 'teeth.' Because data about the normal development of vowels are lacking, it is not clear when this process disappears. Some children apparently continue to neutralize beyond the age when most children are producing vowels correctly (Ingram, 1976). Although neutralization is not commonly found as a problem in children with even the most severe articulation disorders, it is used by some highly unintelligible children (Hodson & Paden, 1981).

VOCALIZATION (VOWELIZATION)

Vocalization is a phonological process that affects /r/ and /l/. Children who distort the onglide /r/ and those who substitute /w/ for /r/ tend to vocalize the offglide /r/ in 'car,' the /ɝ/ in 'bird,' and the /ɚ/ in 'father.' For the offglide /r/ in 'car' and the /ɚ/ in 'father,' children substitute a vowel like /ə/. For the /ɝ/ in 'bird,' they substitute a vowel like /ʊ/. With regard to the offglide /l/ and the syllabic [l̩], apico-alveolar contact does not occur, and a vowel like /o/ or /u/ is substituted, as in /n u d o/ or /n u d u/ for 'noodle.'

UVULARIZATION

Uvularization describes the use of dorso-uvular stops for /k/ and /g/ by hearing-impaired speakers. Hearing-impaired individuals tend to produce /k/ and /g/ sounds that range from an anterior contact at the hard palate to a posterior one at the uvula (Monsen, 1976a). Uvularization should not cause intelligibility problems because the uvular sounds will not be confused with other stops. But the substitutions will be identified as misarticulations (Monsen, 1976a).

PHARYNGEALIZATION AND GLOTTALIZATION

Since the deficient velopharyngeal mechanism of individuals with cleft palates allows air to escape posterior to the closures for bilabial, alveolar, and palatal stops, some individuals produce these sounds using closures posterior to the leaky velopharyngeal port. There are two articulatory closures used, glottal and dorsopharyngeal. In each case, air pressure can be built up by blocking air before it has a chance to escape through the nasal cavity. These problems relating to place of articulation are secondary since they are compensations for inadequate velopharyngeal closures. In using a glottal stop, cleft-palate speakers may or may not make the expected articulatory contact.

MANNER SUBSTITUTIONS

STOPPING

Stopping, affrication, and deaffrication are related phonological processes that involve changes in manner of production of fricatives and affricates by means of the substitution, addition, or deletion of a stop consonant. In addition to the common use of stops for sibilants, as in /tip/ for 'sleep' and /dibrə/ for 'zebra,' substitutions of stops can occur for any fricative, as in /tʌm/ for 'thumb,' /nɑɪp/ for 'knife,' and /dʌpo/ for 'shovel.' Apparently, normally developing children do not generally use stopping beyond the age of three (Ingram, 1976), but it is a commonly used process among older children with unintelligible speech (Hodson & Paden, 1981). Stopping results in the loss of distinction in such minimal pairs as 'sip'/'tip,' 'fat'/'pat,' 'thin'/'tin,' and 'ship'/'tip.' According to Hodson and Paden (1983), liquids and glides may also be replaced by stops.

AFFRICATION

Affrication involves the conversion of a fricative into an affricate, as in /tsop/ for 'soap' and /bɪtʃɪŋ/ for 'fishing.' As far as is known, this process involves only sibilants. Affrication results in the loss of distinction in minimal pairs like 'shop' and 'chop.'

DEAFFRICATION

Deaffrication is the reverse of affrication in that an affricate is converted to a fricative, as in /ʒus/ for 'juice' and /ʃɪn/ for 'chin.' As far as is known, this process involves only the /tʃ/ and /dʒ/ affricates, leading to loss of distinction in minimal pairs like 'shin' and 'chin.' Hodson and Paden (1983) also include the loss of the sibilant in affricates as examples of deaffrication, for example, /tɛɚ/ for 'chair.'

VOICING SUBSTITUTIONS

PREVOCALIC CONSONANT VOICING

As part of normal speech development, children produce voiceless stops that do not differ from voiced stops in VOT, so that adults perceive /b/ for /p/, /d/ for /t/, and /g/ for /k/. Some children persist in these errors and are diagnosed as having misarticulations. Traditionally, errors of this type were classified as substitutions. According to phonological process terminology, however, these errors are examples of prevocalic voicing, which neutralizes the voicing distinction between sounds. This process is not confined to stop sounds; it also applies to prevocalic fricatives, as in /zup/ for 'soup.'

FINAL (POSTVOCALIC) CONSONANT DEVOICING

In using the phonological process of final consonant devoicing, children neutralize the voicing distinction between final stops so that 'pick' and 'pig,' for example, are pronounced /pɪk/. This process is apparently normal for children as old as four years (Hodson & Paden, 1983). Evidence that a child is aware of the voicing distinction takes the form of lengthening the vowel preceding a target voiced stop, as in [pɪ:k] for 'pig.' There are examples of this type of awareness in some children's speech (Ingram, 1976; Compton & Hutton, 1980; Hodson & Paden, 1983).

DISTORTIONS

LISPING

Lisping is a clinical disorder that involves sibilants; traditionally defined, it is the misarticulation of /s/ and /z/ by substituting /θ/ and /ð/ for them. This error is commonly called a frontal lisp, and it was covered under "Place Substitutions," above. The meaning of the word *lisping* has been broadened to include not only these errors of tongue protrusion but any tongue tip deviation that causes a loss of sibilant quality. There are three major types of lisps: protruded, dentalized, and lateralized. In some classification systems these are called frontal, dental, and lateral lisps. In addition to these, some other /s/ and /z/ misarticulations are classified as phonological process problems (see "Stridency Deletion", p. 326).

LATERAL LISP

The lateral lisp is one of the three major types of lisps. Production of the lateral sound /l/ involves putting the tongue in position for the first sound in 'lap' and blowing air out so that it passes over the sides of the tongue. Frication noise, which should have a slushy quality, can be increased by raising the sides of the tongue slightly. Producing the voiced equivalent requires only addition of voicing to the frication noise. Some observers believe that lateral lisping makes /s/ sound like /ʃ/ and /z/ sound like /ʒ/. Lateralizing tends to produce sibilants with less intensity and somewhat lower frequency concentration than normal. Lateral /s, z/ can be produced as bilateral or unilateral sounds, that is, with the air flowing over both sides or just one side of the tongue. Unilateral production involves raising either the right or the left margin of the tongue to block the airflow on that side. The occurrence of unilateral instead of bilateral lisps seems to have no important implications for rehabilitation.

RETROFLEX LISP

The retroflex lisp is not commonly found among native English speakers (Shriberg & Kent, 1982). Although retroflex sibilants are considered distortions in English, they occur as phonemes of some Indian languages (Heffner, 1952). Sounds are produced by arching the tongue tip up and back so that it approximates the palate posterior to the alveolar ridge. The margins of the tongue contact the palate for the retroflex sibilants, and the airflow, while not lateralized, is very diffuse because the tongue constriction opening is wide—more like that for /ʃ, ʒ/ than for /s, z/. This lisp has some of the acoustic characteristics of /ʃ/ and /ʒ/, for example, a lower frequency concentration than is characteristic of /s/ and /z/.

DENTAL LISP

For the dental lisp, the tongue tip is placed very close to the upper teeth so that the airstream is somewhat obstructed as it passes between the upper and lower teeth. This sound is similar to, if not the same as, dentalized allophones of /s, z/. These allophones normally occur in English only when /θ/ and /ð/ precede or follow /s/ and /z/. The use of dentalized variants is considered lisping when the variants occur in the production of sibilants that are not in the context of /θ/ and /ð/. Sound quality varies depending on the degree to which the tongue tip approximates the teeth. These variations may be described as whistling sounds, strident sounds, weakly articulated /ts/ or /dz/ affricates, or weak /s/ and /z/ sounds similar to /θ/ and /ð/. Dentalized /s/ and /z/ still retain their characteristic high-frequency energy, but they are weaker in intensity than the normal sibilants. Unlike the protrusion (frontal) lisp, the dental lisp does not cause the loss of phonemic distinction between sibilants and the /θ/ and /ð/ sounds. For this reason a dental lisp may not be considered as serious a problem as a frontal lisp. In some cases, individuals with a dental lisp have a complex pattern of dentalization that includes the other apico-alveolar sounds /t, d, n, l/. Dentalization of all or any of the apico-alveolar sounds tends to make the dental lisp more noticeable. Since no phonemic substitution is involved, the dental lisp is traditionally described as a distortion, that is, the use of a sound close to the correct one but with an unacceptable sound quality.

DISTORTED (DERHOTICIZED) /r/

Distorting and derhoticizing apply to the /r/ sound described by Ladefoged (1975) as rhoticized when produced normally. *Rhoticization* refers to the r-coloring that is characteristic of the auditory quality of /r/ and includes both the retroflex and the bunched productions used to achieve it. *Derhoticization* implies some degree of loss of r-quality as a result of deviation from the positions necessary for normal production and refers to the misarticulation in which a distorted /r/ substitutes for prevocalic /r/. There are considerable differences of opinion and lack of clarity about the characteristics of distorted /r/. Acoustic evidence and observation suggest that distorted /r/ production starts from the mid central vowel position of /ɜ/ rather than from /ɝ/. The /ɜ/ vowel occurs in New England and Southern American dialects in words like 'bird' and 'sir.' Its production requires a slight lowering of the tongue from the position for /ɝ/ without moving the tongue forward or backward and without changing the lip position. If you vocalize with the tongue in the /ɝ/ position and then in the /ɜ/ position, you can hear the loss of r-coloring, but each vowel still sounds like a central one. If you glide from the /ɜ/ vowel to any other vowel, for example, /e/ or /o/, you will produce the derhoticized versions of the words 'ray' and 'row.'

DELATERALIZING

As in the case of derhoticizing, delateralizing applies to prevocalic glides. In the gliding error, /w/ or /j/ substitutes for /l/ just as /w/ substitutes for /r/. But some children produce /l/ without tongue tip contact by starting from a position close to the /ɪ/ or /ʊ/ vowel. The resulting glides differ from /w/ by not having rounded lips or high back vowel quality and from /j/ by not having high front vowel quality. Although delateralizing may give the impression that no sound replaces /l/, you can reassure yourself that this is not the case by comparing words like 'ate' and 'late' produced by a child. If delateralizing is not present, and the child is omitting /l/, then these words should sound the same. If the child says 'wait' for 'late,' then the problem is gliding rather than delateralizing. Delateralized 'late' does not sound like 'ate' or 'wait.'

NASALIZATION/DENASALIZATION

Some speakers, such as those with cleft palates, nasalize all vowels, no matter what the context. This type of nasalization generally involves a large opening between the oral and nasal cavities during most if not all of the vowels. Because the problem is an articulatory or phonetic one, all vowels and glides are nasalized in all contexts. Nasalized vowels occur in the speech of children demonstrating the phonological process disorder of cluster reduction when they simplify nasal consonant plus stop clusters that occur in words like 'lamp' and 'plant' by deleting the nasal consonant. These children may nasalize the preceding vowel (Compton & Hutton, 1980). Such nasalization should be noted because it provides evidence that the child is aware of the need for a nasal consonant following the vowel.

Denasalization of vowels results if there is blockage of the nasal cavity, as when a speaker has a bad cold. In producing vowels in the context of nasal consonants, the velopharyngeal port may be open, but the blockage in the nasal cavity alters the normal resonance. For vowels, however, it is an unusual phenomenon, extremely difficult to perceive, and clinically of little importance (Compton & Hutton, 1980). Clinically, nasalization and denasalization are called hypernasality and hyponasality, respectively.

Since individuals with cleft palates cannot produce normal velopharyngeal closure, stop production is very difficult because air pressure buildup posterior to the stop closure is precluded by the flow of air through the nasal cavity. Air released after the stop burst also tends to flow out of the nasal cavity. The escape of air during the stop closure may or may not occur, depending on the severity of the cleft-palate problem. Air escaping through the nasal cavity after the burst and nasalization of the vowel is shown by placing the nasal diacritic above the stop and vowel symbols. Because of the loss of air pressure and the flow of air through the nasal cavity, stop sounds produced in cleft-palate speech are very weak.

VOWEL LENGTHENING

Some children who delete or devoice final consonants tend to lengthen the preceding vowel. For example, they may delete or devoice the final consonant in 'bird' and unusually lengthen the /ɝ/ vowel. This variant should be classified as secondary since it is a compensation for the devoiced or deleted final consonant.

IMPLOSIVES/EJECTIVES

Some severely hearing-impaired children substitute implosive and ejective stops for normal ones. As was pointed out in Chapter 5, an implosive stop reverses normal stop production. In it, air bursts into rather than out of the vocal tract when the closure is released. Ejective stops are produced by using double closures, one at the usual place of articulation and another at the vocal folds. Pressure is built up within the vocal tract by raising the level of the larynx to reduce the size of the vocal tract. When the anterior closure at the lips, alveolar ridge, or palate is released, air bursts out of the oral cavity. These stop sounds are highly unusual in English. It may be, as suggested by Monsen (1976a), that they are the consequence of exaggerated attempts to produce vocal fold vibration during the stop closure.

APPENDIX B

Transcription Symbols and Terminology

The transcription system described in this glossary accommodates the needs of clinical phonetics as related to articulatory and phonological disorders. In addition, the system is parsimonious and relatively easy to use. Since the focus of this text is on normal and abnormal variants of American speech, IPA symbols and diacritics (IPA, 1979) have been used as a foundation for the system proposed but with modifications developed by the American tradition of transcription (Pullum & Ladusaw, 1986) and additions specifically chosen for the transcription of disordered speech by the PRDS (Phonetic Representation of Disordered Speech) Group (Grunwell, 1985). The American tradition represents an effort on the part of American scholars to develop a practical system by avoiding the use of special characters, supplementing basic symbols with diacritics rather than new characters, and seeking to provide characters for American English rather than for universal coverage. In devising the proposed symbols, the following principles were used:

1. The system should provide unambiguous symbolization for normal and abnormal variants of American English.
2. The system should utilize the fewest number of different symbols and diacritics possible.
3. Because they are firmly entrenched in the teaching of basic phonetics, IPA symbols should be used for the phonemes of English, and IPA symbols and diacritics should be used for dentalized and retroflex sounds.
4. The system should facilitate writing, typing, and printing symbols as much as possible by using those that are relatively easy to write and are available on standard typewriter or computer keyboards.

In reviewing the presentation of diacritic symbols that follows, refer to Figure B–1 for an indication of where they should be placed in phonetic transcription and to Table B–1 for a list of symbols frequently used to denote variants of English consonants. As much as possible, symbols

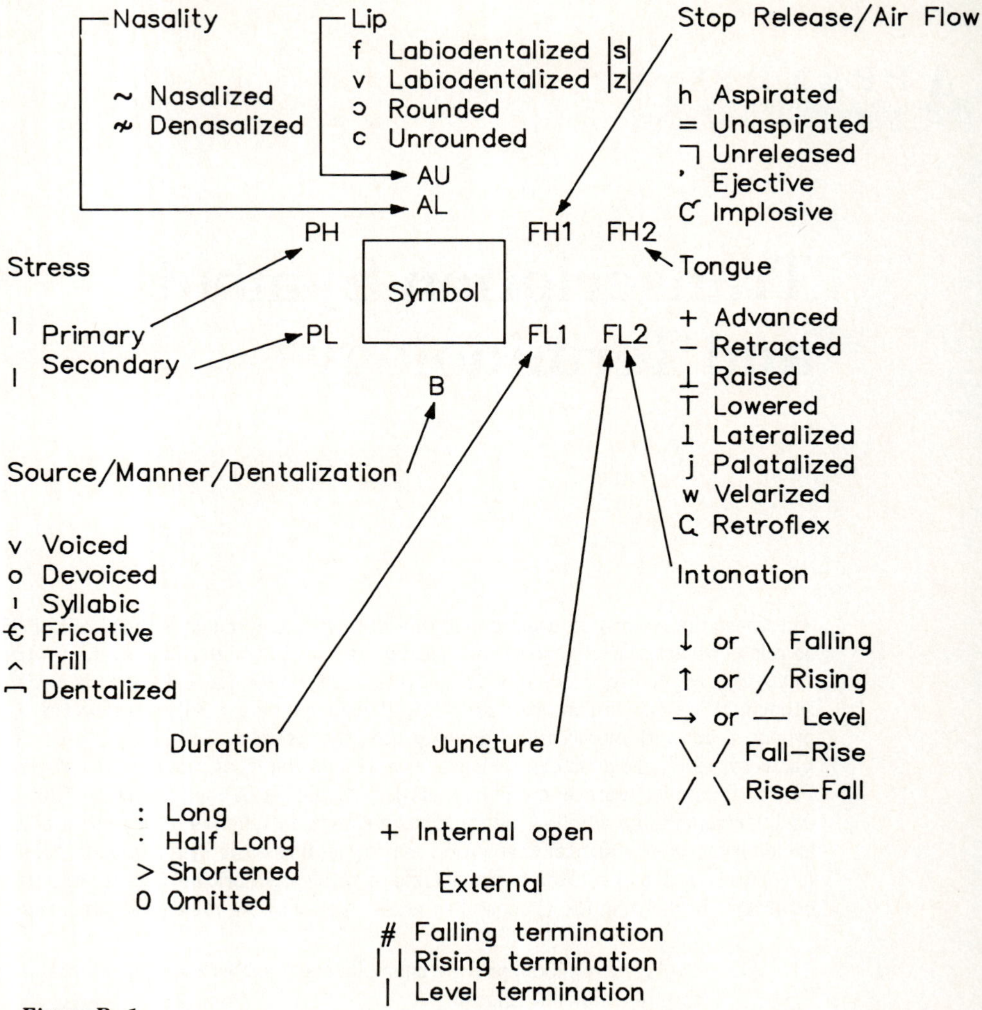

Figure B–1

Diacritics for phonetic transcription and relative locations for placing them in relation to segmental sound symbol. AU = above, upper; AL = above, lower; B = below; PH = preceding, high; PL = preceding, low; FH = following, high; FL = following, low; 1 = first in sequence; 2 = second in sequence. Note that (1) the bar indicating fricative manner goes across the consonant /C/ symbol, (2) the top hook indicating implosive stops is attached to the top of the consonant /C/ symbol, (3) the bottom hook indicating retroflex productions is attached to the bottom of the consonant /C/ symbol, and (4) the /0/ duration symbol replaces any omitted sound.

Table B–1

Symbols and diacritics for indicating consonantal variants.[a] IPA symbols are shown immediately below proposed symbols. 0 indicates no IPA symbol; ″ indicates that IPA uses the same symbol; — indicates impossible or unlikely sound. See Figure B–1.

Place	Manner							
	Nasal	Stop		Fricative		Trill[b]		Liquid/Glide
Bilabial	m	p	b	ɸ	β	p̭	b̭	—
	″	″	″	″	″	0	0	—
Apicolabial	M	P	B	Ᵽ	Ƀ	P̭	B̭	—
	0	0	0	0	0	0	0	—
Labiodental	ɱ	p̪	b̪	f	v	—		—
	″	0	0	″	″	—		—
Labiodentalized	—	—		$\overset{f}{s}$	$\overset{v}{z}$	—		—
	—	—		0	0	—		—
Apico-interdental	— [c]	— [c]		θ	ð	—		—
	0	0	0	″	″	—		0
Apicodental	n̪	t̪	d̪	s̪	z̪	—		l̪
	″	″	″	″	″	—		″
Apico-alveolar	n	t	d	s	z	ṱ	ḓ	—
	″	″	″	″	″	0	r	—
Apico-alveolar lateral	—	—		s^{l}	z^{l}	—		l
	—	—		ɬ	ɮ	—		″
Delateralized	—	—		—		—		$l^{\top}$
	—	—		—		—		0
Apicopalatal (retroflex)	ɳ	ʈ	ɖ	ʂ	ʐ	—		ɭ
	″	″	″	″	″	—		″
Rhotic	—	—		—		—		r
	—	—		—		—		ɹ
Derhoticized[d]	—	—		—		—		$r^{\top}$
	—	—		—		—		0
High Front	—	—		—		—		j
	—	—		—		—		″
Lamino-prepalatal	—	tʃ	dʒ[e]	ʃ	ʒ	—		—
	—	″	″	″	″	—		—
Dorsopalatal	ŋ$^{+}$	k^{+}	g^{+}	ꝁ$^{+}$	ǥ$^{+}$	—		l^{j}
	ɲ	c	ɟ	ç	j	—		ʎ
Dorsovelar	ŋ	k	g	ꝁ	ǥ	—		l^{w}
	″	″	″	x	ɣ	—		ɫ

continued

Table B–1 continued

Place	Manner: Nasal	Stop		Fricative		Trill[b]		Liquid/Glide
High back	–	–		–		–		w
	–	–		–		–		"
Dorso-uvular	ŋ$^-$	k$^-$	g$^-$	ꝁ$^-$	g$^-$	k̭$^-$	g̭$^-$	–
	ɴ	q	ɢ	χ	ʁ	0	ʀ	–
Dorsopharyngeal	–	K	G	Ꝁ	Ǥ	–		–
	–	0	0	ħ	ʕ	–		–
Glottal	–	ʔ		h	ɦ	ʔ̭		–
	–	"		"	"	0		–

[a]Note the proposed multiple use of the following diacritics: (1) superscript [$^+$], which is used to indicate back vowels with advanced (centralized) tongue positions, is also used to change dorsovelar sounds to dorsopalatal ones; (2) superscript [$^-$], which is used to indicate front vowels with retracted (centralized) tongue positions, is also used to change dorsovelar sounds to dorso-uvular ones; (3) superscript [$^\top$], which is used to indicate a vowel or consonant made with a lowered tongue position, is also used to indicate derhoticized or distorted /r/ and delateralized /l/; and (4) subscript [̪], which is used to indicate dentalized apico-alveolar sounds, is also used to indicate labiodental stops.

[b]A very short voiced apico-alveolar trill, commonly referred to as a *flap* and symbolized as [ɾ], is the sound which many phoneticians believe is used in American English for intervocalic /t/ and /d/ in words like 'bitter' and 'bidder.'

[c]IPA has no symbols for interdental sounds other than those for the fricatives; if it is necessary to differentiate interdental and dental sounds, [C̪͆] may be used for the interdentals.

[d]Frequently misspelled as *derhotacized.*

[e]The /tʃ/ and /dʒ/ sounds are affricates involving the release of alveolar stops into lamino-prepalatal fricatives.

for a given category are uniformly placed in a standard position, as proposed by Shriberg and Kent (1982). In some cases, however, it seemed prudent to make exceptions in favor of well-established IPA conventions regarding symbol placement. As indicated in Figure B–1, major symbol categories and their recommended positions, with exceptions noted, are: (1) Nasality—symbols are placed above the sound segment symbols; (2) Lip rounding—symbols are placed above the sound segment symbols, and above the nasality symbols when both are required; (3) Stop release and airflow—symbols are placed to the upper right of the sound segment symbols; (4) Tongue position—symbols are placed to the upper right of the sound segment symbols, and after the stop release and airflow symbols when both are required; (5) Duration—symbols are placed directly to the right of the sound segment symbols; (6) Intonation and juncture—symbols are placed directly to the right of the sound segment symbols, and to the right of duration symbols when both are needed; (7) Manner and voicing—symbols are placed directly below the segmental sound symbols (note that the dentalization symbol is placed here in keeping with IPA practice even though it is a tongue position symbol); and (8) Stress—symbols are placed just to the left of the symbol for the sound segment that begins a syllable. In the indications for placement of symbols that follow, V = vowel and C = consonant.

ARTICULATORY POSITION

LIPS

Rounded: $[\overset{\text{ɔ}}{\text{V}}]$ or $[\overset{\text{ɔ}}{\text{C}}]$

The IPA rounding symbol designates a lip configuration in which the horizontal dimension of the lip opening is about the same as the vertical dimension for a vowel. The /u, ʊ, o, ɔ/ vowels and the /w/ glide are normally rounded in American English; this symbol is used to indicate rounding of other vowels or of a consonant. For example, some speakers may round /ɝ/ and /r/, and the rounding diacritic could be used to indicate these pronunciations. Unrounded vowels may become rounded in English when preceded by /w/, as in 'we,' and consonants may become rounded when followed by /w/, as in 'twin,' or by /u/, as in 'to.' Such allophonic rounding need not be noted in broad transcription. IPA uses the term *labialized* to describe consonants that are rounded and a subscript omega to represent this variant, but in this text, the same symbol is used to indicate rounding for both vowels and consonants. In the IPA system the diacritic for rounding is superscript and follows the sound it modifies. As indicated in Figure B–1, the rounding diacritic is placed above the sound it modifies in this text.

Unrounded: $[\overset{\text{c}}{\text{V}}]$ or $[\overset{\text{c}}{\text{C}}]$

The IPA unrounding symbol designates a lip configuration for a vowel in which the horizontal dimension is greater than the vertical dimension. Since the /u, ʊ, o, ɔ/ vowels and the /w/ glide are the only rounded sounds in American English, this symbol would be used only to indicate unrounding of these sounds. Unrounding might occur when rounded vowels are preceded by normally unrounded sounds like /j/ in 'you.' It is more likely, however, that /u/ will cause the preceding /j/ to round. In the IPA system, the diacritic for unrounding is superscript, following the sound being modified. As indicated in Figure B–1, the unrounding diacritic is placed above the sound it modifies in this text.

Labiodentalized /s/ and /z/: $[\overset{\text{f}}{\text{s}}]$ and $[\overset{\text{v}}{\text{z}}]$

Labiodentalization symbols indicate production of the alveolar sibilant sounds with the lower lip contacting the upper teeth in addition to the usual tongue contact. When these variants occur in environments following /f/, as in 'cuffs,' and /v/, as in 'loves,' they are considered allophones of the /s/ and /z/ phonemes. When they occur in other contexts, the usage is identified as a labiodentalized lisp. Although these variants are often described as labialized sounds, the more precise term *labiodentalized* is used in this text, since *labialized* is used by IPA and many phoneticians to refer to rounded consonants.

TONGUE

Raised: [V˔] or [C˔]

The IPA symbol designates raising of the tongue higher than the normal position for the vowel. For example, [æ˔] denotes that a vowel sounds like one between /æ/ and /ɛ/. Since lingual consonants are all generally made from high tongue positions, this symbol is usually not used with them.

Lowered: [V˕] or [C˕]

The IPA symbol designates lowering of the tongue below the normal position for the vowel or consonant. For example, [ɛ˕] denotes that a vowel sounds like one between /ɛ/ and /æ/. This symbol is also used for modifications of a consonant, specifically, /s/ and /z/ sounds made with the tongue tip oriented toward the lower alveolar ridge rather than the upper one. See the sections on distorted /r/ and delateralized /l/ on page 339.

Advanced: [V$^+$] or [C$^+$]

IPA uses the superscript plus sign to designate advancing the tongue anterior to the normal position for the vowel sound being modified. For example, [ɑ$^+$] indicates that a vowel sound is between /ɑ/ and /a/. For high back vowels the symbol indicates centralization. Such vowels sound like the schwa vowel. For a consonant the diacritic denotes contact by the same part of the tongue as indicated by the consonant symbol, but at a more anterior contact point. As indicated in Table B–1, the superscript plus sign is used with dorsovelar consonant symbols to indicate dorsopalatal nasal, voiceless stop, and voiced stop sounds. IPA uses a lowercase *n* with a leftward hook ([ɲ]), a lowercase *c*, and a dotless lowercase *j* with a crossbar ([ɟ]) to represent these sounds. See "Fricative Indicator," on page 340 for specifics about dorsopalatal and dorsovelar fricatives.

Apicolabial: [M], [P, B], [Ᵽ, Ƀ], [P̭, B̭]

Capitalized equivalents of bilabial stop and nasal symbols designate production of nasal, stop, fricative, and trill sounds with tongue tip and upper lip contact. Apicolabials do not occur normally in any language, but they may be substituted for bilabials and labiodentals by individuals with loss of lip tissue. As indicated in Table B–1, IPA has no symbols for these sounds.

Dentalized and Labiodental: [C̪]

The bridge placed below a consonant symbol is used by IPA to designate production of apico-alveolar consonants, /t, d, n, s, z, l/, with either apico-interdental or apicodental contact. These variants are allophonic when they occur in the context of the apico-interdental fricatives, for example, [t̪] in 'eighth,' [d̪] in 'width,' [n̪] in 'tenth,' [s̪] in 'aesthetic,' [z̪] in 'breathes,' and [l̪] in 'health.' When dentalizing occurs for any of the apico-alveolar sounds in other contexts, the variation is a misarticulation. The subscript bridge symbol is also used in this text below bilabial stop symbols to designate production of labiodental stops, in keeping with the PRDS Group recommendation (Grunwell, 1985). Although this diacritic could be used below the bilabial nasal consonant symbol to represent a labiodental nasal, the IPA symbol shown in Table B–1 for this sound is preferable because it is well known.

Retracted: [V$^-$] or [C$^-$]

The superscript minus sign is used by IPA to designate retracting the tongue posterior to the position for the vowel or consonant being modified. For example, [a$^-$] indicates a vowel that sounds like one between /a/ and /ɑ/. For high front vowels, the diacritic indicates that they are centralized, so that they sound like the schwa vowel. For a consonant, the diacritic denotes contact by the same part of the tongue as indicated by the consonant symbol, but with a more posterior contact point. Dorsovelar symbols with superscript minus signs can be used to represent a dorso-uvular nasal, a dorso-uvular voiceless stop, and a dorso-uvular voiced stop; IPA uses a small capital *N* ([ɴ]), a lowercase *q* ([q]), and a small capital *G* ([ɢ]) for these dorso-uvular sounds. A capital *K* represents a dorsopharyngeal voiceless stop, and a capital *G* represents a voiced dorsopharyngeal stop. These same symbols with a hyphen through the body of the letter indicate dorsopharyngeal voiceless and voiced fricatives. (A nasal sound cannot be made from this position.) IPA uses a lowercase *h* ([ħ]) with a superimposed crossbar and a reversed question mark with no dot ([ʕ]) to represent voiceless and voiced pharyngeal fricatives, but it has no symbols for pharyngeal stop sounds.

Retroflex: [C̢]

A consonant symbol with a rightward tail is used by IPA to designate production of apico-alveolar sounds, /t, d, n, l/, with apicopalatal contact, or apico-alveolar fricatives, /s, z/, with apicopalatal constriction, that is, with the tongue tip arched backward from the position represented by the symbol being modified. These sounds do not occur normally in English except when Indian speakers of English use them because they occur in their native language. The sibilants /s/ and /z/ are pronounced as retroflex by some individuals who misarticulate the sounds. The word *retroflex* is also used to describe one of two tongue positions for /r/, /ɝ/, and /ɚ/ production, the other being a bunched tongue position. No diacritic is necessary to indicate this variation unless one is interested in differentiating the two types of /r/. The retroflex variant could be noted by using the /r/ symbol with a rightward tail ([ɽ]).

Lateralized /s/ and /z/: [sˡ] and [zˡ]

The /s/ and /z/ symbols followed by superscript /l/ designates the modification of these sibilants toward a position like that for /l/ but with a greater constriction so that frication noise is produced. Lateralized /s/ and /z/ sounds are the misarticulations that characterize a lateral lisp. IPA uses a lowercase *l* with a superimposed belt ([ɬ]) to represent a voiceless apico-alveolar lateral fricative, and a ligature of lowercase *l* and /ʒ/ ([ɮ]) to represent a voiced apico-alveolar lateral fricative.

Derhoticized or Distorted /r/: [r˕]

The superscript diacritic for lowered tongue position designates production of /r/ without the retroflex or bunched tongue positions necessary for r-coloring. This misarticulation differs from gliding, in which /w/ substitutes for /r/. With this distortion it is difficult to specify the tongue position, except that it comes close to the /ɜ/ vowel produced by Southerners and New Englanders who delete the r-coloring in their pronunciation of words like 'bird.' IPA has no symbol for this sound.

Delateralized /l/: [l˕]

The superscript diacritic for lowered tongue position designates production of the /l/ sound without the apico-alveolar contact necessary for l-coloring, or lateralizing. The tongue position is close to that for a high back vowel, but the tongue tip approximates the upper alveolar ridge. This misarticulation differs from gliding, in which /w/ or /j/ substitutes for /l/. It also differs from velarized or dark /l/, for which the apico-alveolar contact is maintained but the tongue dorsum is raised toward the palate; dark /l/ sounds occur before back vowels and after any vowel, and are allophonic in English. IPA has no symbol for delateralized /l/.

Palatalized: [Cʲ]

A superscript /j/ following a consonant symbol is used to designate production of an apico-alveolar consonant, /t, d, s, z, l/, with an extended contact or constriction that reaches from the alveolar ridge to the anterior part of the palate. For this contact the tongue blade as well as the tip is involved. Except for /l/, these sounds do not occur in English as dialectal, allophonic, or misarticulated variants. IPA uses a leftward hook attached to a consonant symbol to indicate that it is palatalized. Palatalized /l/ may occur allophonically in words like 'million' [mɪlʲjən] in which the following /j/ influences tongue position. IPA uses a turned lowercase *y* ([ʎ]) to represent a dorsopalatal /l/ and a lowercase *n* with a leftward hook ([ɲ]) to represent a dorsopalatal nasal consonant.

Velarized: [C^{w}]

A superscript /w/ following an apico-alveolar consonant symbol designates production of such sounds with the tongue dorsum raised so as to approximate the posterior part of the palate. Velarized sounds occur as phonemes in other languages. In English, dark /l/ is a velarized sound which occurs allophonically preceding back vowels, as in 'loop,' and following any vowel, as in 'peel' or 'pool.' No other apico-alveolar sound in English has this variant. IPA uses a lowercase *l* crossed by a tilde ([ɫ]) to indicate velarized or dark /l/.

MANNER

Fricative Indicator: [€]

A lowercase stop consonant symbol with a superimposed hyphen designates fricative sounds made from positions represented by bilabial, apicolabial, palatal, velar, uvular, and pharyngeal stop symbols. According to Pullum and Ladusaw (1986), by a general convention, barred stop symbols (symbols with a superimposed hyphen or short dash through the body of the letter) are often used to represent fricatives for which IPA symbols are not used. Such symbols have the advantage of being easy to type with an unmodified typewriter. These fricatives do not normally occur in English, but some cleft-palate speakers produce pharyngeal fricatives. IPA uses additional symbols to represent bilabial, palatal, velar, uvular, and pharyngeal fricatives but has no symbol for apicolabial fricatives.

Trill Indicator: [C̭]

Consonant symbols with a caret below them designate production of trill sounds from articulatory positions represented by bilabial, apicolabial, alveolar, uvular, and glottal stop symbols. Trills do not normally occur in English, but bilabial and apicolabial trills are used by children in vocal play, and the glottal trill or glottal fry is used in speech therapy. IPA uses a lowercase *r* to represent a voiced apico-alveolar trill and a small capital *r* ([ʀ]) to represent a voiced uvular trill but has no symbols for bilabial and glottal trills.

Syllable Indicator: [C̩]

A vertical stroke is used below a consonant to indicate that it is syllabic, in keeping with IPA. This denotes that the consonant is functioning as a vowel, since it is the only sound in a syllable. This occurs frequently for /l/ and /n/ and infrequently for /m/.

AIR PRESSURE AND FLOW

Aspirated: [C^{h}]

Superscript lowercase *h* designates a stop consonant with aspiration, in keeping with IPA. In the production of voiceless stops, the closure release precedes the onset of vocal fold vibration for the following vowel by about 30 msec. During this interval, frication noise and aspiration noise are produced. Aspiration characterizes voiceless stops in English unless they are preceded by /s/. This is an allophonic variation in English. See "Unaspirated," below.

Unaspirated: [C⁼]

A stop consonant symbol with a superscript equal sign designates a stop consonant that is released with little aspiration. In English this stop variant occurs allophonically after /s/, as in 'spy,' 'sty,' and 'sky.' Children with the phonological process disorder of prevocalic voicing, however, do not aspirate voiceless stops in the initial position of words. IPA has no symbol for unaspirated stops.

Unreleased: [C˺]

A superscript corner symbol is used by IPA to designate production of a stop consonant without releasing the closure. This variation is allophonic in English, occurring when stops terminate the first syllable of compound words, for example, the /t/ of 'hotdog,' or when stops terminate the first syllable of a word in which the following syllable begins with a consonant, for example, the /t/ of 'atmosphere.' In word-final position, released and unreleased stops are in free variation, but unreleased stops may be more common.

Ejective: [C']

An apostrophe following a stop consonant symbol designates an ejective stop, in keeping with IPA. In such sounds, air is trapped between a back closure at the vocal folds and a front closure that is labial, alveolar, or velar. Pressure is built up in the vocal tract by raising the larynx. When the anterior closure is released, air bursts out of the cavity. These sounds do not occur normally in English, but they are used by some hearing-impaired individuals in an attempt to produce normal stops.

Implosive: [ɓ], [ɗ], [ɠ]

The hook attached to the top of stop consonant symbols designates implosive stop consonants, in keeping with IPA. Such consonants are formed by producing an anterior closure that is labial, alveolar, or velar. The size of the vocal tract is increased by expanding the lungs or lowering the larynx. The decreased pressure within the vocal tract causes air to burst into the oral cavity when the anterior closure is released. These stops do not occur normally in English, but they are used by some hearing-impaired speakers trying to produce normal stops.

GLOTTAL SOURCE

Voiced: [C̬]

The wedge symbol below a consonant symbol designates voicing of normally voiceless sounds. The diacritic is used only to modify nonnasal consonants, in keeping with IPA. Because each voiceless consonant in English has a voiced cognate, the voiced modifier need only be used when: (1) a part of the consonant is voiced, and (2) doubt exists about the extent to which a voiceless consonant is voiced. This diacritic may also be used to indicate the loss of distinction between /t/ and /d/ by transcribing the stops in 'latter' and 'ladder' as [t̬]. In transcribing prevocalic voicing, 'cat' could be /gæt/ or [k̬æt].

Devoiced: [C̥] or [V̥]

An under-ring below a consonant or vowel symbol designates devoicing of normally voiced sounds. The diacritic can be used to modify consonants and vowels, in keeping with IPA. If used with a vowel, glide, liquid, or nasal, the diacritic indicates partial or complete devoicing. Glides and liquids become devoiced allophonically in English when they are preceded by a voiceless stop. This happens with /j/ in 'cube,' /w/ in 'twin,' /l/ in 'clean,' and /r/ in 'pray.' If used with a voiced stop, fricative, or affricate, the diacritic denotes some degree of devoicing rather than a total change, because the cognate symbol is available to indicate complete devoicing.

RESONANCE

Nasalized or Hypernasal: [Ṽ] or [C̃]

The tilde above a symbol designates nasalizing of a consonant or vowel that is not normally nasalized, as well as greater than normal nasalization in any sound, in keeping with IPA. It is not necessary to use the modifier for nasal consonant symbols or for vowels and liquids that become somewhat nasalized in the context of nasals, because these occurrences are allophonic. But when the nasal resonance of vowels exceeds the norm, or when vowels that are not in the context of nasal consonants have a nasal quality, the nasal modifier should be used. For stops, fricatives, and affricates, the diacritic indicates escape of air through the nasal cavity rather than nasal resonance.

Denasalized or Hyponasal: [Ṽ̸] or [C̸̃]

The tilde with a slash through it is used above a vowel or consonant symbol to designate loss of nasal quality. This diacritic may be used for sounds that are normally nasal, like nasal consonants, or for those that acquire some degree of nasality because of context, as may be the case for vowels and liquids in the context of nasal consonants. The sound is like that of an individual whose cold is blocking the nasal cavities, and it is difficult to pick up from listening to just the vowels. Denasalized consonants sound much like voiced stops made from the same position. 'May' sounds like 'bay,' 'new' sounds like 'do,' and 'bang' sounds like 'bag.' IPA has no symbols for denasalized sounds.

PROSODY

DURATION

Long: [V:] or [C:]

In this text a colon following a vowel or consonant symbol indicates long duration, instead of the upward- and downward-pointing triangles of IPA. It may be used to indicate vowel duration comparable to that preceding voiced consonants, as for /i/ in 'please,' which is an allophonic variant in English. The diacritic may also be used for longer than normal vowel duration produced by children (1) using the phonological process of final consonant devoicing (example: [pɪ:k] for 'pig') or (2) using the phonological process of final consonant deletion (example: [pɪ:] for 'pig'). See "Half-long," below.

Half-long: [V·] or [C·]

As indicated in Figure B–1, a raised period is used to designate a half-long vowel or consonant. It may be used to indicate duration comparable to that in the first syllable of 'pleasing,' as compared with the long vowel duration in 'please' and the short vowel duration in the first syllable in 'pleasingly.' IPA uses a downward-pointing triangle for this variant.

Shortened or Omitted

When the rate of speech production is increased above normal, sounds and syllables generally become very short, or they may be completely omitted. The [>] symbol may be used to indicate unusual shortening of individual sounds; the /0/ symbol indicates omission of a sound. For example, [s>əprɑɪz], /s0prɑɪz/, and /00prɑɪz/ transcriptions indicate shortening of /s/, omission of /ə/, and omission of the first syllable of 'surprise,' respectively.

STRESS

Primary: [ˈC] or [ˈV]

The superior vertical stroke preceding a consonant symbol, as in the first syllable of 'celebrate,' or a vowel symbol, as in the first syllable of 'elevate,' designates the greatest prominence given to a syllable within a word. IPA uses this symbol for the same purpose.

Secondary: [ˌC] or [ˌV]

The inferior vertical stroke preceding a consonant symbol, as in the last syllable of 'celebrate,' or a vowel symbol, as in the first syllable of 'entertain,' designates the next-to-greatest prominence given to a syllable within a word. IPA uses this symbol for the same purpose.

Tertiary or Weak

As in IPA, no diacritic is used for this level of stress, the weakest prominence given to a syllable within a word, for example, the second syllable in 'celebrate.'

JUNCTURE

Internal

The transition between syllables within a word or between adjacent words is referred to as internal juncture. Two types are generally identified, open and close. The plus sign [+] designates open juncture, the transition between syllables in different words, for example, in 'night rate' [nɑɪt+ret] as opposed to 'nitrate' /nɑɪtret/, and the shifting transition that differentiates 'it sprays' [ɪt+sprez] from 'its praise' [ɪts+prez]. Unlike the superscript plus sign used to show tongue advancement, the plus sign used for juncture is on the same level as sound segments. No diacritic is used to mark close juncture, which is the usual transition between sounds and syllables within words, as in 'nitrate.'

External or Terminal

The [#] symbol indicates external or terminal juncture in which the pitch falls at the end of an intonation contour rather than leveling off at level 1. The [||] symbol marks an upward termination of an intonation contour. The [|] symbol shows a leveling off of pitch at the end of an intonation contour rather than a fall or a rise.

INTONATION

[↓] or [\]

The down arrow or the downslant line designates falling intonation, which usually occurs at the end of complete statements and wh- questions. IPA uses a grave accent mark to indicate a high falling tone.

[↑] or [/]

The up arrow or the upslant line designates rising intonation, which usually occurs at the end of yes-or-no questions. IPA uses an acute accent mark to indicate high rising tone.

[→] or [—]

The horizontal arrow or line designates level intonation, which usually occurs at the end of incomplete statements. IPA uses a macron to indicate a high level tone.

[\/]

The downslant-upslant line designates fall-rise intonation, as at the end of cautionary statements. IPA uses a wedge for this tone.

[/\]

The upslant-downslant line designates rise-fall intonation, as at the end of very definite statements. IPA uses a circumflex sign to indicate a rising-falling tone.

APPENDIX C

Tape Log

This log gives the content and location of transcription exercises in the text and the approximate location of the recorded stimuli for each exercise on the four cassette tapes that accompany this book. The transcription exercises in the text indicate the stimuli presented on the tapes and provide forms for transcribing them. Roman numerals I through IV identify the four cassettes, and the two sides of each cassette are identified as A and B. Each transcription exercise on each side of a tape is further identified as a section by an Arabic numeral. Thus, IA1 designates the transcription exercise that is on page 63 of the text and is recorded on tape I, side A and is the first section on that side of the tape. These location codes are listed on pages 346 and 347 for each transcription exercise; they also appear in the heading for each exercise in the text. The length of the exercise and its approximate location on the cassette may be determined from the times presented under "Running Time," which indicates the time it takes to present all of the stimuli in the exercise and "Elapsed Time," which indicates how far into each side of a tape the exercise occurs. For example, exercise IA1S takes 6 minutes and 34 seconds and starts 5 minutes and 41 seconds from the beginning of the first utterance on the tape.

Code and Content	Page	Running Time	Elapsed Time
Chapter 3			
IA1 Front Vowels	63	5:41	00:00–05:41
IA1S /ɪ/ - /ɛ/ Discrimination	65	6:34	05:41–12:15
IA2 Back Vowels	67	5:28	12:15–17:43
IA2S /ɑ/ - /ɔ/ Discrimination	68	7:05	17:43–24:48
IA3 Central Vowels	70	5:20	24:48–30:08
IB1 Offglides	72	6:23	00:00–06:23
IB2 Onglides	73	5:20	06:23–11:43
Chapter 4			
IB3 Prevocalic /r/	96	13:43	11:43–25:26
IB4 Intervocalic /r/	99	3:59	25:26–29:25
IIA1 Intervocalic /r/ Discrimination	101	4:25	00:00–04:25
IIA2 Vocalic /r/	102	3:58	04:25–08:23
IIA3 Prevocalic /l/	103	10:02	08:23–18:25
IIA4 Intervocalic /l/	105	4:39	18:25–23:04
IIA5 Syllabic /l/	107	4:02	23:04–27:06
Chapter 6			
IIB1 Prevocalic Stops	162	5:47	00:00–05:47
IIB2 VOT Distinction	164	9:52	05:47–15:39
IIB3 Postvocalic Stops	166	8:11	15:39–23:50
IIB4 Vowel Duration Distinction	169	5:18	23:50–29:08
IIIA1 Words with Vowels, Glides, and Stops	170	3:25	00:00–03:25
IIIA2 Phonological Processes Affecting Stops	171	5:27	03:25–08:52
Chapter 7			
IIIA3 Fricatives and Affricates	186	14:24	08:52–23:16
Chapter 8			
IIIB1 Normal and Abnormal /s/ and /z/ Variants	210	9:25	00:00–09:25
IIIB2 Words with Vowels, Glides, Stops, and Fricatives	213	3:18	09:25–12:43
IIIB3 Deaffricated and Depalatalized /tʃ/ and /dʒ/	214	3:06	12:43–15:49
IIIB4 Labialization and Stopping of /f/, /v/, /θ/ and /ð/	215	4:27	15:49–20:16

Code and Content	Page	Running Time	Elapsed Time
Chapter 9			
IIIB5 Nasal Consonants	234	3:47	20:16–24:03
IIIB6 Normal and Abnormal Nasal Variants	235	3:08	24:03–27:11
IVA1 Nasalized Vowels and Consonants	237	2:56	00:00–02:56
IVA2 Words with Vowels, Glides, Stops, Fricatives, and Nasals	238	3:25	02:56–06:21
Chapter 10			
IVA3 Assimilations in Adult and Child Speech	255	9:14	06:21–15:35
Chapter 11			
IVA4 Suprasegmentals	292	5:21	15:35–20:56
Appendix E			
IVA5 Reliability Test for Vowels and Consonants	354	7:43	20:56–28:39
IVB1 Reliability Test for /r/ Misarticulations	357	5:14	00:00–05:14
IVB2 Reliability Test for /l/ Misarticulations	358	6:01	05:14–11:15
IVB3 Reliability Test for /s/ and /z/ Misarticulations	360	5:18	11:15–16:33
IVB4 Reliability Test for Phonological Processes	362	6:33	16:33–23:06

APPENDIX D

Transcription Validity, Accuracy, and Reliability

Included in this appendix is information on procedures, standards, techniques, and strategies for achieving transcription validity, accuracy, and reliability. This information not only describes the rationale and procedures used to develop the exercises presented on the Audiotapes to Accompany Phonetic Analysis of Normal and Abnormal Speech but also provides useful guidelines and practice for carrying them out.

TRANSCRIPTION VALIDITY

The validity of a phonetic analysis as an indicator of the misarticulations of an individual is maximized by sampling from continuous speech, but just as the linguistic complexity of the sample increases from sounds in isolation to those in sentences, so does the difficulty of the task. In the exercises prepared for this book there is a range of practice samples, from the relatively easy task of transcribing sounds in minimal contrast nonsense syllables to the relatively difficult task of transcribing sounds in words in sentences.

One problem in transcribing the continuous speech of a child with a severe phonological or articulatory disorder is poor intelligibility. In a clinical situation, you may or may not be aware of the words intended by the speaker whose utterances you are transcribing. This lack of certainty may increase the difficulty of making a phonetic analysis. Knowing what word is intended can help focus your attention on the features of target sounds and the types of errors most likely to occur, but such knowledge can be a drawback if you let it influence your transcription of what was actually said. Oller and Eilers (1975) found that students' transcriptions often included phonetic features expected in target words but not actually present in the utterances transcribed. The exercises offer practice in transcribing both ways. Sometimes you are asked to transcribe sounds produced in minimal contrast contexts with no word intended, and at other times you are asked to transcribe one sound in a word or all the sounds in words as they are produced in complete sentences with prior knowledge of the word intended.

TRANSCRIPTION ACCURACY

TRANSCRIPTION CONDITIONS

It may be necessary to transcribe utterances either directly as they are spoken or indirectly from a tape recording. In either case, every attempt should be made to insure optimum conditions for accurate and reliable transcribing.

Direct Transcribing

If at all possible, direct transcribing should occur in a room that is as noise-free as a recording studio. Special care should be taken to insure that there is a minimum of noise which might interfere with the accurate transcription of even the weakest fricative sounds. If a studio is not available, select the quietest room in the building in which you transcribe and the quietest time of the day. Try to get rid of noise-producing items in the room and position yourself away from any noise sources. Place yourself in front of your subject so that you can see and hear his/her speech.

For reliability testing it is desirable to record the transcription session. Although interjudge reliability can be determined by having a second transcriber in the room, intrajudge reliability can be assessed only by making a recording.

Indirect Transcribing

Ideally, indirect transcribing should involve recordings of speech produced in a recording studio with high-quality recording equipment similar to that used in the preparation of tapes for this book. These recordings were made in an IAC booth at Vanderbilt University which had an optimal signal-to-noise ratio. The microphone used was a Neumann (TLM 170i), and the tape recorder was a Revox (B77 MKII). For purposes of transcribing the tapes to obtain the responses used for the "consensus" and "variants" information included in this text, listening at Vanderbilt was done in a sound-treated room. Listeners heard the stimuli played back on a Sony tape recorder (BM-80) through Sony earphones (MDR-U10). If you cannot obtain a sound-treated room, select the quietest room and the best recording equipment you or your employer can afford. If necessary, go to a store that handles high-quality recording equipment and make sample recordings of speech to see which system gives the best quality that you can afford.

You have the choice of transcribing speech from a tape recording through earphones or a loudspeaker. The choice should be based primarily on the best signal-to-noise ratio you can get for the money you can afford. If you must work in a relatively noisy room, earphones will help reduce the noise. If noise in the room is not a problem, then you can use a loudspeaker. Earphones may become uncomfortable after prolonged use, but you should probably not transcribe speech for extended periods without breaks anyhow.

TRANSCRIPTION GUIDELINES

Ideally, one should transcribe every detail in an individual's speech, but practically speaking, phoneticians generally use guidelines to determine which features must be specified and which ones can be ignored. The guidelines depend on the purpose of the transcription. Since the focus in this book is on articulatory and phonological disorders, the following guidelines are designed to satisfy that focus.

Aspiration

Note its absence in a child's production of the prevocalic voiceless stops /p, t, k/ in words like 'pill,' 'till,' and 'kill,' and its presence or absence in a child's production of these stops when he/she omits a preceding /s/, in words like 'spill,' 'still,' and 'skill.' Absence of aspiration in prevocalic voiceless stops can produce confusion with the voiced cognate, so that 'pill' may sound like 'bill.' When /s/ is omitted before /p, t, k/, the presence or absence of aspiration indicates whether the child is aware of the need to maintain a distinction between s-blend and isolated stops, as in 'spill' [p⁼ɪl] and 'pill' [pʰɪl]. Otherwise, aspiration does not have to be noted, since its occurrence is predictable in English.

Nasality

Note its presence or absence in a child's production of a vowel when he/she omits a postvocalic nasal consonant in such words as 'can' and 'bomb.' In a word like 'lamp,' a child may omit /m/, say /p/, and nasalize /æ/ so that it may seem that the nasal sound is being produced. Transcribe nasality when it is noticeably greater than normal in the production of a vowel or consonant. Otherwise, it is not necessary to indicate the predictable nasality that occurs on vowels in the context of nasal consonants.

Duration

Note prolongation of the following sounds in a child's production of an utterance: (1) a vowel when the following consonant is omitted, as in 'fine' with /n/ deleted, (2) a vowel followed by a consonant that is devoiced, as in 'bad' with /d/ devoiced, and (3) a consonant when the following consonant is omitted, as in 'past' with /t/ deleted. Otherwise, it is not necessary to indicate predictable, contextual differences in vowel duration.

Release of Postvocalic Stops

The release of postvocalic stops is in free variation. It is generally not necessary to indicate release unless it is exaggerated, as in [bædə] 'bad,' or when no release occurs when it might be expected, as in [pæst˺] 'past.'

Devoicing

Note voiced consonants that are produced as voiceless or partially voiceless, particularly those in postvocalic position, that is, so that 'bad' sounds like 'bat.' It is not necessary to indicate predictable devoicing of the glides /w, j, r, l/ that occurs when voiceless consonants precede them, as in 'twelve,' 'cute,' 'try,' and 'please.'

Vowel Distinctions

Note differences in the quality of a vowel produced by an individual and the target vowel in stressed syllables if they are different phonemes, such as /pɪn/ for target /pɛn/ in 'pen,' /hɑt/ for target /hæt/ in 'hat,' /bit/ for target /bɪt/ in 'bit,' /bʊd/ for target /bɝd/ in 'bird,' and /fɑðə/ for target /fɑðɚ/ in 'father.' You should also note prolonged or nasalized vowels, particularly if a normally following consonant is omitted. In unstressed syllables, vowel quality varies among /ə/, /ɪ/, and /i/ in such contexts as the first syllable of 'believe' and between /ɪ/ and /i/ in such contexts as the last syllable of 'baby.' It is limited to /ə/ in such contexts as the first syllable of 'allow' and to /ɪ/ in such contexts as the last syllable of 'magic.' Precise indication of vowel quality is more difficult, but considerably less important, in unstressed than in stressed syllables.

Diphthongization

In English, diphthongization occurs when /e/ and /o/ are followed by voiced consonants, as in [meɪd] 'made' and [koud] 'code,' or when they are in open syllables, as in [meɪ] 'may' and [mou] 'mow,' but not when they are followed by voiceless consonants, as in /met/ 'mate' and /kot/ 'coat.' You need not note this variation.

Stop Termination of Vowels

Note when a vowel is terminated by a stop even if you cannot be sure of the place of articulation. Children may produce a glottal stop, as in /buʔ/ for 'book' or an abrupt termination of the vowel which does not appear to be bilabial, alveolar, or palatal. In the case of a child who appears to eliminate final consonants, make sure he/she is not using what sounds like a stop with an ambiguous place of articulation. If you are not sure of the position, use a stop symbol with a circle around it.

TRANSCRIPTION STRATEGIES

Phonetic transcription is probably part art and part science, so it is not surprising that phoneticians differ as to the best techniques for increasing accuracy of analysis, with little evidence to support any procedure. Based on the experience and background of the authors, the following strategies are recommended:

1. In each utterance, transcribe the sounds you are confident about first. Then concentrate on those that are troublesome.
2. Focus your attention on the sound you are not sure of and listen to it again if you have a tape recording. If not, you can ask the child to repeat the utterance, but keep in mind that the repetition may not be the same as the original.
3. Try to imitate what the individual is saying. If you are a good mimic, this procedure will help you determine what was said.
4. If possible, check your analysis of a sound with that of another phonetician.

TRANSCRIPTION TECHNIQUES

It is not clear what steps phoneticians go through in deciding what they hear in an individual's speech as they transcribe it. Certain techniques seem to be used generally by phoneticians, but no standard process is universally agreed on (Tiffany & Carrell, 1977; Shriberg & Kent, 1982). The following are techniques in a step-by-step procedure for making a phonetic analysis which you may want to follow completely or in part, depending on what seems to work best for you.

1. Count the number of syllables in each produced utterance and determine if it agrees with the number in the target utterance.
2. Identify the vowels, diphthongs, or syllabic consonants that constitute the nucleus of each syllable, using the minimal contrasts of front-back, high-low, tense-lax, and rounded-unrounded to zero in on the vowel.

3. Transcribe the syllable nuclei you are certain of, leaving space for preceding and following consonants.
4. Determine whether each vowel nucleus is initiated and terminated by a consonant or consonant cluster and if a target consonant is deleted.
5. Identify the consonants, using manner, voicing, and place feature analysis to zero in on them and transcribe those you are certain of.
6. Decide which features of the remaining consonants you are uncertain about and how they differ from the target consonants.
7. Transcribe the consonants, using appropriate diacritics to indicate deviations from the targets, if necessary.

TRANSCRIPTION RELIABILITY

It is important for you to determine the reliability of your performance as a transcriber of speech, just as it is important to calibrate the performance of an audiometer or a sound spectrograph. In order to facilitate this procedure, we have included in Appendix E a series of transcription tests to be used for assessing interjudge and intrajudge reliability. These include the following tests: (a) normal vowels and consonants; (b) misarticulations of /r, ɝ, ɚ/; (c) misarticulations of /l/ and [l̩]; (d) misarticulations of /s, z/; and phonological processes.

Listen to these tests on the tapes and transcribe the utterances according to the instructions given. At least one week after this first transcription, transcribe the tests again and compare your transcriptions. Using the formulas provided in Appendix E, calculate the intrajudge reliability.

By comparing your transcriptions with those given in the key, you can also calculate the interjudge reliability. This score provides a measure of your agreement with the panel of experts used in developing the tapes for this book. You can also determine your degree of agreement with anyone else by having him/her do the same reliability test. You might want to have one of your colleagues or your clinical supervisor do this.

APPENDIX E

Procedures and Tests for Assessing Intrajudge and Interjudge Reliability

The following tests are designed to assess your reliability as a transcriber of normal and misarticulated sounds of children. The tests are designed to determine your intrajudge and interjudge reliability (see Chapter 12 and Appendix D). To test intrajudge reliability, you should transcribe the exercises on two different occasions, about one week apart, and then compare your transcriptions for each sound to determine how many of them on the second test agree with those on the first one. To determine interjudge reliability, you can compare your transcriptions for each sound with the consensus given in the key for each test. Formulas for calculating reliability are given in each key. Generally, formulas are provided for determining an overall reliability measure as well as separate measures for determining how reliably you transcribe specific misarticulations. For example, formulas are given for calculating reliability for transcribing /r, ɝ, ɚ/ misarticulations and for calculating reliability for each of these sounds. Tables E–1 to E–5 provide positional distribution of the sounds for each of the tests. When there is no consensus for an utterance, you may score as correct any of the variants given.

LABORATORY ASSIGNMENT

Tape IV, Side A

IVA5: Reliability Test for Normal Vowels and Consonants (Tape running time: 7:43; Elapsed time: 20:56–28:39)

Transcribe all vowels and consonants in each word. You do not need to note allophonic variations such as aspiration or release of final consonants.

1. south ________
2. penny ________
3. boys ________
4. get ________
5. safe ________
6. bat ________
7. mice ________
8. bounce ________
9. boom ________
10. should ________
11. sister ________
12. fishing ________
13. duck ________
14. coins ________
15. church ________
16. guide ________
17. size ________
18. comb ________
19. map ________
20. neat ________
21. father ________
22. dozen ________
23. boat ________
24. zipper ________

25. daughter ________________
26. cab ________________
27. nod ________________
28. hog ________________
29. judging ________________
30. tagging ________________
31. cover ________________
32. thumb ________________
33. matter ________________
34. fighter ________________
35. packing ________________
36. fading ________________
37. tub ________________
38. path ________________
39. money ________________
40. dummy ________________
41. measure ________________
42. this ________________
43. shady ________________
44. hog ________________
45. head ________________
46. towns ________________
47. choice ________________
48. join ________________
49. van ________________
50. gave ________________
51. coffee ________________
52. zap ________________
53. sadder ________________
54. could ________________
55. today ________________
56. shot ________________
57. penny ________________
58. chin ________________
59. tomato ________________
60. pin ________________

****

Consensus: 1. /saʊθ/ 2. /pɛni/ 3. /bɔɪz/ 4. /gɛt/ 5. /sef/ 6. /bæt/ 7. /maɪs/ 8. /baʊnts/ 9. /bum/ 10. /ʃʊd/ 11. /sɪstɚ/ 12. /fɪʃɪŋ/ 13. /dʌk/ 14. /kɔɪnz/ 15. /tʃɝtʃ/ 16. /gaɪd/ 17. /saɪz/ 18. /kom/ 19. /mæp/ 20. /nit/ 21. /faðɚ/ 22. /dʌzən/ 23. /bot/ 24. /zɪpɚ/ 25. /dɔɾɚ/ 26. /kæb/ 27. /nad/ 28. /hag/ 29. /dʒʌdʒɪŋ/ 30. /tægɪŋ/ 31. /kʌvɚ/ 32. /θʌm/ 33. /mæɾɚ/ 34. /faɪtɚ/ 35. /pækɪŋ/ 36. /feɾɪŋ/ 37. /tʌb/ 38. /pæθ/ 39. /mʌni/ 40. /dʌmi/ 41. /mɛʒɚ/ 42. /ðɪs/ 43. /ʃedi/ 44. /hɔg/ 45. /hɛd/ 46. /taʊnz/ 47. /tʃɔɪs/ 48. /dʒɔɪn/ 49. /væn/ 50. /gev/ 51. /kɔfi/ 52. /zæp/ 53. /sæɾɚ/ 54. /kʊd/ 55. /tude/ 56. /ʃat/ 57. /pɪni/ 58. /tʃɪn/ 59. /təmeto/ 60. /pɪn/

Variants: 1. /saθ/ 4. /gɪt/ 7. /maɪs/ 8. /baʊns/ 11. [sɪs̪tɚ] 22. [dʌzn̩] 25. /datɚ/ 28. /hɔg/ 36. /fedɪŋ/ 44. /hag/ 51. /kafi/ 53. /sædɚ/ 57. /pɛni/

$$\% \text{ reliability (stops)} = \frac{\text{total number of stop agreements}}{58}$$

$$\% \text{ reliability (nasals)} = \frac{\text{total number of nasal agreements}}{28}$$

$$\% \text{ reliability (fricatives)} = \frac{\text{total number of fricative agreements}}{46}$$

$$\% \text{ reliability (vowels)} = \frac{\text{total number of vowel agreements}}{84}$$

Table E–1
Positional distribution of target sounds on reliability test for normal vowels and consonants.

	Consonants				Vowels	
	Prevocalic	Intervocalic	Postvocalic	Totals		
Stops						
/p/	5	1	2	8	/i/	7
/t/	5	5	6	16	/ɪ/	12
/k/	6	1	1	8	/e/	6
/b/	5	0	2	7	/ɛ/	4
/d/	4	4	5	13	/æ/	10
/g/	3	1	2	6	/u/	2
Totals	28	12	18	58	/ʊ/	2
Nasals					/o/	3
/m/	5	2	3	10	/ɔ/	3
/n/	2	3	8	13	/ɑ/	4
/ŋ/	0	0	5	5	/ə/	2
Totals	7	5	16	28	/ʌ/	8
Fricatives					/ɚ/	9
					/ɝ/	1
/f/	4	1	1	6	/ɑɪ/	4
/θ/	1	0	2	3	/ɑʊ/	3
/s/	5	1	4	10	/ɔɪ/	4
/ʃ/	3	1	0	4	Total	84
/tʃ/	3	0	1	4		
/h/	3	0	0	3		
/v/	1	1	1	3		
/ð/	1	1	0	2		
/z/	2	1	4	7		
/ʒ/	0	1	0	1		
/dʒ/	2	1	0	3		
Totals	25	8	13	46		

Tape IV, Side B
Sections 1–4: Reliability Tests
IVB1: Reliability Test for /r, ɝ, ɚ/ Misarticulations (Tape running time: 5:14; Elapsed time: 00:00–05:14)

Transcribe only the sounds produced for the target /r/, /ɝ/, and /ɚ/. The target sound to listen for follows each word.

1. bird /ɝ/ ________
2. raid /r/ ________
3. sorry /r/ ________
4. ray /r/ ________
5. rake /r/ ________
6. garage /r/ ________
7. sister /ɚ/ ________
8. bird /ɝ/ ________
9. curb /ɝ/ ________
10. sugar /ɚ/ ________
11. red /r/ ________
12. parade /r/ ________
13. rot /r/ ________
14. red /r/ ________
15. merry /r/ ________
16. sorry /r/ ________
17. mother /ɚ/ ________
18. doctor /ɚ/ ________
19. ray /r/ ________
20. curve /ɝ/ ________
21. carrot /r/ ________
22. merry /r/ ________
23. father /ɚ/ ________
24. read /r/ ________
25. rope /r/ ________
26. mother /ɚ/ ________
27. parade /r/ ________
28. parade /r/ ________
29. father /ɚ/ ________
30. dairy /r/ ________
31. bird /ɝ/ ________
32. rot /r/ ________
33. fern /ɝ/ ________
34. curb /ɝ/ ________
35. mother /ɚ/ ________
36. ray /r/ ________
37. dairy /r/ ________
38. parrot /r/ ________
39. doctor /ɚ/ ________
40. father /ɚ/ ________
41. bird /ɝ/ ________
42. curb /ɝ/ ________
43. harry /r/ ________
44. raid /r/ ________
45. rot /r/ ________
46. dairy /r/ ________
47. raid /r/ ________
48. rake /r/ ________
49. rock /r/ ________
50. bird /ɝ/ ________

****

Consensus: 1. /ʊ/ 2. /r/ 3. /r/ 4. /w/ 5. [r˔] 6. /w/ 7. /ɚ/ 8. /ʊ/ 9. /ɝ/ 10. /ə/ 11. /r/ 12. [r˔] 13. [r˔] 14. /r/ 15. /w/ 16. /w/ 17. /o/ 18. /ɚ/ 19. [r˔] 20. /ɝ/ 21. /r/ 22. /r/ 23. /o/ 24. [r˔] 25. /r/ 26. /ə/ 27. /r/ 28. /w/ 29. /ə/ 30. [r˔] 31. /ʊ/ 32. /w/ 33. /ɝ/ 34. /ʊ/ 35. /ə/ 36. /r/ 37. /r/ 38. [r˔] 39. /ɚ/ 40. /ɚ/ 41. /ʊ/ 42. /ʊ/ 43. [r˔] 44. [r˔] 45. /r/ 46. /w/ 47. /w/ 48. /w/ 49. [r˔] 50. /ɝ/

Variants: 5. /w/ 10. /ʊ/ 16. [r˔] 17. /ʊ/ 19. /w/ 42. /ɜ/ 44. /w/ 49. /w/

Table E–2
Positional distribution of sounds on reliability test for /r, ɝ, ɚ/ misarticulations.[a]

	Prevocalic	Intervocalic	Vocalic	Totals
r/r	6	5	–	10
w/r	4	5	–	10
r^{T}/r	6	4	–	10
ɝ/ɝ	–	–	4	4
ɚ/ɚ	–	–	4	4
ʊ/ɝ	–	–	6	6
ə/ɚ	–	–	4	4
o/ɚ	–	–	2	2
Totals	16	14	20	50

[a] In the first column, the sound preceding the slash was the produced sound, and the sound following the slash was the target sound.

$$\%\ \text{reliability /r, ɝ, ɚ/} = \frac{\text{total number of agreements}}{50}$$

$$\%\ \text{reliability /r/} = \frac{\text{total number of /r/ agreements}}{30}$$

$$\%\ \text{reliability /ɝ, ɚ/} = \frac{\text{total number of /ɝ, ɚ/ agreements}}{20}$$

IVB2: Reliability Test for /l/ and [l̩] Misarticulations (Tape running time: 6:01; Elapsed time: 05:14–11:15)

Transcribe only the sounds produced for the target /l/ and [l̩] in each of the words. The target sound to listen for follows each word.

1. leaf /l/ ________
2. lag /l/ ________
3. lawn /l/ ________
4. lake /l/ ________
5. feel /l/ ________
6. saddle [l̩] ________
7. nail /l/ ________
8. yellow /l/ ________
9. belly /l/ ________
10. hello /l/ ________
11. pillow /l/ ________
12. lot /l/ ________
13. noodle [l̩] ________
14. less /l/ ________
15. leak /l/ ________
16. lot /l/ ________
17. billy /l/ ________
18. yellow /l/ ________
19. feel /l/ ________
20. cattle [l̩] ________
21. yellow /l/ ________
22. yellow /l/ ________
23. tail /l/ ________
24. cattle [l̩] ________

25. leg /l/ ____________
26. lot /l/ ____________
27. lot /l/ ____________
28. silly /l/ ____________
29. wheel /l/ ____________
30. medal [l̩] ____________
31. let /l/ ____________
32. billy /l/ ____________
33. hilly /l/ ____________
34. sally /l/ ____________
35. sail /l/ ____________
36. kettle [l̩] ____________
37. let /l/ ____________
38. let /l/ ____________
39. yellow /l/ ____________
40. hello /l/ ____________
41. noodle [l̩] ____________
42. tail /l/ ____________
43. lock /l/ ____________
44. billy /l/ ____________
45. billy /l/ ____________
46. let /l/ ____________
47. lot /l/ ____________
48. yellow /l/ ____________
49. feel /l/ ____________
50. cattle [l̩] ____________
51. yellow /l/ ____________
52. lot /l/ ____________
53. lot /l/ ____________
54. billy /l/ ____________
55. feel /l/ ____________
56. nail /l/ ____________
57. saddle [l̩] ____________
58. cattle [l̩] ____________
59. lot /l/ ____________
60. yellow /l/ ____________

****

Consensus: 1. /l/ 2. /w/ 3. /j/ 4. [l˔] 5. /o/ 6. [l̩] 7. /l/ 8. /l/ 9. /w/ 10. /j/ 11. /l/ 12. /l/ 13. /o/ 14. /j/ 15. /w/ 16. /l/ 17. /l/ 18. /w/ 19. /l/ 20. [l̩] 21. /j/ 22. [l˔] 23. /o/ 25. /l/ 26. /w/ 27. /j/ 28. /l/ 29. /o/ 30. /o/ 31. [l˔] 32. /j/ 33. /w/ 34. /l/ 35. /l/ 36. [l̩] 37. /l/ 38. /w/ 40. /j/ 41. /o/ 42. /o/ 43. /l/ 44. /w/ 45. [l˔] 46. /j/ 47. /l/ 48. /l/ 49. /o/ 51. /l/ 52. [l˔] 53. /j/ 54. /l/ 55. /l/ 56. /l/ 57. [l̩] 58. [l̩] 59. /w/ 60. /j/

Variants: 21. [l˔] 22. /l/ 24. /o/; /ə/; /ʊ/ 29. /l/ 39. /w/; /l/; [l˔] 50. /o/; /ə/; /ʊ/ 56. [l˔] 60. [l˔]

$$\% \text{ reliability /l/ and [l̩]} = \frac{\text{total number of agreements}}{60}$$

$$\% \text{ reliability /l/} = \frac{\text{total number of /l/ agreements}}{50}$$

$$\% \text{ reliability [l̩]} = \frac{\text{total number of [l̩] agreements}}{10}$$

Table E–3
Positional distribution of sounds on reliability test for /l/ and [l̩] misarticulations.[a]

	Prevocalic	Intervocalic	Postvocalic	Syllabic	Totals
l/l	7	8	5	–	20
w/l	5	5[b]	0	–	10
j/l	5	5	0	–	10
l˔/l	3	2	0	–	5
o/l	0	0	5	–	5
l̩/l̩	0	0	0	5	5
o/l̩	0	0	0	5	5[c]
Totals	20	20	10	10	60

[a] In the first column, the sound preceding the slash was the produced sound, and the sound following the slash was the target sound.
[b] Note variants for yellow in 39.
[c] Note variants for cattle in 24 and 50.

IVB3: Reliability Test for /s, z/ Misarticulations (Tape running time: 5:18; Elapsed time: 11:15–16:33)

Transcribe only the sounds produced for the target /s/ and /z/ in each of the words. The target sound to listen for follows each word.

1. toss /s/ ________
2. supper /s/ ________
3. days /z/ ________
4. messy /s/ ________
5. sign /s/ ________
6. razor /z/ ________
7. zap /z/ ________
8. please /z/ ________
9. sit /s/ ________
10. sap /s/ ________
11. sick /s/ ________
12. messy /s/ ________
13. reason /z/ ________
14. laws /z/ ________
15. zipper /z/ ________
16. zoo /z/ ________
17. sang /s/ ________
18. blouse /s/ ________
19. days /z/ ________
20. puss /s/ ________
21. bossy /s/ ________
22. freeze /z/ ________
23. sap /s/ ________
24. razor /z/ ________
25. zap /z/ ________
26. blouse /s/ ________
27. zap /z/ ________
28. tease /z/ ________
29. zoom /z/ ________
30. dozen /z/ ________
31. freezer /z/ ________
32. send /s/ ________
33. mess /s/ ________
34. face /s/ ________
35. face /s/ ________
36. aside /s/ ________
37. soak /s/ ________
38. zap /z/ ________
39. ways /z/ ________
40. zipper /z/ ________
41. puss /s/ ________
42. blouse /s/ ________

43. please /z/ ________ 46. raising /z/ ________ 49. dozen /z/ ________

44. wiser /z/ ________ 47. peace /s/ ________ 50. ways /z/ ________

45. icy /s/ ________ 48. rosy /z/ ________

****

Consensus: 1. /s/ 2. [s^l] 3. [z^l] 4. /t/ 5. /θ/ 6. [z^l] 7. [z̪] 8. /z/ 9. /s/ 10. [s̪] 11. /t/ 12. /t/ 13. /ð/ 14. /ð/ 15. /d/ 16. /ð/ 17. [s^l] 18. /θ/ 19. [z^l] 20. [s^l] 22. /t/ 23. [s̪] 24. [z^l] 25. [z̪] 26. /θ/ 27. /z/ 28. /ð/ 29. /d/ 30. [z^l] 31. /t/ 32. /t/ 33. /t/ 34. /θ/ 35. /θ/ 36. /s/ 37. /s/ 38. /z/ 39. /ð/ 40. [z^l] 41. [s^l] 42. /θ/ 43. /z/ 44. /d/ 45. /t/ 46. /z/ 47. /s/ 48. /z/ 49. [z^l] 50. /ð/

Variants: 7. /z/ 10. /θ/ 14. /θ/ 16. /z/ 17. /ʃ/ 18. /ð/ 21. [s̪]; /θ/; /s/ 23. /ʃ/ 25. /z/ 26. /ð/ 31. /d/ 34. [s̪] 35. [s̪] 37. [s̪] 41. /ʃ/ 42. /ð/ 43. /ð/ 45. /ts/

$$\%\ \text{reliability } /s,\ z/ = \frac{\text{total number of agreements}}{50}$$

$$\%\ \text{reliability } /s/ = \frac{\text{total number of } /s/ \text{ agreements}}{24}$$

$$\%\ \text{reliability } /z/ = \frac{\text{total number of } /z/ \text{ agreements}}{26}$$

Table E–4
Positional distribution of sounds on reliability test for /s, z/ misarticulations.

	Prevocalic	Intervocalic	Postvocalic	Totals
Voiceless				
/s/	2	1	2	5
[s̪]	2	1[a]	0	3
[s^l]	2	0	2	4
/θ/	1	0	5	6
/t/[b]	2	4	2	8
Voiced				
/z/	2	2	2	6
[z̪]	2	0	0	2
[z^l]	1	4	2	7
/ð/	1	1	4	6
/d/	2	1	0	3
Totals	17	14	19	50

[a] Note variants for bossy in 21.
[b] Note /t/ for /z/ in freeze (22) and freezer (31).

IVB4: Reliability Test for Phonological Processes (Tape running time: 6:33; Elapsed time: 16:33–23:06)

Transcribe the vowels and consonants in each of the words. The target sounds follow each word.

1. coat /k o t/ ________
2. fishing /f ɪ ʃ ɪ ŋ/ ________
3. cow /k ɑ ʊ/ ________
4. shoes /ʃ u z/ ________
5. soap /s o p/ ________
6. thank you /θ æ ŋ k j u/ ________
7. match /m æ t ʃ/ ________
8. paper /p e p ɚ/ ________
9. shoe /ʃ u/ ________
10. dog /d ɔ g/ ________
11. sweater /s w ɛ t ɚ/ ________
12. feather /f ɛ ð ɚ/ ________
13. feather /f ɛ ð ɚ/ ________
14. lamb /l æ m/ ________
15. thumb /θ ʌ m/ ________
16. nose /n o z/ ________
17. yellow /j ɛ l o/ ________
18. Santa /s æ n t ə/ ________
19. lamb /l æ m/ ________
20. yellow /j ɛ l o/ ________
21. fishing /f ɪ ʃ ɪ ŋ/ ________
22. stop /s t ɑ p/ ________
23. table /t e b ə l/ ________
24. soap /s o p/ ________
25. coat /k o t/ ________
26. thumb /θ ʌ m/ ________
27. spoon /s p u n/ ________
28. string /s t r ɪ ŋ/ ________
29. bridge /b r ɪ d ʒ/ ________
30. table /t e b ə l/ ________
31. thumb /θ ʌ m/ ________
32. dog /d ɔ g/ ________
33. Santa /s æ n t ə/ ________
34. nose /n o z/ ________
35. cow /k ɑ ʊ/ ________
36. fishing /f ɪ ʃ ɪ ŋ/ ________
37. doggie /d ɔ g i/ ________
38. thumb /θ ʌ m/ ________
39. paper /p e p ɚ/ ________
40. pie /p ɑ ɪ/ ________
41. thick /θ ɪ k/ ________
42. shoe /ʃ u/ ________
43. string /s t r ɪ ŋ/ ________
44. doggie /d ɔ g i/ ________
45. bridge /b r ɪ d ʒ/ ________
46. shoes /ʃ u z/ ________
47. dog /d ɔ g/ ________
48. tree /t r i/ ________
49. feather /f ɛ ð ɚ/ ________
50. match /m æ t ʃ/ ________

****

Consensus: 1. /kok/ 2. /fɪtsɪn/ 3. /tɑu/ 4. /ʃuʃ/ 5. /sop/ 6. /fæŋkju/; /pæŋkju/; both indicate labialization 7. /mætʃ/ 8. /bepə/; /p⁼epə/; both indicate prevocalic voicing 9. /su/ 10. /dɑk/ 11. /fwɛtə/ 12. /fɛðɚ/ 13. /fɛðɚ/ 14. /læm/ 15. /θʌm/ 16. /noz/ 17. /lɛlo/ 18. /sæntə/ 19. /næp/ 20. /jɛlo/ 21. /fɪsɪŋ/ 22. /bɑp/ 23. /pebo/ 24. /hop/ 25. /kot/ 26. /fʌm/ 27. /pum/; /pub/; both indicate labial assimilation 28. /nɪŋ/ 29. /brɪdz/ 30. /tebəl/ 31. /nʌp/ 32. /dɔg/ 33. /nænə/ 34. /nos/ 35. /kɑu/ 36. /fɪʃɪŋ/ 37. /dɑdi/ 38. /sʌm/ 39. /pepɚ/ 40. /tɑɪ/ 41. /fɪk/ 42. /ʃu/ 43. /strɪə/ 44. /dɔgi/ 45. /brɪdʒ/ 46. /ʃuz/ 47. /gɔg/ 48. /fwi/ 49. /fɛvə/; /bɛvə/; both indicate labial assimilation 50. /mæts/

Variants: 2. /tʃ/ 6. /dæŋkju/ 8. /pepə/ 10. /bɑk/ 11. /hwɛtə/ 12. /fɛzɚ/ 19. /læp/ 24. /pop/ 26. /pʌm/ 27. /pu/ 35. /tɑu/ 41. /θɪt/ 49. /bɛθə/

$$\% \text{ reliability} = \frac{\text{total number of agreements}}{50}$$

Table E–5
Distribution of misarticulations on reliability test for phonological processes.

	Plus	Minus[a]	Totals
Labial assimilations/labialization	9[b]	3	12
Alveolar assimilations/fronting/apicalization	5[c]	3	8
Palatal and velar assimilations/backing	4[d]	4	8
Palatalization/depalatalization	5[e]	4	9
Voicing/manner changes	7[f]	6	13
Totals	30	20	50

[a]"Minus" indicates normal productions of words in which processes were used in other productions of them.
[b]See Consensus 6, 11, 22, 23, 26, 27, 41, 48, and 49.
[c]See Consensus 3, 17, 37, 38, and 40.
[d]See Consensus 1, 4, 24, and 47.
[e]See Consensus 2, 9, 21, 29, and 50.
[f]See Consensus 8, 10, 19, 28, 31, 33, and 34.

REFERENCES

Allen, G. (1984). Some tips on tape recording speech/language samples. *Journal of the National Student Speech-Language-Hearing Association, 12,* 10–17.

Baer, W. P., & Winitz, H. (1968). Acquisition of /v/ in "words" as a function of the consistency of /v/ errors. *Journal of Speech and Hearing Research, 11,* 316–333.

Bauer, H. R., & Kent, R. D. (1987). Acoustic analyses of infant fricative and trill vocalizations. *Journal of the Acoustical Society of America, 81,* 505–511.

Benjamin, B. J., & Greenwood, J. L. (1983). A comparison of three phonological assessment procedures. *Journal of Childhood Communication Disorders, 7,* 19–27.

Bernstein, L. E. (1983). Perceptual development for labeling words varying in voice onset time and fundamental frequency. *Journal of Phonetics, 11,* 383–393.

Bernthal, J. E., & Bankson, N. W. (1988). *Articulation and phonological disorders.* Englewood Cliffs, NJ: Prentice-Hall.

Best, C. T., & Wilkenfeld, D. (1988). Phonologically motivated substitutions in a 20–22 month old's imitations of intervocalic alveolar stops. *Journal of the Acoustical Society of America, 84,* (Suppl. 1), 114 (abstract).

Blache, S. E., Parsons, C. L., & Humphreys, J. M. (1981). A minimal-word-pair model for teaching the linguistic significance of distinctive feature properties. *Journal of Speech and Hearing Disorders, 46,* 291–296.

Bloomer, H. H. (1971). Speech defects associated with dental malocclusions and related abnormalities. In L. E. Travis (Ed.), *Handbook of speech pathology and audiology* (pp. 715–766). New York: Appleton-Century-Crofts.

Blumstein, S. E., & Stevens, K. N. (1979). Acoustic invariance in speech production: Evidence from measurements of the spectral characteristics of stop consonants. *Journal of the Acoustical Society of America, 66,* 1001–1017.

Bond, Z. S., & Wilson, H. F. (1980). /s/ plus stop clusters in children's speech. *Phonetica, 37,* 149–158.

Bronstein, A. J. (1960). *The pronunciation of American English.* New York: Appleton-Century-Crofts.

Brungard, M. (1961). *Effect of consistency of articulation of* [r] *and* [s] *on gains made with and without therapy.* Unpublished doctoral dissertation, Pennsylvania State University.

Calvert, D. R. (1980). *Descriptive phonetics.* New York: Thieme-Stratton.

Carter, E. T., & Buck, M. (1958). Prognostic testing for functional articulation disorders among children in the first grade. *Journal of Speech and Hearing Disorders, 23,* 124–133.

Carterette, E., & Jones, M. (1974). *Informal speech: Alphabetic and phonemic texts with statistical analyses and tables.* Berkeley: University of California Press.

Catford, J. C. (1977). *Fundamental problems in phonetics.* Bloomington: Indiana University Press.

Chermak, G. D., & Schneiderman, C. R. (1986). Speech timing variability of children and adults. *Journal of Phonetics, 13,* 477–480.

Chiat, S. (1989). The relation between prosodic structure, syllabification and segmental realization: Evidence from a child with fricative stopping. *Clinical Linguistics and Phonetics, 3,* 223–242.

Chomsky, N., & Halle, M. (1968). *The sound pattern of English.* New York: Harper and Row.

Collins, M., Rosenbek, J. C., & Wertz, R. T. (1983). Spectrographic analysis of vowel and word duration in apraxia of speech. *Journal of Speech and Hearing Research, 26,* 224–230.

Compton, A. J., & Hutton, S. (1980). *Phonetics for children's misarticulations.* San Francisco: Carousel House.

Costello, J., & Onstine, J. M. (1976). The modification of multiple articulation errors based on distinctive feature theory. *Journal of Speech and Hearing Disorders, 41,* 199–215.

Cruttenden, A. (1986). *Intonation.* Cambridge: Cambridge University Press.

Crystal, D. (1982). *Clinical linguistics.* Vienna: Springer-Verlag.

Curtis, J. F., & Hardy, J. C. (1959). A phonetic study of misarticulation of /r/. *Journal of Speech and Hearing Research, 2,* 244–257.

Daniloff, R. G., Wilcox, K., & Stephens, M. I. (1980). An acoustic-articulatory description of children's defective /s/ productions. *Journal of Communication Disorders, 13,* 347–363.

Delattre, P. C., & Freeman, D. C. (1968). A dialect study of American r's by X-ray motion picture. *Linguistics, 44,* 29–68.

Delattre, P. C., Liberman, A. M., & Cooper, F. S. (1955). Acoustic loci and transitional cues for consonants. *Journal of the Acoustical Society of America, 27,* 769–773.

Dew, D., & Jensen, P. J., (1977). *Phonetic processing: The dynamics of speech.* Columbus: Merrill.

Dickson, D. R. (1962). An acoustic study of nasality. *Journal of Speech and Hearing Research, 5,* 103–111.

Diedrich, W. M. (1983). Stimulability and articulation disorders. In J. Locke (Ed.), *Seminars in speech and language: Vol. 4, Assessing and treating phonological disorders: Current approaches* (pp. 297–311). New York: Thieme-Stratton.

Diedrich, W. M., & Bangert, J. (1980). *Articulation learning.* San Diego: College-Hill.

Dinnsen, D. A. (1984). Methods and empirical issues in analyzing functional misarticulation. In M. Elbert, D. A. Dinnsen, & G. Weismer (Eds.), *Phonological theory and the misarticulating child* (ASHA Monographs No. 22, pp. 5–17). Rockville, MD: ASHA.

Dinnsen, D. A., & Elbert, M. (1984). On the relationship between phonology and learning. In M. Elbert, D. A. Dinnsen, & G. Weismer (Eds.), *Phonological theory and the misarticulating child* (ASHA Monographs No. 22, pp. 59–68). Rockville, MD: ASHA.

DiSimoni, F. G. (1974). Influence of consonant environment on duration of vowels in the speech of three-, six-, and nine-year-old children. *Journal of the Acoustical Society of America, 55,* 362–363(L).

Donegan, P. J., & Stampe, D. (1979). The study of natural phonology. In D. A. Dinnsen (Ed.), *Current approaches to phonological theory* (pp. 126–173). Bloomington: Indiana University Press.

Dyson, A. T. (1986). Development of velar consonants among normal two-year-olds. *Journal of Speech and Hearing Research, 29,* 493–498.

Dyson, A. T. (1988). Phonetic inventories of 2- and 3-year-old children. *Journal of Speech and Hearing Disorders, 53,* 89–93.

Dyson, A. T., & Robinson, T. W. (1987). The effect of phonological analysis procedure on the selection of potential remediation targets. *Language, Speech, and Hearing Services in Schools, 18,* 364–377.

Edwards, M. L., & Shriberg, L. D. (1983). *Phonology: Applications in communicative disorders.* San Diego: College-Hill.

Elbert, M., & Gierut, J. A. (1986). *Handbook of clinical phonology: Approaches to assessment and treatment.* San Diego: College-Hill.

Elbert, M., & McReynolds, L. (1978). An experimental analysis of misarticulating children's generalization. *Journal of Speech and Hearing Research, 21,* 136–150.

Elbert, M., Shelton, R., & Arndt, W. (1967). A task for evaluation of articulation change: 1. Development of methodology. *Journal of Speech and Hearing Research, 10,* 281–288.

Faircloth, M. A., & Faircloth, S. R. (1970). An analysis of the articulatory behavior of a speech-defective child in connected speech and in isolated-word responses. *Journal of Speech and Hearing Disorders, 35,* 51–61.

Farquhar, M. S. (1961). Prognostic value of imitative and auditory discrimination tests. *Journal of Speech and Hearing Disorders, 26,* 342–347.

Fischer, R. M., & Ohde, R. N. (1985). Vowel constriction effects on the perception of F_1 offset and vowel duration cues for word final stop consonant voicing. *Journal of the Acoustical Society of America, 78* (S1), S (68) A.

Fischer, R. M., & Ohde, R. N. (1986, November). *Rate of frequency change as a cue to voicing perception.* Paper presented at the meeting of the American Speech-Language-Hearing Association, Detroit.

Fitch, H. L., Halwes, T., Erickson, D. M., & Liberman, A. M. (1980). Perceptual equivalence of two acoustic cues for stop-consonant manner. *Perception and Psychophysics, 27,* 343–350.

Flege, J. E. (1988). The development of skill in producing word-final English stops: Kinematic parameters. *Journal of the Acoustical Society of America, 84,* 1639–1652.

Fletcher, S. G. (1989). Palatometric specifications of stop, affricate, and sibilant sounds. *Journal of Speech and Hearing Research, 32,* 736–748.

Gallagher, T. M. (1975). The relationship between lexical boundaries and speech production behavior in children. *Journal of Phonetics, 3,* 35–39.

Gallagher, T. M., & Shriner, T. H. (1975a). Contextual variables related to inconsistent /s/ and /z/ production in the spontaneous speech of children. *Journal of Speech and Hearing Research, 18,* 623–633.

Gallagher, T. M., & Shriner, T. H. (1975b). Articulatory inconsistencies in the speech of normal children. *Journal of Speech and Hearing Research, 18,* 168–175.

Galligan, R. (1987). Intonation with single words: Purposive and grammatical use. *Journal of Child Language, 14,* 1–21.

Ganong III, W. F. (1980). Phonetic categorization in auditory word perception. *Journal of Experimental Psychology: Human Perception and Performance, 6,* 110–125.

Gierut, J. A. (1989). Maximal opposition approach to phonological treatment. *Journal of Speech and Hearing Disorders, 54,* 9–19.

Greenlee, M. (1974). Interacting processes in the child's acquisition of stop-liquid clusters. *Papers and Reports on Child Language Development, 7,* 85–100.

Grunwell, P. (1985). *Phonological assessment of child speech.* San Diego: College-Hill.

Grunwell, P. (1988). Phonological assessment, evaluation and explanation of speech disorders in children. *Clinical Linguistics & Phonetics, 2,* 221–252.

Haggard, M., Summerfield, Q., & Roberts, M. (1981). Psychoacoustical and cultural determinants of phoneme boundaries: Evidence from trading f_0 cues in the voiced-voiceless distinction. *Journal of Phonetics, 9,* 49–62.

Heffner, R-M. S. (1952). *General phonetics.* Madison: University of Wisconsin Press.

Henderson, F. M. (1938). Accuracy in testing the articulation of speech sounds. *Journal of Educational Research, 31,* 348–356.

Hillenbrand, J., Ingrisano, D. R., Smith, B. L., & Flege, J. E. (1984). Perception of the voiced-voiceless contrast in syllable-final stops. *Journal of the Acoustical Society of America, 76,* 18–26.

Hodson, B. W. (1986). *The assessment of phonological processes—Revised.* Danville, IL: Interstate.

Hodson, B. W., & Paden, E. P. (1981). Phonological processes which characterize unintelligible and intelligible speech in early childhood. *Journal of Speech and Hearing Disorders, 46,* 369–373.

Hodson, B. W., & Paden, E. P. (1983). *Targeting intelligible speech.* San Diego: College-Hill.

Hoffman, P. R., & Schuckers, G. H. (1978). Audio-recording effects upon judgment reliability of children's /r/ misarticulation. *Perceptual and Motor Skills, 47,* 451–456.

Hoffman, P. R., Schuckers, G. H., & Daniloff, R. G. (1989). *Children's phonetic disorders: Theory and treatment.* Boston: College-Hill.

Hoffman, P. R., Schuckers, G. H., & Ratusnik, D. L. (1977). Contextual-coarticulatory inconsistency of /r/ misarticulation. *Journal of Speech and Hearing Research, 20,* 631–643.

Hogg, R., & McCully, C. B. (1987). *Metrical phonology: A coursebook.* Cambridge: Cambridge University Press.

House, A. S. (1961). On vowel duration in English. *Journal of the Acoustical Society of America, 33,* 1174–1178.

House, A. S., & Fairbanks, G. (1953). The influence of consonant environment upon the secondary acoustical characteristics of vowels. *Journal of the Acoustical Society of America, 25,* 105–113.

Hudgins, C. V., & Numbers, F. C. (1942). An investigation of the intelligibility of the speech of the deaf. *Genetic Psychology Monographs, 25,* 289–392.

Hyman, L. M. (1975). *Phonology: Theory and analysis.* New York: Holt, Rinehart & Winston.

Ingram, D. (1976). *Phonological disability in children.* New York: Elsevier.

Ingram, D. (1978). The production of word-initial fricatives and affricates by normal and linguistically deviant children. In A. Caramazza and E. B. Zurif (Eds.), *Language acquisition and language breakdown* (pp. 63–85). Baltimore: Johns Hopkins University Press.

Ingram, D. (1981). *Procedures for the phonological analysis of children's language.* Baltimore: University Park Press.

International Phonetic Association (1979). Revised chart for *The principles of the International Phonetic Association. Journal of the International Phonetic Association, 8,* insert.

Jakobson, R., Fant, G., & Halle, M. (1951). *Preliminaries to speech analysis.* Cambridge, MA: MIT Press.

Jakobson, R., & Halle, M. (1956). *Fundamentals of language.* The Hague: Mouton.

Johnson, H. P., & Hood, S. B. (1988). Teaching chaining to unintelligible children: How to deal with open syllables. *Language, Speech, and Hearing Services in Schools, 19,* 211–220.

Jones, D. (1956). *An outline of English phonetics.* New York: Dutton.

Kelso, J. A. S., Saltzman, E. L., & Tuller, B. (1986). The dynamical perspective on speech production: Data and theory. *Journal of Phonetics, 14,* 29–59.

Kenney, K. W., Prather, E. M., Mooney, M. A., & Jeruzal, N. C. (1984). Comparisons among three articulation sampling procedures with preschool children. *Journal of Speech and Hearing Research, 27,* 226–231.

Kent, R. D. (1976). Anatomical and neuromuscular maturation of the speech mechanism: Evidence from acoustic studies. *Journal of Speech and Hearing Research, 19,* 421–447.

Kent, R. D. (1982). Contextual facilitation of correct sound production. *Language, Speech, and Hearing Services in Schools, 13,* 66–76.

Kent, R. D., & Forner, L. L. (1980). Speech segment durations in sentence recitations by children and adults. *Journal of Phonetics, 8,* 157–168.

Kent, R. D., & Rosenbek, J. C. (1982). Prosodic disturbance and neurologic lesion. *Brain and Language, 15,* 259–291.

Kewley-Port, D. (1982). Measurement of formant transitions in naturally produced stop consonant-vowel syllables. *Journal of the Acoustical Society of America, 72,* 379–389.

Kewley-Port, D. (1983). Time-varying features as correlates of place of articulation in stop consonants. *Journal of the Acoustical Society of America, 73,* 322–335.

Khan, L. M. (1982). A review of 16 major phonological processes. *Language, Speech, and Hearing Services in Schools, 13,* 77–85.

Khan, L. M., & Lewis, N. P. (1986). *Khan-Lewis phonological analysis.* Circle Pines, MN: American Guidance Service.

Klatt, D. H. (1975). Voice onset time, frication, and aspiration in word-initial consonant clusters. *Journal of Speech and Hearing Research, 18,* 686–706.

Klein, H. B. (1984). Learning to stress: A case study. *Journal of Child Language, 11,* 375–390.

Kowal, S., O'Connell, D. C., & Sabin, E. J. (1975). Development of temporal patterning and vocal hesitations in spontaneous narratives. *Journal of Psycholinguistic Research, 4,* 195–207.

Krause, S. E. (1982a). Developmental use of vowel duration as a cue to postvocalic stop consonant voicing. *Journal of Speech and Hearing Research, 25,* 388–393.

Krause, S. E. (1982b). Vowel duration as a perceptual cue to postvocalic consonant voicing in young children and adults. *Journal of the Acoustical Society of America, 71,* 990–995.

Kurowski, K., & Blumstein, S. E. (1984). Perceptual integration of the murmur and formant transitions for place of articulation in nasal consonants. *Journal of the Acoustical Society of America, 76,* 383–390.

Ladefoged, P. (1975). *A course in phonetics.* New York: Harcourt Brace Jovanovich.

Ladefoged, P. (1989). Personal communication.

Lapko, L. L., & Bankson, N. W. (1975). Relationship between auditory discrimination, articulation stimulability and consistency of misarticulation. *Perceptual and Motor Skills, 40,* 171–177.

Lehiste, I. (1970). *Suprasegmentals.* Cambridge, MA: MIT Press.

Lehman, M. E. (1988). *On the development of speech perception and production: Evidence from the vowel duration cue to final consonant voicing.* Unpublished doctoral dissertation, University of Michigan.

Leonard, L. B. (1973). Some limitations in the clinical application of distinctive features. *Journal of Speech and Hearing Disorders, 38,* 141–143.

Leonard, L. B., Schwartz, R. G., Allen, G. D., Swanson, L. A., & Frome-Loeb, D. (1989). Unusual phonological behavior and the avoidance of homonymy in children. *Journal of Speech and Hearing Research, 32,* 583–590.

Liberman, A. M. (1957). Some results of research on speech perception. *Journal of the Acoustical Society of America, 29,* 117–123.

Liberman, A. M., Cooper, F. S., Shankweiler, D. P., & Studdert-Kennedy, M. (1967). Perception of the speech code. *Psychological Review, 74,* 431–461.

Liberman, A. M., Delattre, P. C., Cooper, F. S., and Gerstman, L. J. (1954). The role of consonant-vowel transitions in the perception of the stop and nasal consonants. *Psychological Monographs, 68* (8, Whole No. 379), 1–13.

Liberman, A. M., & Mattingly, I. G. (1985). The motor theory of speech perception revised. *Cognition, 21,* 1–36.

Lindblom, B. (1983). Economy of speech gestures. In P. F. MacNeilage (Ed.), *The production of speech* (pp. 217–245). New York: Springer-Verlag.

Lisker, L., & Abramson, A. S. (1967). Some effects of context on voice onset time in English stops. *Language and Speech, 10,* 1–28.

Locke, J. L. (1979). The child's processing of phonology. In W. A. Collins (Ed.), *Minnesota symposium of child psychology: Vol. 12* (pp. 83–119). Hillsdale, NJ: Lawrence Erlbaum.

Lowe, R. J. (1986). Phonological process analysis using three position tests. *Language, Speech, and Hearing Services in Schools, 17,* 72–79.

Lund, N. L., & Duchan, J. F. (1978). Phonological analysis: A multifaceted approach. *British Journal of Disorders of Communication, 13,* 119–126.

MacKay, I. (1987). *Phonetics: The science of speech production.* Boston: Little, Brown.

Macken, M. A. (1980). The child's lexical representation: The "puzzle-puddle-pickle" evidence. *Journal of Linguistics, 16,* 1–17.

Macken, M. A., & Barton, D. (1980). The acquisition of the voicing contrast in English: A study of voice-onset time in word-initial stop consonants. *Journal of Child Language, 7,* 41–74.

Mader, J. (1954). The relative frequency of occurrence of English consonant sounds in words in the speech of children in grades one, two, and three. *Speech Monographs, 21,* 294–300.

Madison, C. L. (1979). Articulatory stimulability reviewed. *Language, Speech, and Hearing Services in Schools, 10,* 185–190.

Malmberg, B. (1963). *Phonetics.* New York: Dover.

Massaro, D. W., & Cohen, M. M. (1983). Phonological context in speech perception. *Perception and Psychophysics, 34,* 338–348.

Maxwell, E. M. (1981a). The use of acoustic phonetics in phonological analysis. *Journal of the National Student Speech-Language-Hearing Association, 9,* 20–37.

Maxwell, E. M. (1981b). *A study of misarticulation from a linguistic perspective.* Unpublished doctoral dissertation, Indiana University. (Available from Indiana University Linguistics Club, Bloomington, IN.)

Maxwell, E. M., & Rockman, B. K. (1984). Procedures for linguistic analysis of misarticulated speech. *ASHA Monographs, 22,* 69–91.

Maxwell, E. M., & Weismer, G. (1982). The contribution of phonological, acoustic, and perceptual techniques to the characterization of a misarticulating child's voice contrast for stops. *Applied Psycholinguistics, 3,* 29–43.

Mazza, P. L., Schuckers, G. H., & Daniloff, R. G. (1979). Contextual-coarticulatory inconsistency of /s/ misarticulation. *Journal of Phonetics, 7,* 57–69.

McDonald, E. T. (1964a). *A deep test of articulation.* Pittsburgh: Stanwix House.

McDonald, E. T. (1964b). *Articulation testing and treatment: A sensory motor approach.* Pittsburgh: Stanwix House.

McGlone, R. E., & Profitt, W. R. (1974). Comparison of lingual pressure patterns in lisping and normal speech. *Folia Phoniatrica, 26,* 389–397.

McReynolds, L. V., & Bennett, S. (1972). Distinctive feature generalization in articulation training. *Journal of Speech and Hearing Disorders, 37,* 462–470.

McReynolds, L. V., & Engmann, D. L. (1975). *Distinctive feature analysis of misarticulations.* Baltimore: University Park Press.

Meyers, S. C., & Freeman, F. J. (1985). Mother and child speech rates as a variable in stuttering and disfluency. *Journal of Speech and Hearing Research, 28,* 436–444.

Miller, J. L., & Liberman, A. M. (1979). Some effects of later-occurring information on the perception of stop consonant and semivowel. *Perception and Psychophysics, 25,* 457–465.

Miller, W. L., & Hamlet, S. L. (1988). Nasal consonants in esophageal speech. *Journal of Speech and Hearing Disorders, 53,* 108–111.

Moll, K. L. (1962). Velopharyngeal closure on vowels. *Journal of Speech and Hearing Research, 5,* 30–37.

Monsen, R. B. (1974). Durational aspects of vowel production in the speech of deaf children. *Journal of Speech and Hearing Research, 17,* 386–398.

Monsen, R. B. (1976a). Second formant transitions of selected consonant-vowel combinations in the speech of deaf and normal-hearing children. *Journal of Speech and Hearing Research, 19,* 279–289.

Monsen, R. B. (1976b). The production of English stop consonants in the speech of deaf children. *Journal of Phonetics, 4,* 29–41.

Monsen, R. B. (1978). Toward measuring how well hearing-impaired children speak. *Journal of Speech and Hearing Research, 21,* 197–219.

Moore, W. H., Burke, J., & Adams, C. (1976). The effects of stimulability on the articulation of /s/ relative to cluster and word frequency of occurrence. *Journal of Speech and Hearing Research, 19,* 458–466.

Naeser, M. A. (1970a). *Influence of initial and final consonants on vowel duration in CVC syllables* (Technical Report No. 130). Madison: Research and Development Center for Cognitive Learning, University of Wisconsin.

Naeser, M. A. (1970b). *The American child's acquisition of differential vowel duration* (Technical Report No. 144). Madison: Research and Development Center for Cognitive Learning, University of Wisconsin.

Norris, M., Harden, J. R., & Bell, D. M. (1980). Listener agreement on articulation errors of four- and five-year-old children. *Journal of Speech and Hearing Disorders, 45,* 378–389.

Ohde, R. N. (1984). Fundamental frequency as an acoustic correlate of stop consonant voicing. *Journal of the Acoustical Society of America, 75,* 224–230.

Ohde, R. N. (1985). Fundamental frequency correlates of stop consonant voicing and vowel quality in the speech of preadolescent children. *Journal of the Acoustical Society of America, 78,* 1554–1561.

Ohde, R. N. (1988a). The development of cues to the perception of the [m] - [n] distinction in CV syllables. *Journal of the Acoustical Society of America, 84* (S1), S (154) A.

Ohde, R. N. (1988b). Revisiting stop-consonant perception for two-formant stimuli. *Journal of the Acoustical Society of America, 84,* 1551–1555.

Ohde, R. N., McCarver, M. E., & Sharf, D. J. (1989). Perceptual and acoustic characteristics of distorted /r/. *Journal of the Acoustical Society of America, 86* (S1), S (48) A.

Ohde, R. N., & Sharf, D. J. (1977). Order effect of acoustic segments of VC and CV syllables on stop and vowel identification. *Journal of Speech and Hearing Research, 20,* 543–554.

Ohde, R. N., & Sharf, D. J. (1981). Stop identification from vocalic transition plus vowel segments of CV and VC syllables: A follow-up study. *Journal of the Acoustical Society of America, 69,* 297–300.

Oller, D. K., & Eilers, R. E. (1975). Phonetic expectation and transcription validity. *Phonetica, 31,* 288–304.

Ostreicher, H. J., & Sharf, D. J. (1976). Effects of coarticulation on the identification of deleted consonant and vowel sounds. *Journal of Phonetics, 4,* 285–301.

Paden, E. P., & Moss, S. A. (1985). Comparison of three phonological analysis procedures. *Language, Speech, and Hearing Services in Schools, 16,* 103–109.

Parker, F. (1976). Distinctive features in speech pathology: Phonology or phonemics? *Journal of Speech and Hearing Disorders, 41,* 23–39.

Paynter, E. T., & Bumpas, T. C. (1977). Imitative and spontaneous articulatory assessment of three-year-old children. *Journal of Speech and Hearing Disorders, 42,* 119–125.

Pentz, A., Gilbert, H. R., & Zawadzki, P. (1979). Spectral properties of fricative consonants in children. *Journal of the Acoustical Society of America, 66,* 1891–1893.

Perkell, J. S. (1969). *Physiology of speech production: Results and implications of a quantitative cineradiographic study.* Cambridge, MA: MIT Press.

Peterson, G. E., & Lehiste, I. (1960). Duration of syllable nuclei in English. *Journal of the Acoustical Society of America, 32,* 693–703.

Pickett, J. M. (1980). *The sounds of speech communication: A primer of acoustic phonetics and speech perception.* Baltimore: University Park Press.

Pindzola, R. H., Jenkins, M. M., & Lokken, K. J. (1989). Speaking rates of young children. *Language, Speech, and Hearing Services in Schools, 20,* 133–138.

Pisoni, D. B. (1981). Some current theoretical issues in speech perception. *Cognition, 10,* 249–259.

Pollack, E., & Rees, N. S. (1972). Disorders of articulation: Some clinical applications of distinctive feature theory. *Journal of Speech and Hearing Disorders, 37,* 451–461.

Potter, R. K., Kopp, G. A., & Green, H. C. (1947). *Visible speech.* New York: Van Nostrand.

Prather, E., & Whaley, P. (1984). Articulation training based on coarticulation. In H. Winitz (Ed.), *Treating articulation disorders for clinicians by clinicians.* Baltimore: University Park Press.

PRDS Group (1983). *The phonetic representation of disordered speech.* London: King's Fund.

Pullum, G. K., & Ladusaw, W. A. (1986). *Phonetic symbol guide.* Chicago: University of Chicago Press.

Raphael, L. J. (1972). Preceding vowel duration as a cue to the perception of the voicing characteristic of word-final consonants in American English. *Journal of the Acoustical Society of America, 51,* 1296–1303.

Raphael, L. J., & Bell-Berti, F. (1975). Tongue musculature and the feature of tension in English vowels. *Phonetica, 32,* 61–73.

Repp, B. H. (1984). Categorical perception: Issues, methods, findings. In N. J. Lass (Ed.) *Speech and language: Advances in basic research and practice: Vol. 10* (pp. 243–335). New York: Academic.

Repp, B. H. (1986). Perception of the [m] - [n] distinction in CV syllables. *Journal of the Acoustical Society of America, 79,* 1987–1999.

Ritterman, S. I., Zook-Herman, S. L., Carlson, R. L., & Kinde, S. W. (1982). The pass/fail disparity among three commonly employed articulatory screening tests. *Journal of Speech and Hearing Disorders, 47,* 429–433.

Rositzke, H. A. (1939). Vowel-length in General American speech. *Language, 15,* 99–109.

Russell, G. O. (1928). *The vowel.* Columbus: Ohio State University Press.

Ryan, B. (1969). *The prediction of articulation proficiency of children in first grade.* Paper presented at the annual meeting of the American Speech and Hearing Association, Chicago.

Sander, E. K. (1972). When are speech sounds learned? *Journal of Speech and Hearing Disorders, 37,* 55–63.

Scott, D. A., & Milisen, R. (1954). The effectiveness of combined visual-auditory stimulation in improving articulation. *Journal of Speech and Hearing Disorders, Monograph Supplement, 4,* 51–56.

Shadden, B. B., Asp, C. W., Tonkovich, J. D., & Mason, D. (1980). Imitation of suprasegmental patterns by five-year-old children with adequate and inadequate articulation. *Journal of Speech and Hearing Disorders, 45,* 390–400.

Sharf, D. J. (1962). Duration of post-stress intervocalic stops and preceding vowels. *Language and Speech, 5,* 26–30.

Sharf, D. J., & Benson, P. J. (1982). Identification of synthesized /r - w/ continua for adult and child speakers. *Journal of the Acoustical Society of America, 71,* 1008–1015.

Sharf, D. J., & Hemeyer, T. (1972). Identification of place of consonant articulation from vowel formant transitions. *Journal of the Acoustical Society of America, 51,* 652–658.

Sharf, D. J., & Lehman, M. E. (1984). Relationship between the speech characteristics and effectiveness of telephone interviewers. *Journal of Phonetics, 12,* 219–228.

Sharf, D. J., & Ohde, R. N. (1981). Physiologic, acoustic, and perceptual aspects of coarticulation: Implications for the remediation of articulatory disorders. In N. J. Lass (Ed.), *Speech and language: Advances in basic research and practice: Vol. 5* (pp. 153–247). New York: Academic.

Sharf, D. J., & Ohde, R. N. (1983). Perception of distorted "r" sounds in the synthesized speech of children and adults. *Journal of Speech and Hearing Research, 26,* 516–524.

Sharf, D. J., Ohde, R. N., & Lehman, M. E. (1986, November). *Acoustic characteristics of distorted /r/ in real and synthesized speech.* Paper presented at the meeting of the American Speech-Language-Hearing Association, Detroit.

Sharf, D. J., Ohde, R. N., & Lehman, M. E. (1988). Relationship between the discrimination of /w-r/ and /t-d/ continua and the identification of distorted /r/. *Journal of Speech and Hearing Research, 31,* 193–206.

Shriberg, L. D. (1972). Articulation judgments: Some perceptual considerations. *Journal of Speech and Hearing Research, 15,* 876–882.

Shriberg, L. D., & Kent, R. D. (1982). *Clinical phonetics.* New York: John Wiley & Sons.

Shriberg, L. D., & Kwiatkowski, J. (1980). *Natural process analysis (NPA): A procedure for phonological analysis of continuous speech samples.* New York: John Wiley & Sons.

Siegel, G. M. (1962). Experienced and inexperienced articulation examiners. *Journal of Speech and Hearing Disorders, 27,* 28–35.

Siegel, G. M., & Winitz, H., & Conkey, H. (1963). The influence of testing instruments on articulatory responses of children. *Journal of Speech and Hearing Disorders, 28,* 67–76.

Singh, S. S., & Singh, K. S. (1976). *Phonetics: Principles and practices.* Baltimore: University Park Press.

Sloat, C., Taylor, S. H., & Hoard, J. E. (1978). *Introduction to phonology.* Englewood Cliffs, NJ: Prentice-Hall.

Smith, B. L., & McLean-Muse, A. (1986). Articulatory movement characteristics of labial consonant productions by children and adults. *Journal of the Acoustical Society of America, 80,* 1321–1328.

Smith, B. L., & McLean-Muse, A. (1987). Effects of rate and bite block manipulations on kinematic characteristics of children's speech. *Journal of the Acoustical Society of America, 81,* 747–754.

Smith, B. L., Sugarman, M. D., & Long, S. H. (1983). Experimental manipulation of speaking rate for studying temporal variability in children's speech. *Journal of the Acoustical Society of America, 74,* 744–749.

Smith, B. L., Wasowicz, J., & Preston, J. (1987). Temporal characteristics of the speech of normal elderly adults. *Journal of the Acoustical Society of America, 30,* 522–529.

Smith, C. R. (1973). Residual hearing and speech production in deaf children. *C.U.N.Y. Communications Sciences Laboratory Research Report No. 4.*

Smith, M. W., & Ainsworth, S. (1967). The effects of three types of stimulation on articulatory responses of speech defective children. *Journal of Speech and Hearing Research, 10,* 333–338.

Smith, N. V. (1973). *The acquisition of phonology: A case study.* Cambridge: Cambridge University Press.

Snow, K. (1963). A detailed analysis of articulation responses of "normal" first grade children. *Journal of Speech and Hearing Research, 6,* 277–290.

Snow, K., & Milisen, R. (1954). The influence of oral versus pictorial presentation upon articulation testing results. *Journal of Speech and Hearing Disorders, Monograph Supplement, 4,* 29–36.

Sommers, R. K., Leiss, R. H., Delp, M. A., Gerber, A. J., Fundrella, D., Smith, R. M., Revucky, M. V., Ellis, D., & Haley, V. A. (1967). Factors related to the effectiveness of articulation therapy for kindergarten, first, and second grade children. *Journal of Speech and Hearing Research, 10,* 428–437.

Stampe, D. (1972). *A dissertation on natural phonology.* Unpublished doctoral dissertation, University of Chicago.

Stephens, M. I., & Daniloff, R. G. (1977). A methodological study of factors affecting the judgment of misarticulated /s/. *Journal of Communication Disorders, 10,* 207–220.

Stetson, R. H. (1951). *Motor phonetics* (2nd ed.). Amsterdam: North-Holland.

Stoel-Gammon, C. (1985). Phonetic inventories, 15–24 months: A longitudinal study. *Journal of Speech and Hearing Research, 28,* 505–512.

Stoel-Gammon, C., & Dunn, C. (1985). *Normal and disordered phonology in children.* Baltimore: University Park Press.

Swisher, W. E. (1973). *An investigation of physiologically and acoustically facilitating phonetic environments on the production and perception of defective speech sounds.* Unpublished doctoral dissertation, University of Wisconsin.

Templin, M. C. (1947a). A non-diagnostic articulation test. *Journal of Speech Disorders, 12,* 392–396.

Templin, M. C. (1947b). Spontaneous versus imitated verbalization in testing articulation in preschool children. *Journal of Speech and Hearing Disorders, 12,* 293–300.

Templin, M. C., & Darley, F. L. (1969). *The Templin-Darley tests of articulation.* Iowa City: Bureau of Educational Research and Service, University of Iowa.

Tiffany, W. R., & Carrell, J. (1977). *Phonetics: Theory and application.* New York: McGraw-Hill.

Toombs, M. S., Singh, S., & Hayden, M. E. (1981). Markedness of features in the articulatory substitutions of children. *Journal of Speech and Hearing Disorders, 46,* 184–191.

Turton, L. J. (1973). Diagnostic implications of articulation testing. In W. D. Wolfe & D. J. Goulding (Eds.), *Articulation and learning* (pp. 195–218). Springfield, IL: Charles C Thomas.

Van Riper, C. (1978). *Speech correction: Principles and methods* (6th ed.). Englewood Cliffs, NJ: Prentice-Hall.

Van Riper, C., & Irwin, J. V. (1958). *Voice and articulation.* Englewood Cliffs, NJ: Prentice-Hall.

Vihman, M. M. (1981). Phonology and the development of the lexicon: Evidence from children's errors. *Journal of Child Language, 8,* 239–264.

Vihman, M. M., Ferguson, C. A., & Elbert, M. (1986). Phonological development from babbling to speech: Common tendencies and individual differences. *Applied Psycholinguistics, 7,* 3–40.

Walsh, H. (1974). On certain practical inadequacies of distinctive feature systems. *Journal of Speech and Hearing Disorders, 39,* 32–43.

Weiner, F. F. (1979). *Phonological process analysis.* Baltimore: University Park Press.

Weiner, F. F. (1981). Treatment of phonological disability using the method of meaningful minimal contrast: Two case studies. *Journal of Speech and Hearing Disorders, 46,* 97–103.

Weismer, G. (1984). Acoustic analysis strategies for the refinement of phonological analysis. *ASHA Monographs, 22,* 30–52.

Weismer, G., Dinnsen, D., & Elbert, M. (1981). A study of the voicing distinction associated with omitted, word-final stops. *Journal of Speech and Hearing Disorders, 46,* 320–328.

Weismer, G., & Elbert, M. (1982). Temporal characteristics of "functionally" misarticulated /s/ in 4- to 6-year-old children. *Journal of Speech and Hearing Research, 25,* 275–287.

Winitz, H. (1963). Temporal reliability in articulation testing. *Journal of Speech and Hearing Disorders, 28,* 247–251.

Winitz, H. (1969). *Articulatory acquisition and behavior.* New York: Appleton-Century-Crofts.

Winitz, H. (1975). *From syllable to conversation.* Baltimore: University Park Press.

Winitz, H., LaRiviere, C., & Herriman, E. (1975). Variations in VOT for English initial stops. *Journal of Phonetics, 3,* 41–52.

Wolf, C. G. (1973). The perception of stop consonants by children. *Journal of Experimental Child Psychology, 16,* 318–331.

Wright, H. N. (1954). Reliability of evaluations during basic articulation and stimulation testing. *Journal of Speech and Hearing Disorders Monograph Supplement, 4,* 19–27.

Wright, V., Shelton, R. L., & Arndt, W. B. (1969). A task for evaluation of articulation change: III. Imitative task scores compared with scores for more spontaneous tasks. *Journal of Speech and Hearing Research, 12,* 875–884.

Zawadzki, P. A., & Kuehn, D. P. (1980). A cineradiographic study of static and dynamic aspects of American English /r/. *Phonetics, 37,* 253–266.

Zehel, Z., Shelton, R. L., Arndt, W. B., Wright, V., & Elbert, M. (1972). Item context and /s/ phone articulation test results. *Journal of Speech and Hearing Research, 15,* 852–860.

Zlatin, M. A., & Koenigsknecht, R. (1975). Development of the voicing contrast: Perception of stop consonants. *Journal of Speech and Hearing Research, 18,* 541–553.

Zlatin, M. A., & Koenigsknecht, R. (1976). Development of the voicing contrast: A comparison of voice onset time in stop perception and production. *Journal of Speech and Hearing Research, 19,* 93–111.

Zue, V. W. (1976). *Acoustic characteristics of stop consonants: A controlled study.* Unpublished doctoral dissertation, Massachusetts Institute of Technology. (A revised version was published as MIT Lincoln Laboratory Technical Report No. 523.)

Zue, V. W., & Laferriere, M. (1979). Acoustic study of medial /t, d/ in American English. *Journal of the Acoustical Society of America, 66,* 1039–1050.

DEFINED TERMINOLOGY INDEX

This index indicates the chapter where each term was first defined in a Glossary.

AUTHOR INDEX

SUBJECT INDEX